AF702366

Praise for the previous edition of this book

"The book is fascinating. It gives great insights into the organ functions and also uses an interesting approach to explain the mental and emotional factors in causing disease. My students find the book indispensable."

- Brandon Fuller, Acupuncture Chair,
East West College of Natural Medicine,
Sarasota, Florida.

"The book is an excellent alternative to the Maciocia textbook, *The Foundations of Chinese Medicine,* and my students find it very useful in their studies."

- Fanyi Meng, Programme leader,
BSc Acupuncture Course,
Lincoln College, UK.

"We have come across many books on Chinese Medicine and particularly like this book's approach of blending the Western and Chinese understanding of the organs, to make it clear that both systems describe the same organs."

- Sam Patel, Joint Principal,
The International College of Oriental
Medicine, UK.

Acupuncture Today and in Ancient China

Fletcher Kovich, Lic.Ac.

CuriousPages Publishing
Bristol, United Kingdom

Published 2019 by CuriousPages Publishing, Bristol, United Kingdom

First published June 2019
Updated 9 June 2020

ISBN 978-1-9164830-6-4 (hardback)
ISBN 978-1-9164830-7-1 (paperback)

This book does not serve as a manual on how to do acupuncture or acupressure. Such treatments, whether by needling, moxibustion, cupping or pressure, should always be performed by a qualified Chinese Medicine acupuncturist.

The author is involved in an ongoing research project to obtain objective experimental data that validates the key aspects of this book's intelligent tissue hypotheses on what the meridians are, what acupuncture is and how it works. Details of the latest published papers and experimental datasets can be found at: **www.curiouspages.com/research.**

The cover photo was taken in the Northern part of the Philippine island of Negros.

Contents

Chapter 1. Introduction

A brief history of Chinese medicine

The early seeds of Chinese medicine can be traced back to the Shang Empire (1800-1600 BC). Like other early cultures around the world, at this period in China the belief was that illness was a state caused by the evil intentions of a third party, such as a curse from another person or from an ancestor, which then caused bad things to happen.[1] This could include physical signs or symptoms but also bad luck—and such bad luck was considered a part of the "illness". For example, a toothache was thought of as a "tooth illness" that was caused by a curse. A common remedy was to make an offering to the displeased ancestor to attempt to placate them and hence lift the curse.[2] And to this day, making offerings to ancestors remains culturally important in China, though the motivation is now more related to securing good luck for the family. In a similar way, another factor believed to cause illness was the wind, where the wind itself was thought of as having evil intentions.[3]

It was believed that each person had two souls, the "corporal soul" (the *po* 魄), which entered the body at birth and departed the body at death; and the "ethereal soul" (the *hun* 魂), which entered the body some time after birth, could temporarily leave the body during periods of sleep, and after death wondered alone through space and time.[4] From about 770 BC, the early demonic medicine of China perceived these unattached souls (or spirits or demons) as inherently evil and constantly striving to hurt people.[5]

The earliest surviving record of needles being used in the context of "acupuncture" dates from the 5th century BC. Sun Ssu-miao cited the earlier physician Pien Chio, from the 5th century BC, who recommended the exact location of thirteen puncture points for the needle treatment of demon-related illnesses, the points being given names such as "demon camp", "demon hearts" and "demon hall".[6] This suggests that initially acupuncture may have been used in the context of expelling demons from the body.

In the closing years of the Chou period (481-221 BC, known as the Warring States period), less significance was given to the influence of dead ancestors, but illness (and misfortune) was still seen as being largely caused by demons. And shaman-like practitioners, called *wu*, were used to exorcise the demons.[7]

The concept of "yin" and "yang"

During the last centuries of the Chou period (around the 4th century BC) there was a move by Chinese intellectuals to explain worldly phenomena as natural occurrences, without referring to mysterious forces such as gods or ancestors. Empirical evidence seemed to suggest that many phenomena in the world could be grouped into pairs, where opposing forces appeared to act between the pair, so that as one of the pair became stronger, the other became weaker—such as in the alternation between day and night. And the principle could be applied to every physical and functional aspect of a person's body, including their organs. The terms *yin* 陰 and *yang* 陽 were used to describe these opposing forces—the terms originally meaning "shady side of a hill" and "sunny side of a hill" respectively (p.345).[8]

The five phase doctrine

Around the time that the *yin-yang* doctrine first appeared, a second natural philosophy that would influence Chinese medicine thinking was created, known as the five phases. Its creator is thought to be Tsou Yen (circa 350-270 BC),[9] who arranged natural phenomena into five categories, rather than two. According to Tsou's doctrine, all phenomena may exist in any one of five states, and these five states (or phases of existence) may transform into one another in an organized cycle, with the progress determined by one of several relationships that were thought to exist between the five phases. To name the phases, Tsou chose five natural substances: water, wood, fire, earth, and metal (p.263).

The Huang Di Nei Jing

Probably the oldest surviving document describing the comprehensive application of the *yin-yang* and five phase doctrines in Chinese medicine, is the *Huang Di Nei Jing* (The Yellow Emperor's Classic of Internal Medicine—*Nei Jing* for short). The document is a series of scrolls containing a collection of separate essays by different authors, the earliest probably dating back to the 2nd century BC.[10] The document is divided into two parts, the *Su Wen* and the *Ling Shu*, and these terms alone are usually now used to refer to these separate parts of the *Nei Jing*.

Already, by this early stage, the documents feature different schools of thought, each favouring either the five phase or the *yin-yang* doctrine; and even the *yin-yang* doctrine was also further divided into either four or six phases by some schools. There is clear disagreement between the differing schools, sometimes providing contradictory explanations for the same phenomena.[11] And the disagreements also extended to such subjects as the detail of each organ's role in metabolism (p.33).

The Nan Jing

Another important classic text is the *Nan Jing* (The Classic of Difficult Issues). This was compiled a few centuries after the *Nei Jing*, probably in the 1st or 2nd centuries AD,[12] and clarifies and expands upon many of the issues introduced in the *Nei Jing*.

The common foundations

Despite these differing doctrines and the disagreements in other areas, some of the knowledge described is common to every faction within Chinese medicine and has remained stable for over two thousand years. This is the knowledge gained from practical observation, rather than from theorizing, and includes

- the details of the main meridians and acupuncture points (acupoints);
- the organs they relate to;
- the signs and symptoms produced when a particular organ is stressed;
- the facial colour, tone of voice, and scent also produced when each organ is stressed;
- the mental and emotional factors that impede the organ functions; and
- the lifestyle factors that promote either good or ill health.

All this knowledge was acquired over two thousand years ago and remains the same today.

The evolution of medical knowledge

In 1973, fourteen medical scripts were unearthed from the Ma-wang-tui graves near Hunan. The graves date back to 168 BC, and the scripts help to clarify some aspects of the evolution of medical knowledge leading up to the *Nei Jing*.

The *Ma-wang-tui* scripts describe only eleven main meridians which were said to flow *independently* of each other, and only four of them were said to be linked to internal organs. And it was considered that the signs and symptoms a patient suffered were associated with a certain meridian, and that it was the meridian itself that was ill, rather than the illness being associated with an organ. It was thought the illness consisted of either a deficiency or surplus of the contents of either the upper or lower section of the meridian.[13]

But by the time of the *Nei-jing*, the full twelve meridians were described, each connecting to a separate organ; and all the meridians were now thought to flow *into* one another in a continuous cycle. It was now also recognised that the same signs and symptoms mentioned above were associated with illnesses in certain organs (rather than in the meridian), and that these illnesses were merely *reflected* in signs in each organ's related meridian (i.e. the "movement" of the organ's "influences" in the meridian).

The introduction of needles

It is also notable that the *Ma-wang-tui* scripts (pre 168 BC) contained no indication that needles could be used to puncture the various "holes" on the meridians to achieve therapeutic effects. Instead, the use of moxibustion (the burning on the skin of powdered mugwort plants) was recommended as the sole method for influencing the contents of the meridians. The earliest surviving documented account of the use of needles for therapeutic effect is in Ssu-ma Chien's biography (of 90 BC) of the earlier physician Shun-yu I. Legal documents survive recording two trials of Shun-yu I, in 167 and 154 BC. He was accused of malpractice due to his use of needles and asked to explain their use, which suggests the practice was unfamiliar to his accusers.[14]

By the time the *Nei Jing* was compiled, only shortly after Shun-Yu I's lifetime, acupuncture was adopted, in addition to moxibustion and blood letting, as the dominant therapeutic technique. This suggests that the use of needles in acupuncture became widespread somewhere between the life of Shun-Yu I (around 160 BC) and the composition of the various chapters of the *Nei Jing*, very shortly after this.[15]

The terms used in Chinese medicine

The *Nei Jing* constitutes a sophisticated system that describes how the body works, becomes ill, and may be treated. Yet in ancient China, there was only a rudimentary knowledge of the body's internal anatomy. The dissection of corpses for medical education was not culturally acceptable, though it was still occasionally performed. [16] At that time though, this rudimentary knowledge of internal anatomy was not sufficient to provide a physiological explanation for the signs and symptoms of ill health that the physicians observed (as recorded throughout the *Nei Jing*). Their ingenious solution was to instead devise a system of anatomy and physiology using the analogy of their state's administrative and military systems.[17]

The new administrative systems (emerging after the conclusion of the Warring States period) had to now organize, feed and manage large populations—in the newly unified, stable and peaceful China. And the collective population of a large state was seen as being analogous to a single person's body.

Grain fed the state and kept it alive, just as it does a person. There were massive storage facilities to store the grain, which were akin to the organs in a person's body that tended to store resources; hence the term *zang* 脏 was used to refer to such an organ, which is translated as "depot" or "long-term depot".

In the state, there were also centres of consumption, largely the palaces, where the grain was processed and consumed; and these were akin to a person's organs that tended to process the grain to extract the resources from it; hence the term *fu* 腑 was used to refer to such an organ, which is translated as "palace" or "short-term repository".[18]

To allow the resources to be exchanged between the depots and palaces, they were linked by a system of transportation channels, or conduits, which were termed the *jing* 經 and *luo* 絡. The term *jing mai* 經脈 referred to the main vessels that linked every depot and palace, and translates as "conduit vessel". Today, these are usually known as either "meridians" or "channels". The term *luo mai* 絡脈 referred to the secondary vessels which were thought to branch off from the main vessels, and translates as "network vessel". Today, these are usually known as "collaterals" or sometimes "*luo* channels"[19] (all these terms are further clarified on page 29).

The term *jing* was a direct reference to the large rivers in China (*jing shui*) running from the mountains and into the countryside, bringing nourishment to the land.[20]

Irrigation played a vital role in China throughout its history. Authors from the 3rd to the 1st centuries BC stressed the importance of opening clogged waterways, draining floods, and irrigating the soil, to ensure the productivity (or health) of the land.[21] And these concepts were applied to the body, where it was seen as vitally important to keep the flow of substances through *its* conduits clear, which then ensured the health of the person; whereas any blockages in the conduits (meridians) were seen as being one of the major causes of illness.[22]

The *Nei Jing* texts abound with descriptions of how to identify the depletion or repletion in a particular organ (one of the *depots* or *palaces*) which is responsible for a health problem, and of the blockages in conduits or network vessels which give rise to pain or discomfort. And to this day, acupuncture treatments are often described as "dredging a meridian" to clear its flow—just as ditches are dredged to clear a problem in the health of the state.[23]

In the body, each of the organs (the *depots* and *palaces*) were considered to have a different function; and to characterize these functions, they were compared to those of the officials of state. Chapter 8 of the *Su Wen* describes them as follows.

The heart was equated to the ruler (or emperor); the lungs to a chancellor or mentor who functioned to provide order and moderation; the liver to a general who provided planning and deliberation; the gallbladder to a "rectifier" who was responsible for making decisions and judgements; the small intestine to the official who received "what had been perfected" and transformed it further; the large intestine to the official who "transmitted [things] along the way" thereby producing "changes and transformations"; and so on. And it was said that "…All these twelve officials must not lose contact with each other. Hence, if the ruler is enlightened, his subjects are in peace.… If the ruler is not enlightened, then the twelve officials are in danger. This causes the paths to be obstructed and impassable."[24]

Just as the state was protected from outside invaders by its military, so the body was seen as being protected in the same way. Pathogens (such as wind) may "hit" the body, and to protect us, the body possessed guards (*wei* 衛) who were responsible for fending off the attack. And, as in military strategy, when the body was weak, it was then that invaders would take advantage. And this same principle also applied inside the body. When any of the organs became weak, the other organs in a position to do so would take advantage and "subdue" (*ke* 克) their neighbours or "seize" (*sheng* 生) their territory.[25] According to the five phase doctrine, this notion produces the "control" (*ke*) and "generation" (*sheng*) sequences that were thought to exist between the main organs (p.263).[26]

The *Nei Jing* was the first medical text to describe the workings of the body using the analogy of a state's administrative and military apparatus.[27] And other advances also included changed notions regarding pathogens and illness. Wind was still considered to be a major cause of illness, but it was no longer seen as having evil intent. The wind was simply one of several natural phenomena that could cause illness (as well as heat, cold, dampness and dryness), but it was not inevitable that you would fall ill when exposed to these pathogens; this depended on your body's ability to resist the pathogen, and was no longer down to mere fate.[28]

Over the two millennia since the compilation of the *Nei Jing*, Chinese physicians have argued over the meanings (and even the validity) of many passages. The most contentious issues have been the change to reading pulses only at a patient's wrist, rather than palpating certain locations on every meridian (p.299), and the application of the five phase doctrine to medicine (p.267).[29]

Through all this time, there have been separate schools of thought in acupuncture, some choosing to apply only certain aspects of the *Nei Jing*, while others focus on other aspects; and this same approach exits today, with numerous different styles of acupuncture being practised. The fundamental knowledge tends to be the same in all schools (that is, the bullet points listed on page 15 above) and the main differences tend to be in the approach to forming a diagnosis, selecting the acupoints to use, and in needling technique.

Who invented acupuncture?

Today's acupuncture schools tend to refer back to the *Nei Jing* as the source of all key knowledge on the subject, which is understandable. This is how I was trained, and the ancient systems and terminology have a beauty and charm to them, and when applied in practice, acupuncture works as well today as it always has done. After all, the ancient Chinese invented acupuncture, so surely their writings convey the subject.

At first glance, this might appear so. But an important fact usually overlooked is that acupuncture is not manmade. It was not invented by the ancient Chinese, nor by anyone else. The phenomenon (that is, what happens in the body when an acupoint is stimulated, and how this affects the organs and other systems), this phenomenon has always been present in the body, and may even have been present from the earliest stages of evolution. It is said to exist in all life forms, including plants; and in an animal embryo, the *primo vascular system* (which is geographically related to the meridian system) is the first system to form, even before the vascular or nervous systems do, which then form *around* the primo vessels (p.321).

It is true that (according to the surviving texts) the ancient Chinese were the first to discover how to *activate* this acupuncture system. But the mechanisms in the body that are utilized have always been present, from millions of years before humans evolved.

What the ancient Chinese *did* discover is the information in the bullet list on page 15 above; that is, the signs and symptoms each organ produces when stressed, the accompanying diagnostic signs, the meridian pathways, and the main causes of disease, including mental and emotional factors. All this information is fact based, since it was gained from practical observation, rather than from theorizing; and over two thousand years later, it still forms the core of Chinese acupuncture.

The challenges for acupuncturists today

The training of acupuncturists today is based on the *Nei Jing*, but apart from its fact-based core content, its other content is notoriously difficult to understand, since it is either metaphorical or uses theories that are incompatible with today's medical terminology—theories to attempt to explain how the body works, how people become ill and how acupuncture works to treat those illnesses. Apart from the challenge of understanding these theories, another big obstacle is that many of them are simply untrue, which only makes it even harder for them to be understood and accepted.

One way this book helps is by demonstrating how to determine which of the *Nei Jing* content is fact-based, which is metaphorical and not intended to be interpreted literally, and which is simply untrue (Chapters 2, 3 and 14).

This makes learning Chinese acupuncture easier, but when practising acupuncture, another great challenge then arises. How on earth do you explain to patients what their condition is and how acupuncture works to treat it? Much of the vocabulary you learnt as an acupuncture student would be incomprehensible to them—and also to anyone outside of Chinese medicine.

However, since the phenomenon of acupuncture is a natural part of the body and was not invented by the ancient Chinese, it ought to be possible to explain it in relation to today's *anatomy and physiology*,* so that everyone can understand what it is, how it works, and what conditions it can treat. This is the other challenge undertaken by this book. It uses terms and concepts familiar to today's readers to explain how acupuncture works, to describe all the common health conditions treated by it, and their causes—including mental and emotional causes.

This makes the entire subject much easier to understand and learn, and enables acupuncturists to use terms and concepts familiar to their patients to communicate about the patient's condition and any aspect of the treatment.

* Note that when this term is used in this book, this is referring *only* to the scientific study of anatomy and physiology. It is not in any way referring to the pharmaceutical approach to healthcare, which is an entirely separate activity. That activity utilizes knowledge from contemporary physiology (often misguidedly), but this does not mean that contemporary physiology *is* the pharmaceutical approach to healthcare. These two should not be confused, nor equated to one another.

My journey in writing this book

In my early thirties, acupuncture transformed my health and life. The treatments were like nothing I had ever experienced and they had unexpected effects, rejuvenating my energy (overnight I felt like a nineteen-year-old again), and even appearing to awaken feelings and sensibilities within me which I had long since forgotten existed. After a few weeks, I was a different person.

Years later, I trained in Chinese acupuncture and started my own practice. I found the treatments routinely had the same dramatic effect on many of my patients, curing serious conditions they suffered for years and transforming their lives. Naturally, I felt the desire to spread the word to as many people as possible. But several obstacles stood in the way, the most significant being that it simply was not possible to tell patients how acupuncture worked, nor to communicate this to other healthcare workers, scientists or the media.

Today we think about healthcare in terms of how the nervous system or the chemistry of the body communicates between the main organs, and we look for disruptions in these systems to explain health problems. We also rely entirely on the contemporary terms for diseases, whether or not we know what those terms mean. For example, the Greek suffix "-itis" is often added to the Latin or Greek term for a part of the body to indicate there is swelling in that area, giving us labels such as "tendonitis", "tonsillitis", "bronchitis", "appendicitis" and so on. We are familiar with these terms and imagine they describe the condition—even though the terms merely mean there is swelling in a particular location. They do not in any way describe *why* there is swelling, and often the reason may not even be known. Or we may be told the problem is with the chemistry of our body—that perhaps there is an imbalance in our hormones. Whether or not this describes the cause of our problem, rather than being merely an indicator of it, does not matter. We are familiar with the concept, so we feel we understand it. This is the way we are used to thinking about our bodies and illness.

In contrast, as mentioned above, acupuncturists today are still trained using terms and concepts that originated in the *Nei Jing* (though they have often been modified or added to), so when talking about acupuncture, these are the terms acupuncturists tend to use. For example, I might say to a patient that their migraine symptoms were produced by "Liver chi stagnation" (a term used in today's Chinese medicine). To understand this, the patient would naturally attempt to convert the term into the concepts they were used to, and might imagine I was saying they had a liver disease of some sort. They might reply "But my doctor did a blood test last week which revealed no problem with my liver," and give me a puzzled look.

To clarify, I might then use Chinese medicine concepts to describe the disease mechanism and say something along the lines of: "The *yin* of your kidney is deficient, which means the *yang* of your liver is not restrained, enabling it to rise up into your head and produce your migraine symptoms." Again, the patient would attempt to convert this into the concepts they were used to, perhaps trying to imagine hormonal imbalances or physical abnormalities in their organs or bodily structures. But such Chinese medicine concepts do not ordinarily translate into the terms of contemporary anatomy and physiology, so the patient would, understandably, be left baffled. And this same situation also meant that other healthcare workers, scientists and the media also had no idea what acupuncture was or how it worked, which has generated much prejudice and widespread misunderstanding, even causing some people to claim the system has no physical effect and is an intricate hoax.

It was clear to me that acupuncture worked (and had a far more powerful effect on my own health than any other healthcare system I had tried), but even when trained as an acupuncturist, I still had no idea *how* it worked—in terms of contemporary anatomy and physiology. What was physically happening in the patient's body during and after an acupuncture treatment? There was no explanation for this. And it was partly my burning desire to spread the word about acupuncture, and partly the need to satisfy my own insatiable curiosity that drove me to find an explanation.

My first few years of research were fruitless. I had a large store of unusual firsthand experiences to draw upon (some explained in this book), together with my experiences of the effects of acupuncture on patients and on myself, and of course knowledge of the *Nei Jing*. The task was to use contemporary medical concepts to devise an explanation of how acupuncture worked, such that it accounted for all these experiences. I spent several years trying to imagine a control system, similar to the nervous or hormonal systems, or some way that acupuncture might interact with these systems. It seemed logical that acupuncture did this, since this is how we are used to thinking about how the body works. But none of the systems I devised seemed credible.

Then one day I realized that acupuncture was not a control system at all, and instead it achieved its effects by utilizing the resonance that exists between each of the abdominal organs and specific locations on the body.[30]

As described throughout this book, the signs and symptoms of an illness are caused by the improper function of an organ, due to the organ being stressed in some way. And due to the resonance that exists between that organ and a specific bodily location (a particular acupoint), this causes that location to become tender. By stimulating one of these tender locations, this same resonance is utilized but in reverse, which encourages the associated organ to cancel out the improper function in itself that caused the location to become tender. The organ function returns to normal and the signs and symptoms clear.

This hypothesis then needed to be tested experimentally. Fortunately, I had a background in electronics and programming, which meant I was able to begin the research myself. I spent the following two years designing the experiments and equipment necessary to demonstrate this resonance.

Measuring the electrical impedance at acupoints had been done since the 1950's (p.322). It was found that when an organ was diseased, the impedance at its related acupoints dropped notably. This seemed like a good starting point. By studying the impedance at key acupoints in real time (taking 1,000 samples per second), I found that the tissue at an acupoint adopted microscopic patterns that mirrored the real-time states in the related organ (p.333).

It transpired that all organ states were constantly being conveyed to every part of the body on electromagnetic waves; and that all bodily tissue intelligently interpreted this information. It is even possible that it was this process that initially caused the body to evolve in response to the organ functions, and hence also caused the tissue that now constitutes the meridians, to evolve so that each meridian now emphasized the information from its related organ (p.353).

Thus, the "intelligent tissue" hypothesis resulted. This process of bodily tissue constantly interpreting organ information conveyed on electromagnetic waves, is able to explain why, in response to organ stress, acupoints become tender, and meridian phenomena also result, such as boils, red or cold skin, or even shooting pains. Then, when one of these tender acupoints is needled, this causes the tissue at the acupoint to release this borrowed stress and revert to normal function, which transformation is communicated back to the related organ via the same electromagnetic waves, causing the organ to also revert to normal function.

Key experimental results are summarized starting on page 323. But before this, the book primarily focuses on the clear communication of what Chinese acupuncture is, how it works, how it is practised, and what it can treat.

The layout of this book

Chapter 2 describes the *Nei Jing* notions of metabolism (how the organs transform the food we eat into useable resources), explaining which notions are fact based and which are untrue; and also explains and translates the key Chinese medicine terms, such as *chi* 氣.

Chapter 3 describes the varying notions of *chi* through the history of Chinese medicine, including the 1970's reinterpretation of it. It also suggests an approach that may enable practitioners who are familiar with the 1970's concept of *chi*, to be able to accept the new "intelligent tissue" explanation for all meridian phenomena.

Chapters 4 to 10 are dedicated to the individual organs, and describe the organ functions by referring to the practical observations of the *Nei Jing*, and also comparing these with contemporary physiology, so that the key aspects of the Chinese medicine organ systems and disease mechanisms can be clearly understood.

Chapters 11 and 12 cover painful meridian symptoms and the mental and emotional factors in causing disease.

Chapter 13 provides detailed case histories covering many common conditions, from diagnosis through to the outcome of the treatments; and these are referred to throughout the above organ chapters.

Chapter 14 describes which of the *Nei Jing* content is factual, which is metaphorical, and which is simply untrue. Many *Nei Jing* passages and theories are analysed, demonstrating an approach that can be used to identify the fact based content, so that students are then able to more fruitfully study the *Nei Jing* for themselves.

Chapters 15 and 16 discuss issues related to pulse diagnosis and the treatment of viral or bacterial infections.

Chapter 17 summarizes the scientific evidence for the structures that underlie the meridians (the primo vessels), describes their physiological purpose, and also describes the latest research on the intelligent tissue hypothesis.

Chapter 18 describes evidence related to the body's use of electrical energy—since this is thought to play a part in enabling acupuncture to achieve its effects.

Chapter 19 describes why the meridians and acupoints are located where they are, relates this to the "intelligent tissue" notions, and introduces a new definition of a meridian.

Chapter 20 describes how information about the organ functions is encapsulated in the body's electrical current. This information is thought to play a key role in the two-way communication between the organs and the acupoints, which then enables acupuncture to correct organ malfunctions. The intelligent tissue hypothesis is then described in detail and compared with other hypotheses on how acupuncture works.

Chapter 2. Chinese medicine metabolism and physiology

Translation of key Chinese medicine terms

One of the commonest Chinese medicine terms is also one of the hardest concepts to translate into English. This is the term *chi* 氣. As suggested by Unschuld, this concept was used in Chinese medicine when it was moving away from the notion that demons were responsible for causing illness.[1] Instead it was now considered that environmental factors (such as wind, cold, or dampness) were responsible. These were referred to using the concept of *chi*. In this context, the term encompassed a range of ideas, such as: wind, breath, vapours, or the clouds in the sky. Its character 氣 is made up by placing the pictogram for "rising vapour" above the pictogram for "rice" or "millet", so that the entire character means "vapours rising from food". And these same "vapours" were also thought to be present in the body, either as a pathogen (such as the essence of "harmful wind" that had penetrated the skin) or as a nourishing element, such as the vapours extracted from the food we eat. The English translation of *chi* 氣 favoured by Unschuld is therefore "finest matter influences" or simply "influence".

This concept was depicted nicely by Yü Shu, writing in 1067 (more than a millennium after the *Nei Jing*), when he said that the influences passing from the lungs and heart "resemble mist gently flowing into all the meridians".[2]

As Unschuld points out, this concept is entirely different from the contemporary notion of energy, which is how *chi* is often translated in today's Chinese medicine. But such a notion did not exist in ancient China and only obscures the term's intended meaning. For this reason, this book follows Unschuld's translation of *chi* as "influence", so as to more accurately capture the term's intended meaning.

How the body processes food

As mentioned above, the ancient Chinese had no concept of energy as we think of it today, yet they had intricate notions about how ingested food was converted by the organs to provide the resources the body needs.

Separating fact from metaphor and supposition

Some aspects of Chinese medicine were discovered through practical observation and are therefore fact based. For example, this includes all the signs and symptoms that occur when any organ is stressed, and also the causes of disease, including mental and emotional factors. These are all still remarkably accurate today, and to have worked these out over 2,000 years ago was impressive. But other aspects were created theoretically and tend to be either metaphorical, or based on unreliable suppositions about how the body might work. In ancient China, there was no useful information about the body's internal anatomy, physiology, or its chemistry. Therefore, the intellectuals had to, in effect, make their best guess about how the body might work, and they developed a range of theories to explain how the organs transformed ingested food into useable resources. But when considered alongside today's fact-based knowledge of anatomy and physiology (as far as it has so far progressed), most of these ancient *Nei Jing* ideas are simply untrue.

Overview of Chinese medicine metabolism

Food and liquids are taken in by the stomach, which extracts "food influence" from them. The lungs then extract "clear influence" from the air to create a third type of vapour which nourishes the lungs and heart and enables them to carry out their functions.

Liquids are also extracted from ingested food and transformed into blood. In ancient China, there was no notion of a separate blood circulatory system, nor of the heart acting like a pump (p.43). Instead the "meridian" network was the only known circulatory system, and it was assumed that all substances circulated within it.[3] Therefore, the blood was thought to circulate within the "meridians", while the various types of influence also travelled either within (along with the blood) or outside of the "meridians", much like a vapour or mist encircling each "meridian".

To confuse matters, the *Nei Jing* notion of a "meridian" was different from today's notion. In the *Nei Jing*, the "meridians" were thought to be deep, artery-like tubes; whereas today, they are considered to be more akin to pathways on the skin. This is explained on page 29 below. (Whenever the term "meridian" is given in quotes in this text, this refers to the *Nei Jing* notion, rather than to today's notion. However, in the *Nei Jing* extracts, quotes are not used, since it is already clear the term is being used in the *Nei Jing* context.)

Once food influence was extracted by the stomach, it then divided into two parts. The food influence (like all other influence) was thought to be a vapour-like substance, and this contained some vapours that were more active and aggressive (the *yang* portion) and some that were more restful and supportive (the *yin* portion). The supportive portion of the vapour was known as "constructive influence" and this circulated within the "meridians" to every part of the body, having a nutritive action. Whereas the more active portion of the vapour was known as "defensive influence" and this circulated on the outside of the "meridians" and warmed the muscles and skin.

The purpose of the blood was seen as purely nutritive. The blood provided nutrition to every part of the body—the muscles, joints, and organs—which meant there were two factors that nourished the body, the blood and the constructive influence, both flowing together in the "meridians".

External pathogens, known as "harmful wind"* or "uninvited guests", would enter the body through the skin. In form, these were similar to the vapours the digestion extracted from food and would travel through the body in the same way. The "defensive influence" had the role of warming the skin and muscles, and as long as the defensive influence was strong enough, then the harmful wind would not be able to penetrate the skin. But if a person's defensive influence was depleted, the harmful wind could penetrate. The wind (in the form of a harmful vapour) would reach the "meridians" and lodge there, causing local discomfort. If not cleared by treatment, this harmful vapour would then travel along the "meridians" and eventually lodge within the organs, causing serious illness.[4]

There was also thought to be a constitutional influence (another type of vapour) which was passed on to us from our parents. It was thought to be stored in the kidneys† and circulated to the organs, so as to provide an extra vital stimulus that the organs needed to function properly. This influence, while stored in the kidneys, may be supplemented each day by the vapours extracted from ingested food.

* In the *Nei Jing*, a wind pathogen was known as "evil wind", where "evil" was simply understood to mean "harmful", rather than meaning that it had any intent of its own. But because the word "evil" now has other connotations, I think it is less misleading to translate it as "harmful".

† When the term "kidneys" is used in Chinese medicine, this refers to three structures collectively: they kidneys, adrenal glands, and gonads (p.153).

The Chinese terms for these various "influences"

The Chinese term for food influence is *gu chi* 穀氣. Alternative translations are "grain influence" or "valley influence".

The term for clear influence (extracted from the air we breathe) is *qing chi* 清氣.

The term *zong chi* 宗氣 refers to the influence formed in the lungs and heart. *Zong chi* is variously translated as "chest influence", "stem influence", "pectoral influence", or "gathering influence".

The term for constructive influence is *ying chi* 營氣, which is also translated as "nourishing influence" or "camp influence".

The term for defensive influence is *wei chi* 衛氣, which is also translated as "protective influence" or "guard influence".

The term used for the constitutional influence varied between different texts. In the *Su Wen* and the *Ling Shu*, the term *jing chi* 精氣 was used, which is translated as "essence influence"; or the term *jing* 精 was also used alone and is variously translated as "pure essence", "seminal essence", "congenital essence", "acquired essence", or simply "essence".[5] But in the slightly later *Nan Jing*, the term *yuan chi* 原氣 was now used, which is translated as "original influence" or "primary influence".

The above influences are present in the "meridians", which circulate them; and when combined together they were known as "true influence". The Chinese term *zhen chi* 真氣 was used to describe true influence.[6]

The terms for body liquids

The liquids in the body were termed the *jin* 津 liquids and the *ye* 液 liquids. These were defined as follows.

> **Extract from *Ling Shu*, Chapter 30**
> That which is released to flow out of the skin structures, when a person sweats profusely, that is what is called "*jin* liquid" ... When grains enter the body and fill it with the [influences], then a viscous liquid pours into the bones, enabling the [joints] to bend and stretch. The [influences] flow out to fill the brain with marrow and they provide the skin with dampness. That is what is called "*ye* liquid".[7]

Hence, the *jin* are the finer liquids, and the *ye* are the more viscous liquids, including marrow, and even the brain, since "marrow" (being a product of the kidneys) was thought to fill up the spinal cord and also the brain (p.163).

Summary of contemporary metabolism

None of the above terms can be accurately translated into the terms used in contemporary metabolism, since the two systems are entirely different. To help highlight these differences, contemporary metabolism is summarized below.

The lungs extract oxygen from air and this is transported in the blood.

The stomach, pancreas, gallbladder, and small intestine (in combination) extract nutrients from our diet, and these are also transported in the blood.

One of the most important nutrients is glucose, which is the body's main fuel (p.386). But this cannot directly provide the body's cells with energy. The glucose, along with oxygen, is transported (via the blood) into every cell, where these two substances are used to create the molecule ATP; and this molecule is then further processed to release energy into the cell, enabling the cell to perform its functions (p.336). Therefore glucose, by itself, is unusable by the body; it requires oxygen to be present in every cell of the body to enable the glucose to be made use of.

Our defence against pathogens is provided by the active components of the immune system, such as lymphocytes (p.212), and the combat largely takes place systemically, in the blood.

Other uses of the term "influence"

Organ influence

This term is also often used in association with an organ, such as in the phrase "lung influence" (lung *chi*) or "liver influence" (liver *chi*), for example. To understand such phrases as the ancient Chinese meant them, it is necessary to realize that Chinese medicine organ physiology was conceived theoretically, rather than discovered through practical observation of organ tissue. The "organs" were considered to be metaphorical centres of activity akin to administrative roles within the Chinese state.

Within this metaphorical system, the term "lung influence" (lung *chi*), for example, could be interpreted to mean literally that: the nature or degree of the lungs' influence amongst the other organs and on the body in general. In other words, how the lungs interact with the other organs and with the body.

An organ's influence was considered akin to a vapour or mist that emanates from that organ. There is no equivalent of this in contemporary physiology, but there is a close analogy. When an organ's function is weak, its interactions with the other organs and the tissue of the body would be affected, such that its usual effects would be proportionally weaker. Likewise, when an organ's "influence" (the vapour emanating from it) is weak, its effects on the other organs and on the body would *also* be weaker than usual. Therefore, such phrases as "lung influence" (lung *chi*) could be considered analogous to that organ's function—in contemporary physiology.

In today's Chinese medicine, the phrase is also used to describe conditions related to the organs. For example, the term "Lung chi deficiency" (or, lung influence deficiency) is used to describe a common lung condition characterised by weak function. This term could be translated as "poor lung function", which is the translation used in this book.

Meridian influence

The term "influence" (*chi*) is also used in relation to the "meridians". As said above, it is often assumed that the influence of each organ flows along its related "meridian" (along with the various other forms of influence). The intended meaning of this notion would have been along the lines of the following. Something akin to a vapour flowed within each organ's related "meridian", and this vapour (the organ's influence) contained the "essence" of that organ (much like steam contains the scent of the food being cooked), which might change in character to reflect various conditions in the organ. These conditions might include the organ (the "administrative centre") becoming "full" or "empty" or over-energetic (having an excess of *yang*) or too sluggish (being deficient in *yang*), and so on.

The organ's influence was able to produce effects at any place along the "meridian", effects which reflected these various states within the organ. And the nature of an organ's influence could be affected at various "holes" (acupoints) along the "meridian", so that if the influence was currently "full" in nature (for example), this "fullness" could be reduced by letting some of the influence out through this "hole" in the "meridian", and hence bring the influence level back to normal. This was imagined as being akin to unblocking an irrigation ditch, so that the related administrative centre (the organ) could resume its proper role in organizing the state—so that the fields were irrigated and the products transported to nourish the state (the entire person).[8]

By applying the above analogy (that an organ's influence is analogous to its function), stimulating an organ's influence (its *chi*) at one of these "holes" along that organ's "meridian" had the effect of normalizing the organ's function.

Parallels with the intelligent tissue hypothesis

Interestingly, when considering the term *chi* as it was originally intended (in contrast to the 1970's trend of equating it to energy), the above descriptions then become remarkably reminiscent of the intelligent tissue hypothesis (p.372). The hypothesis explains (in relation to contemporary anatomy and physiology) how an organ's function is able to influence any location along its related meridian[*], and

[*] As said on page 24, in this book's text, when the term "meridian" is placed within quotes, this refers

how stimulation of that location is able to rectify malfunctions in the organ. And this influence is produced, not by some physical substance that flows along the meridian, but by the details of the organ's function that are captured in an electrical wave—something as ethereal as the steam rising from food.

Pathogenic influence

The term "influence" (*chi*) was also applied to any other substances that enter the body. For example, after drinking wine, or any other form of alcohol, this clearly had an effect on us, and this was understood in terms of the "wine influence" (wine *chi*) circulating in the body. This, like any other form of influence, was in the form of a vapour that contained some essence of the wine, which circulated in the "meridians", interacting with the other influences and, finally, with the organs. And it was the interaction of these various vapours that was thought to produce the effect (heating us up, etc).

> **Extract from *Su Wen*, Chapter 45**
> Huang Di: Heat recession, how does this condition come about?
>
> Qi Bo: When wine enters the stomach, then the [collaterals] are full, while the [meridians] are depleted. ... The [influence] has assembled in the [pancreas*] and cannot disperse. The [influence] of the wine and the [influence] of the grain strike at each other. Heat abounds in the centre. Hence, heat is everywhere in the body. The interior is hot and the urine is red. Now, when the [influence] of wine abounds and is fierce and when the [influence] of the kidneys is weak, the *yang* [influence] dominates alone. Hence, it is therefore that the hands and the feet are hot.[9]

The same applied to other pathogens, such as cold. When we were exposed to a cold wind, this was thought to enter us in the form of "cold influence" (cold *chi*), which, again, was a vapour that contained some essence of the coldness. And this vapour circulated in the "meridians", interacting with other influences and with the "meridians" themselves, which is what was thought to account for the results.

> **Extract from *Su Wen*, Chapter 39**
> When cold [influence] settles outside the vessels, then the vessels become cold. When the vessels are cold, then they shrink. When they have shrunk, then the vessels are curved and tense. When they are curved and tense, then they pull on the small [collaterals] outside. Hence, sudden pain results. When they are given heat, then the pain stops immediately.[10]

The wind could also be thought of as simply a "harmful" wind which entered us and caused harm. In this case the pathogen was known as "evil influence" (*xie chi*) 邪氣. Again, this was in the form of a vapour that contained some essence of the wind, which then circulated in the "meridians", interacting with the other influences to produce its various effects. During treatment, it could be released through certain "holes" in the "meridians" (i.e. acupoints), but if left to travel around the body, it would attach itself to

to the *Nei Jing* notion; whereas when the term is used without quotes, this refers to today's notion of a meridian. These two are quite different; see page 29.

* Usually called the spleen in Chinese medicine; see page 61.

various structures, causing local signs and symptoms.

> **Extract from *Su Wen*, Chapter 56**
> The first emergence of the one hundred diseases must begin in the skin and its hair. When the evil strikes there, then the interstice structures open. When they are open, then the evil enters the [collaterals] and settles there. If it stays there and is not made to leave, it will be transmitted into the [meridians]. If it stays there and is not made to leave, it will be transmitted into the [*yang* organs (*fu*)] where it accumulates in the intestines and in the stomach. ... When the evil has entered the [collaterals], then the [collaterals] abound with evil and their colour changes. ... When it stays in the region of sinews and bones, [if] it consists of plenty of cold, then this causes sinew cramp and the bones to have pain.[11]

These other applications of the concept of influence (*chi*) demonstrate beyond any doubt that the *Nei Jing* authors considered all such substances in the body to consist of vapour-like substances that circulate in the "meridians". This is entirely different to the interpretation of the term *chi* that has been adopted in today's Chinese medicine (i.e. the notion of it equating to energy). This subject is explained in detail in Chapter 3 (p.49).

What was the *Nei Jing* notion of a "meridian"?

Throughout the *Nei Jing*, the authors appeared to share the same notion of what "meridians" were. But this is different from today's notion of a meridian, and this may cause confusion when reading texts from the *Nei Jing*, or any text that quotes *Nei Jing* passages.

Bloodletting was then common, and this was let from vessels just beneath the skin, which were consistently called the "collaterals" and the "tertiary network vessels". In today's anatomical terms, it is clear that these are the superficial veins and arterioles that can be seen through the skin (p.31).

It was thought that these vessels then travelled deeper into the muscle and connected with larger vessels, which they called *jing mai* 經脈, or "meridians", and that the same blood (and influences, *chi*) flowed in all these vessels.

Was this idea based on practical observation or was it purely theoretical? Dissection of bodies was occasionally performed (p.16), which is probably what informed the above observation. When dissecting a corpse and following the path of a superficial vein or arteriole, it would have travelled deeper and joined onto a larger vessel (either an artery or a deep vein*). These were larger tube-like vessels, through which the same blood flowed. From this description, it seems clear that these vessels are what the *Nei Jing* authors meant by "meridians". In other words (in today's terminology) the arteries and deep veins.

But there is another practical observation that they may have had in mind. The practitioners from the time of the *Nei Jing* would have been able to detect the same "pathways on the skin" that practitioners can today, but perhaps they only viewed these as being shadows of the actual "meridians", which were these larger, artery-like tubes that lay deep

* Note that arteries are the main vessels that travel from the heart and that veins are the main vessels that transport deoxygenated blood back to the heart. See page 177.

beneath the skin and were not visible through the skin. Hence, they may have imagined that these *pathways on the skin* indicated the exact route that the deep "meridians" took around the body.

It may be that the entire body was not dissected to trace the actual route of all the arteries and deep veins. Instead, perhaps dissection was only carried out at the wrist (for example), where the deeper vessels appeared to follow the course of those *pathways on the skin* (here, the radial and ulnar arteries would have seemed to be aligned with the lung- and heart-related *pathways*). Having discovered this, the dissectors then perhaps only assumed that these deeper vessels lay deep to these surface *pathways* throughout the entire body. And when needling an acupoint on one of the *pathways on the skin* anywhere on the body, they may have imagined that when the needle penetrated the muscle beneath, it was penetrating the "meridian", which lay in the muscle directly beneath the *pathway on the skin.*

Today, it is these *pathways on the skin* that we call the meridians, and we regard the system of arteries and veins to be a separate circulatory system, unrelated to the meridians.

It is difficult to avoid projecting today's beliefs onto the words in the *Nei Jing,* but the *Nei Jing* only makes sense when the "meridians" are viewed as being these artery-like tubes deep beneath the skin's surface which followed the exact routes of those *pathways on the skin.* The *Nei Jing* authors would have imagined that

- vapours (i.e. influences, or *chi*) flowed within these tubes;
- they contained the same blood as the superficial veins;
- the "meridians" tended to flow vertically along the limbs, while the collaterals (superficial veins) branched off from these and tended to travel horizontally (p.31); and
- the "meridians" consisted of tubes which could be constricted by cold, which then impeded the flow of blood and influences (p.37).

When visualizing such a system of vessels (though the deeper "meridians" are imaginary), every *Nei Jing* passage that refers to this system then makes sense, which further reinforces the notion that this was the system they had in mind. However, this entire system was misguided theory. Of course, arteries and deep veins exist, but not in the locations they imagined (aligning with every *pathway on the skin*), and not having the imagined function; for example, no vapours extracted from food flowed through this network (since the network does not even exist).

But as with most *Nei Jing* passages, the knowledge they gained from practical observations (rather than from theorizing) was usually fact based. The existence and pathways of the meridians (i.e. the *pathways on the skin*) were probably discovered through practical observation (by sensitive practitioners being able to feel their presence, just as practitioners can today), therefore the *Nei Jing* notion of the pathways of the "meridians" is true.

Today a meridian is defined (according to this book) as a tract of distal tissue affected by organ function (p.355). It does not therefore have a dedicated anatomical structure of its own, and it is not possible for any physical substance (or vapour of any sort) to flow within it.

What are "collaterals", "tertiary network vessels" and "blood vessels"?

These are referred to throughout the *Nei Jing*, and over the millennia since, there has been uncertainty about what these terms refer to.

The *Nei Jing* authors considered the "meridian" network to be the sole circulatory system in the body, which circulated both blood and influences simultaneously. The blood circulatory system known today (with arteries, veins and capillaries circulating blood which was pumped by the heart) was then unknown (p.42).

The "meridians", or "conduit vessels" *(jing mai)* 經脈, were considered to be the part of the network that tends to run vertically in the body. But the *Nei Jing* authors also described vessels branching off from these, in a sideways direction, which they called the collaterals, or "network vessels" (*luo mai*) 絡脈. And branching off from the collaterals, were said to be the "tertiary network vessels" 孫絡.

Bloodletting was then a common form of therapy, along with acupuncture. And it is from here that the confusion stems.

From the following *Nei Jing* passages, it seems clear that the "collaterals" and the "tertiary network vessels" refer to the superficial veins (or arterioles*) that can be seen, often travelling diagonally to the meridians, and sometimes crossing them. These were where blood was let from. The "meridians" were thought to lie more deeply beneath the skin, so that the blood within them could not be seen, but that these extra vessels travelled nearer to the skin's surface, so that the blood *could* be seen within them.

The term "blood vessel" 血脈 (*xue mai*) was also frequently used in the *Nei Jing*, which adds to the confusion. But with the above points being made clear, I believe the term "blood vessel" was often used to simply mean the vessels that blood was let from. That is, the collaterals and tertiary network vessels. But confusingly, the term could also refer to the "meridians", since the same blood was thought to flow within the "meridians".

The important points to realize are that the *Nei Jing* authors considered

- all these vessels to be separate parts of the same circulatory system and to be thus interconnected;
- that the same blood and influences flowed through every part of the network;
- that the blood circulatory system known today was then unknown; and
- that when blood was let from the superficial veins, it was considered to be flowing out of the "meridian" network as a whole.

The following extracts demonstrate these points.

Extract from *Ling Shu*, Chapter 17

The [meridians] constitute a lining. Those branch courses extending sidewise, they form a network [i.e. the collaterals]. Those diverging from this network, they are the tertiary network vessels. If the tertiary net-

* "Arteries" flow from the heart, and "veins" transport deoxygenated blood *back* to the heart. The arteries branch off into smaller arteries, and the smallest of these are called "arterioles". Hence the vessels that are visible beneath the skin might be either veins or arterioles, depending on the direction of flow. However, for brevity's sake this book usually refers to these vessels simply as superficial veins.

work vessels abound with blood, a punishment is to be swiftly initiated [i.e. to swiftly let blood]. Those vessels where it abounds, they are to be drained. Those that are depleted, they are to be supplemented by means of liquid medication.[12]

This passage portrays the clear notion of letting blood from the superficial veins, which are the "tertiary network vessels". Today, these vessels are often interpreted to be finer versions of meridians (i.e. the *pathways on the skin*—p.29). But if they were, it would not be possible to let blood from them. And also, in my own clinical experience, I have never encountered any meridians other than the main meridians that bear the acupoints, so that these "vessels" that "extend sidewise" from the main "meridians" could only be superficial veins.

Extract from *Ling Shu*, Chapter 1

As for the blood vessels, they lie diagonally to the transport [acupoints]. If one looks at them, they appear distinctly clear. If one presses them, they appear distinctly hard.[13]

Here, the term "blood vessels" could only be referring to the superficial veins that "lie diagonally to the" acupoints (i.e. diagonally to the meridians). Therefore, here the term "blood vessel" is being used as an alternative term for the collaterals. Hence the collaterals correspond to the superficial veins that can be seen through the skin; and the "meridians" were thought to run deeply, such that they are not visible from the surface.

The following extract is in the context of "obstruction-illness", which is known today as "bi syndrome" (p.219).

Extract from *Ling Shu*, Chapter 81

In the blood vessels, the [constructive and defensive influence] flow without cease.... In the case of cold [influence] settling inside the [meridians and collaterals], the blood will cease to flow. When the blood ceases to flow, it fails to penetrate the [meridians and collaterals]. As soon as it fails to penetrate the [meridians and collaterals], the [constructive and defensive influence] will [accumulate] there. This cannot be reverted. Hence obstruction-illness with swelling results.[14]

Here, the term "blood vessel" is being used to refer to every type of vessel, the "meridians" and also the collaterals. This was probably because all these vessels were thought to transport the same blood.

The first line in the above quote makes it clear that blood and influences were thought to flow in the same vessels—the "meridians" and collaterals. The passage goes on: when "cold influence" settles inside the "meridians", the blood ceases to flow. When this ceases to flow, it "fails to penetrate the meridians and collaterals", which causes the constructive and defensive influence to "accumulate there" (i.e. a "blockage" results in the "meridian").

The fact that blood was considered to flow in the "meridians" as well as in the collaterals, makes it clear that "collaterals" refers to the superficial veins (as known today) and that "meridians" refers to those imaginary artery-like tubes (which were inspired by the literal arteries that are known today, but imagined to take different paths—p.29).

Extract from *Ling Shu*, Chapter 39

Huang Di: I wish to be informed of the unusual [diseases] that are not in the [meridians].

Qi Bo: They are in the blood [collaterals].

Huang Di: When the blood [collaterals] are pierced and the patient falls to the ground, why is that? When the blood shoots out, why is that? When the blood is emitted in small quantities only, and is dark and turbid, why is that? ... How can this be seen?

Qi Bo: When the blood vessels are filled to abundance, when they run hard across and are of red colour, and ascend and descend without a regular location, with the small ones being thin like a needle, and the big ones resembling a sinew, if in such a situation a drainage is performed...[15]

The chapter that the above extract is taken from is called "The blood [collaterals]" and the entire chapter is about the practice of letting blood. This title, taken together with the content, leaves no doubt that the term "collaterals" or "*luo* channels" refers to the superficial veins.

The phrase "when the blood collaterals are pierced" refers to incising the superficial veins to let blood. In the *Nei Jing*, "pierced" means either using a needle to perform acupuncture on the meridians (i.e. the *pathways on the skin*), or using a specialized "needle" (p.289) to let blood from the collaterals (i.e. the superficial veins).

After the above extract, Chapter 39 of the *Ling Shu* continues to theorize about why various outcomes occur during bloodletting—such as the patient falling to the ground or their complexion turning green. This content is analysed on page 295.

How accurate are the *Nei Jing* notions of metabolism and physiology?

The following quotations demonstrate the key notions in Chinese medicine metabolism and physiology. Different chapters from the *Su Wen* and *Ling Shu* were probably written by different authors,[16] and the conflicting notions between the different quotes are notable. The validity of each notion is discussed in the *Conclusions* section below (p.40).

Extract from *Ling Shu*, Chapter 16

For the WAY of the [constructive influence (*ying chi*)], the intake of grain is its most precious function. The grain enter the stomach. The [influences] are forwarded to the lung. They flow into the centre, and they disperse toward the outside. The [pure, essential elements of beverages and food] pass through the [meridians]. It always circulates, without cease.... The influences pour out of the [lung meridian] into the [large intestine meridian]. Upward they pour into the stomach meridian; downward they pass to the instep... [and the text goes on to describe the complete circuit of the 12 "meridians", ending back at the lung "meridian", then progressing into the lung itself, then back out to the lung "meridian" again to restart the whole circuit.][17]

The above passage conveys the notion that nutrition (in the form of vapours) is extracted from ingested food by the stomach, transferred to the lungs, then circulated in the "meridians". If it is accepted that the "meridians" were thought to be deep (imaginary) artery-like tubes (p.29), then the passage confirms that influences were thought to circulate in these tubes, and that the (imaginary) "meridians" took the same paths as those *pathways on the skin* (what we today think of as the meridians).

From the viewpoint of contemporary physiology, it is also implied that this "nutrition" involved glucose but no oxygen, since the lungs' role in extracting oxygen from the air is dealt with separately, and given a different significance (see the extract from *Ling Shu* Chapter 71 on page 36 below).

Extract from *Ling Shu*, Chapter 60

That from which man receives his [influences], that is the grain. Where the grain flows, that is the stomach. The stomach is the sea where water and grain, the [influences] and the blood gather.... The [influences] and the blood leaving the stomach, they follow the [meridians]. These channels constitute the [big passageways] linking the [organs].[18]

This passage appears to convey the notion that the blood is formed in the stomach; that both the blood and the influences flow in the "meridians"; that these substances flow directly *from* the stomach *to* the "meridians", rather than via the lungs; and that (in terms of contemporary metabolism) none of these elements involve the presence of oxygen.

Extract from *Ling Shu*, Chapter 62

The stomach is the sea supplying [all the organs]. Its clear [influences] flow upward into the lung. The [influences] of the lung move along the [lung meridian]. Their movement follows the [inhaling and exhaling of breath].[19]

In contrast to the previous passage, this passage conveys the clear notion that the food influences from the stomach, travel to the lungs *before* progressing to the "meridians".

Extract from *Ling Shu*, Chapter 47

The [meridians] serve to transmit blood and [influences]; they nourish the *yin* and *yang* realms. They moisten the sinews and the bones and they make the joints flexible. The [defensive influence (*wei chi*)] serves to warm the partings of the flesh. They fill the skin, fatten the skin structures, and are responsible for their opening and closing.[20]

Again, the notion is conveyed that both the blood and the influences (*chi*) flow in the "meridians". Added to this is the notion that the defensive influence (*wei chi*) warms the flesh, etc. Neither of these notions is literally true, but the *Conclusions* section below (p.40) discusses this and suggests how they might be interpreted.

The passage also states that both the blood and influences provide the body with nourishment, and implies that the blood nourishes the *yin* realms (or aspects) and the influences the *yang* aspects. One possible interpretation of this is that both the blood and influences were thought to nourish every type of tissue, only the *yin* aspect is nourished by the blood, while the *yang* aspect is nourished by the influences.

Extract from *Su Wen*, Chapter 10

When man lies down the blood returns to the liver. When the liver receives blood, one can see. When the feet receive blood, one can walk. When the palms receive blood, they can grasp. When the fingers receive blood, they can hold.[21]

Again, this passage indicates that the blood serves a nourishing role, enabling the muscles to work (so we can walk, grasp, hold) and even enabling the senses to work, such as sight. This, of course, is all literally true, for without a blood supply, no part of the body would survive for long; and when the quality of the blood is reduced, signs and symptoms may develop in all the tissue mentioned in the passage (such as numbness or weak tremors in the limbs, blurred vision, or "floaters"; p.83).

Interestingly, the first sentence in the quote is also literally true. In contemporary physiology, the liver serves as a reservoir for blood, and when at rest, a proportion of the blood returns to the liver (p.100). Over two thousand years ago, this notion could not have been based on practical observation, so must have been deduced by logic alone. To have correctly deduced this (using scanty clues, and those based mainly on metaphor and supposition, much of which was not literally true) was impressive.

A Chinese anatomy chart from around 1590 AD states that "The body of the liver is solid; it cannot be compared to the intestines, stomach, and bladder. As a result, it is unable to store blood as the ancients stated".[22] It is interesting that the "ancients" got the facts right (working from pure logic) but that this later author (his observations being clearly gained from dissection) got the facts wrong. But this would not have been known until recent physiology studies "discovered" the fact that the liver stores the blood.

Extract from *Su Wen*, Chapter 43

The [constructive influence (*ying chi*)], that is the essence [influence] of water and grain. When it is harmoniously balanced in the five [*yin* organs (*zang*)], and when it is dispersed throughout the six [*yang* organs (*fu*)], then it can enter the vessels.... The [defensive influence (*wei chi*)], that is the violent [influence] of water and grain. This [influence] is fast and unrestrained and cannot enter the vessels. Hence, it moves inside the skin and in the partings of the flesh.[23]

This passage seems to be saying that the constructive influence (*ying chi*) is generated by the harmonious blending of the food influence (*gu chi*) *by* the five *yin* organs (*zang*); and only after being "dispersed throughout the six *yang* organs (*fu*)", is it able to enter the vessels (the "meridians"). This is certainly a different notion to that of the influences being passed directly to the "meridians" by the stomach, or even via the lungs, but now includes the processing of these influences by *all* the organs (*yin* and *yang*) before the influences may emerge at the "meridians". This now seems to provide a third alternative version of basic metabolism.

Extract from *Su Wen*, Chapter 21

The [influence] of food enters the stomach. The stomach spreads essence to the liver. Excessive [influence] flows into the sinews.

The [influence] of food enters the stomach. The turbid [part of the influence] turns to the heart. Excessive essence flows into the vessels. The [influence] in the vessels flows through the [meridians]. The [influence] in the [meridians] turns to the lung. The lung invites the one hundred vessels to have an audience with it. [The lungs] transport essence to the skin and the body hair. The hair vessels unite the essence and they move [influence] to the [yang organs]....

Beverages enter the stomach. Overflowing essence [influence] is transported upward to the [pancreas*]. The [pancreas influence] spreads the essence, which turns upward to the lung. The [lung] frees and regulates the paths of the water, it transports the water downward to the urinary bladder.[24]

This passage also seems to favour the notion that the food influence from the stomach is transferred *directly* to the *yin* organs (*zang*), which then enables each organ to perform its functions (though only selected functions are mentioned). This thereby enables the liver to maintain the sinews; the heart to maintain the "vessels" (i.e. the "meridians" and collaterals), which are also closely associated with the lungs, so that this also enables the lungs to maintain the skin and body hair. And the pancreas is described as *only* processing the water ("beverages"), rather than the food, and thereby assisting the lungs to maintain the water passages.

Extract from *Ling Shu*, Chapter 56

The stomach is the sea of [all the organs]. All water and grain enter the stomach. All the [organs] are supplied with [influences] by the stomach. Each of the five flavours proceeds to its preferred [*yin* organ (*zang*)]. The sour flavour of the grains at first proceeds to the liver. The bitter flavour of the grains at first proceeds to the heart. The sweet flavour of the grains at first proceeds to the [pancreas]. The acrid flavour of the grains at first proceeds to the lung. The salty flavour of the grains at first proceeds to the kidneys. When the [influence] of the grains and the *jin* and *ye* liquids have assumed their movements, and when the [constructive and defensive influences] widely penetrate the body, then the food is transformed to waste which is transmitted to be released downward one by one.[25]

This passage also suggests that the food influence from the stomach is transferred directly to all the organs.

Interestingly, this theoretical passage also accounts for the factual observation of the associations between the five flavours and their respective *yin* organs (*zang*). It was noticed that each of these flavours appeared to benefit a particular *yin* organ (*zang*), and the theory accounted for this by suggesting each of the five flavours proceeded to its "preferred" organ.

Extract from *Ling Shu*, Chapter 71

The five grains enter the stomach. The dregs, the *jin* and *ye* liquids and the [chest influence (*zong chi*)] are separated to enter three channels. The [chest influence] collects in the chest, it leaves the chest through the windpipe. It penetrates the heart vessels, and it is responsible for ex- and inhalation. The [constructive influence (*ying chi*)] seeps out as *jin* and *ye* liquids, and they pour into the vessels. There they are transformed to blood, serving to nourish the four limbs. Internally they pour into the five [*yin* organs (*zang*)] and the six [*yang* organs (*fu*)]... The [defensive influence (*wei chi*)] appears as the wild and fast ones among the aggressive [influence]. At first it moves into the region of the partings of the flesh and the skin in the four limbs. It never rests.[26]

This passage states that the blood is manufactured in the "vessels", which term is used to mean the "meridians" and collaterals. In other passages, it is stated that the blood is manufactured in the stomach (see *Ling Shu*, Chap-

* Also called the spleen in Chinese medicine; see page 61.

ter 60, p.34). And again it is also notable that the notion of constructive influence (*ying chi*), which was theorized to provide nourishment to the organs and also the entire body, does not (in terms of contemporary metabolism) allow for the presence or involvement of oxygen to release that nourishment.

Extract from *Su Wen*, Chapter 39

The flow in the [meridians] does not stop. It circulates without break. When cold [influence] enters the [meridians], stoppage and retardation result. The contents of the [meridians] are impeded to the degree that they fail to flow. When the cold [influence] settles outside the [meridians], then the blood is diminished; when it settles inside the [meridians], then the [influences] cannot pass through. Hence, there is sudden pain.[27]

This passage again conveys the notion that both blood and influences (*chi*) are circulated in the "meridians"; and also graphically depicts the notion that the "meridians" were thought to be tube-like structures, through which the contents flowed, and (here and elsewhere[*]) it is implied that these tubes could contract due to cold, which could then prevent the contents (both blood and influences) from flowing through them.

Extract from *Ling Shu*, Chapter 18

Man receives his [influence (*chi*)] from the grain. The grain enters the stomach, and from there its [influences] are transmitted to the lung. This way, all [organs] receive [influences]. Their clear parts become the [constructive influence (*ying chi*)]. The turbid parts become the [defensive influence (*wei chi*)]. The [constructive influence] is in the vessels. The [defensive influence] is outside the vessels. They circulate without stop.[28]

Again this passage opts for the stomach–lungs–"meridian" route, and also appears to imply that the constructive and defensive influences are a product of the influence transferred from the stomach—perhaps each being a subdivision of this. But it is not clear where this division might take place, whether in the stomach, the lungs, somewhere between them, or even somewhere after the lungs. The passage does not contain enough detail to determine this. One possibility is that this detail was not in the mind of the author (that he simply had not thought about such things) so that future commentators are left to argue amongst themselves on this issue.

Extract from *Nan Jing*, Section 30

Man receives his [influence] from the grains. The grains enter the stomach, from which they are transmitted further to [all the organs]. All the [organs] are supplied with [influences] by the stomach. The clear portion turns into constructive influence [*ying chi*]; the turbid portion turns into protective influence [*wei chi*]. The constructive influence proceeds inside the vessels; the protective influence proceeds outside the vessels.[29]

This passage repeats the detail from Chapter 18 of the *Ling Shu*, but now states that the stomach supplies all the other organs with influences directly, rather than this being done via the lungs. Some commentators saw this as having little significance while others took great exception to the change:

[*] The extract from Chapter 39 of the *Su Wen* on page 28 states that the vessels "shrink" when cold.

Hua Shou (in 1361), pointed out the differences between this passage and the passage in Chapter 18 of the *Ling Shu*, but stated "That is a minor difference."[30]

Hsü Ta-Chun (in 1727), took great exception with this variance from the *Ling Shu* text. He wrote

> In [the *Ling Shu*], following the sentence "the grains enter the stomach" are the four words "which transmits them to the lung".* Then the text continues: "From there [all the organs] receive their influences". The meaning of this passage is quite clear. Here now, in the *Nan Jing*, those four words are omitted. How could the stomach introduce anything directly into the [other organs]? The consequences of this passage are very significant... That amounts to a distortion of the pattern of the transmission of the influences through the [organs].[31]

And Chang Shih-hsien (in 1510), added significant new details of his own, stating

> The grains enter the stomach, from which their essential influences flow out to be transported upward to the [pancreas]. The influences of the [pancreas] distribute the essential influences further to [all the other organs]. They all are supplied with the influences of the grains in the stomach.[32]

The detail added in the last quotation above, now brings Chinese medicine metabolism much nearer to contemporary metabolism. We now know that the digestion of most of the glucose in the diet is begun by the pancreas, which then enables the small intestine to absorb the glucose into the blood (p.387). Once in the blood stream, the glucose is directly supplied to every structure in the body, including the other organs.

This modification was suggested in 1510, but by 1727, Hsü Ta-Chun was still insisting that every word of the *Nei Jing* (compiled around the 2nd century BC) should be interpreted literally.

However (from the viewpoint of contemporary metabolism), this modified model of Chinese medicine metabolism still has no awareness that oxygen was also needed to be supplied in the blood, alongside the glucose, to enable the cells to extract from the glucose the nutrition they need (what we now know is energy released during the transformation of ATP—p.336).

The role of the *san jiao*

A further complication added to Chinese medicine metabolism and physiology is the involvement of the *san jiao* organ (also called the "triple burner"). From its first mention in the *Nei Jing*, around two thousand years ago, this organ has been surrounded with controversy—with commentators and authors arguing about its functions and form (p.214). The organ is said to be divided into three sections, corresponding to the upper, central, and lower parts of the torso. In one interpretation, each of these sections simply serves as a summary of the functions of the organs in that part of the torso, so that the upper section summarizes the functions of the lungs and heart; the central section, the stomach and pancreas; and the lower section, the kidneys, intestines and bladder.[33] This is probably the easiest way to think of the *san jiao* in the following extracts. However, the *san jiao* being such an ill-defined organ, adding its role to

* Though this phrase contains six English words, the original Chinese contains only four characters.

Chinese medicine metabolism and physiology only casts a further veil of uncertainty.

Extract from *Ling Shu*, Chapter 56

When the grains have just entered the stomach, their finest essence at first is emitted by the stomach's two [sections of the *san jiao*] to moisten the five [*yin* organs (*zang*)]. They move in two separate streams, along the paths of the [constructive influence (*ying chi*)] and [defensive influence (*wei chi*)].[34]

The wording of the first sentence of this extract is vague and hence confusing, and the following are two examples of commentators' attempts to clarify it.

Ren Gu'an (in the 17th century) wrote

The five types of grain enter the stomach. The waste, the liquids, and the [chest influence (*zong chi*)] move into three separate channels.... The liquids pour into the five [*yin* organs (*zang*)], where they generate the [constructive influence (*ying chi*)] and the [defensive influence (*wei chi*)]. The [chest influence (*zong chi*)], finally, collect in the chest and control [breathing].[35]

The above passage avoids referring to the *san jiao*, so avoids the uncertainties in that way. And note that the passage also favours the notion that the constructive and defensive influences are manufactured in the five *yin* organs (*zang*), similar to the notion expressed in Chapter 43 of the *Su Wen* (see the extract on page 35).

A 1980 Taiwanese edition of the *Ling Shu* clarifies the passage

When water and grain enter the stomach and once they have passed digestion in the central [section of the *san jiao* (i.e. the stomach and pancreas)], they leave the stomach upward via the upper [section of the *san jiao* (i.e. the heart and lungs)], and downward via the lower [section of the *san jiao* (i.e. the kidneys and intestines)], and then pour into the five [*yin* organs (*zang*)] and supply the entire body with nourishment.[36]

The approach of the above commentator seems to be to (in effect) construct a new passage based on ideas gleaned from other *Nei Jing* chapters. However, the resultant interpretation is no less vague than the original *Ling Shu* extract, which may reflect the inherent vagueness of the *san jiao*.

Extract from *Ling Shu*, Chapter 81

The stomach and the intestines receive grain; the upper [section of the *san jiao* (i.e. the heart and lungs)] releases [the influences]. It is to them to supply the partings of the flesh with warmth, and to nourish the bones and the joints, as well as to penetrate the skin structures. The [influences] released from the central [section of the *san jiao* (i.e. the stomach and pancreas)] are like dew.* They ascend and pour into the mountain gorges and valleys and they provide dampness to the tertiary vessels.† When the *jin* and *ye* liquids are balanced, they will transform to red blood. When the blood is

* " 'Like dew' is to say: they drip like a liquid. In the same manner as rain and dew moisten herbs and trees, they are able to nourish the entire body." (cited by Unschuld, 2016, p.763, footnote 2).

† The "mountain gorges and valleys" are the spaces between the muscles; and the "tertiary vessels" are the small network vessels [i.e. veins] which were thought to branch off from the "meridians". These are defined in *Su Wen* Chapter 58 (Unschuld, 2011, Vol II, pp.55-56).

> balanced, then the tertiary vessels are filled to the extent that they spill over. The spill over flows into the network vessels. As soon as the network vessels are filled, their contents will flow into the [meridians].[37]

This passage states that the blood is manufactured from the body fluids (extracted from ingested food), and that the manufacture takes place in the "tertiary vessels" (i.e. the superficial veins).

> **Extract from *Ling Shu*, Chapter 18**
> The [influence] of the central [section of the *san jiao* (i.e. the stomach and pancreas)], they too emerge from the stomach opening; they emerge from behind the upper [section of the *san jiao* (i.e. the heart and lungs)]. The [influence] received there are discharged as dregs, steamed as *jin* and *ye* body liquids, and transformed to fine essence. The latter pours upward into the lung [meridian] where it is transformed to blood which in turn is supplied to the entire body. There is nothing more precious! Hence it may pass only through the [meridians]. It is called [constructive influence (*ying chi*)].[38]

This passage, again, states that the blood is manufactured from body fluids and that the manufacture takes places in the "meridians"; but this time a very specific location is given: the lung "meridian". It is stated that the blood is then supplied to the whole body—through the complete "meridian" network, presumably beginning at the lung "meridian". Thus the passage also repeats the theory that blood circulates in the "meridians". And, confusingly, the extract ends by referring to this circulating blood as constructive influence (*ying chi*). It is true that "constructive influence" and blood are both generally theorized to nourish the body simultaneously, and perhaps this was the concept the passage's author had in mind.

Finally, in some contemporary Chinese medicine textbooks, it is even stated that "The transformation of [food influence (*gu chi*)] into blood takes place in the heart," though there is no *Nei Jing* source to support this notion. And the same contemporary author also claims that "The heart is responsible for the circulation of blood just the same as in Western Medicine".[39] This same claim is repeated by other contemporary textbooks,[40] though there is no basis for the claim in either the *Nei Jing* or the *Nan Jing*.

Such statements are possibly made to attempt to reconcile these aspects of Chinese medicine with contemporary anatomy and physiology; though, however well-meant, their only effect is to make it even more difficult to appreciate the Chinese medicine of the *Nei Jing*, which is already muddled enough.

Conclusions

The *Nei Jing* (which comprises the *Su Wen* and the *Ling Shu*) is a collection of ancient scrolls which today still forms the basis of the training of Chinese medicine acupuncturists. Much of the content of the *Nei Jing* is factual. This tends to be the content discovered through practical observation. But other content was arrived at by theorizing, and much of this is either metaphorical and not intended to be interpreted literally, or is simply untrue. To fully appreciate the beauty of Chinese medicine it is necessary to be clear about which elements of the *Nei Jing* are fact based, which are metaphorical, and which are untrue.

It may also be helpful to keep in mind that many of the *Nei Jing* chapters were written by different authors,[16] which may explain why the above extracts often contradict one another, particularly when expressing mere theories, rather than practical observations.

The intake of food and air

The *Nei Jing* authors (or their ancestors) noticed that we are sustained by the intake of food, drink and air, which are all essential to our survival; and that food and drink enter the stomach, while the lungs receive the air. All these observations were true.

It was deduced that the stomach then extracted something from the food, and the lungs extracted something from the air,[41] and that these extracted substances (in the form of vapours) were utilized in the body. Again, in essence, this was true—if we overlook the notion of vapours circulating in the body which contain some essence of the original substance, and instead assume that this notion of vapours being utilized in the body is analogous to the transport systems known today.

So far, the picture is fairly clear. But from this point onwards in the metabolism, comprehending the intended meaning becomes more difficult, because there are two versions to consider—the original *Nei Jing* version, and the version adopted by today's Chinese medicine.

Today's version

In today's Chinese medicine, it is usually stated that these two extracted substances, food influence (*gu chi*) and clear influence (*qing chi*), are combined in the lungs to produce a third substance, chest influence (*zong chi*).

This statement is probably informed by today's knowledge. In contemporary physiology, the stomach (and the pancreas, gallbladder, and small intestine working together) extract glucose from ingested food; the lungs extract oxygen from the air we breathe; and these are then combined to produce ATP, which releases the energy that drives every cell in the body (p.336). However the combining takes place in the cells, remotely, rather than in the lungs, as stated by today's Chinese medicine. This is the first incorrect fact.

But further, in none of the various versions of Chinese medicine metabolism, is the equivalent of oxygen (clear influence) transported in the "meridians" at all (and the "meridians" were the only known circulatory system, so there was no other way to circulate it). And chest influence (*zong chi*), which is the only Chinese medicine substance that *could* be considered analogous to ATP (albeit generated in the lungs—according to today's Chinese medicine), is not present throughout the "meridian" network—and hence throughout the body.

The *Nei Jing* authors simply did not realize that "oxygen" was required by every part of the body to release the nutritive value of "glucose" (or food influence); and their various models of metabolism reflect this mistake.

The Nei Jing version

In all the extracts from page 33 onwards, and in any other similar *Nei Jing* passages, or indeed in the original full chapters that the extracts were taken from, chest influence (*zong chi*) is not described as resulting from the combining of air and food influence. It is simply stated that the inhaled air is stored in the lungs and heart; that (in *some* versions) food influence is "steamed" from the stomach up into the lungs*; and that the combined functioning of the heart and lungs relies on chest influence. That is, the heart and lungs work closely together (p.183), and chest influence represents the functioning of these two organs in the same way that any other organ's influence is said to represent the functioning of those organs (p.26). Nowhere is there the specific notion that inhaled air and food influence are combined, which thereby *creates* chest influence. This is a notion adopted by today's Chinese medicine, probably informed by today's knowledge of metabolism.[42]

Putting aside today's knowledge, there was no reason for the *Nei Jing* authors to think that the products of the stomach and lungs needed to be combined. We only eat about three times a day, but breathe continuously, so it was not obvious that the products of eating and breathing needed to be combined in the body. And considering the other *Nei Jing* notions of metabolism, there was also no reason for them to imagine that clear influence (or "oxygen") needed to be present in any part of the body except the lungs. They had no knowledge of chemistry, or of how cells work, what energy drives them, nor even of the *existence* of cells (as we know them today), so how could they have imagined the need for oxygen everywhere in the body?

It would be wrong to project contemporary knowledge onto the *Nei Jing* texts. It is possible that the *Nei Jing* authors simply regarded breathing as something the lungs do but that the air played no part in the metabolic processes in the body. Likewise, in today's Chinese medicine, the notion that the lungs expel "waste influence" is projected onto the *Nei Jing* texts, simply because we now know that this happens (in the expelling of carbon dioxide). But there is no indication in the texts that the *Nei Jing* authors believed this, nor that it had ever occurred to them (p.124). This notion is one of the many contemporary ideas that have been wrongly attributed to the *Nei Jing* texts by today's Chinese medicine textbooks.[43] This issue highlights a further pitfall in the interpretation of ancient medical texts—the tendency to project today's knowledge onto them.

The manufacture and transport of blood

It was imagined that blood was made by combining two types of liquid that the stomach separated from the food we ate, was manufactured either within the "meridian" network or in the stomach itself (depending on which text you choose to follow) and was circulated in the "meridians". Every aspect of these descriptions is either untrue or largely untrue.

The *Nei Jing* notions about blood manufacture were largely untrue; there was an element of truth in that our diet does supply the raw materials that go to make up the nutritional part of blood, but their notion of how blood is produced is simply untrue (it is not manufactured in the "meridians", nor in the stomach).

* Their notion of organ physiology was metaphorical; it assumed the stomach "cooked" the food to produce such "steam" (i.e. the vapours that are food influence); see endnote 41 in this chapter.

The notion of blood

The *Nei Jing* authors regarded blood as a red liquid that spilled from the body when we were wounded, or could be deliberately released by incising the collaterals (i.e. the superficial veins). They were familiar with palpating the pulse at many locations on the body, locations where a meridian existed near to an artery or vein (p.299); and the pulse was not associated with a pumping action in the heart (Unschuld makes it clear that the *Nei Jing* texts contain no indication that either the heart or the lungs were thought to perform any kind of pump-like or bellow-like function[44]). Instead the pulse was simply regarded as a "movement in the 'meridian' " that could be monitored to indicate various states about the function of the organ associated with that particular "meridian".

To put this in perspective, it should be noted that in the West, it was not until 1628 that William Harvey discovered the function of the heart and the existence of the blood circulatory system.[45]

In contemporary physiology, blood is not simply a nutritive substance. It consists of plasma (about 55%) and cells (about 45%), which together contain

- water (about 90% of plasma is water);
- plasma proteins (such as antibodies, clotting factors);
- minerals;
- nutrients, including glucose, vitamins, amino acids, fatty acids (mainly extracted from digested foods);
- hormones (for cellular communication);
- enzymes;
- gasses such as oxygen, carbon dioxide;
- red blood cells, or *erythrocytes* (which transport oxygen); and
- white blood cells, or *leukocytes* (which perform immune functions, such as killing microbes or removing waste materials, such as dead cells).[46]

Therefore the blood is made up of many different elements, which are manufactured in separate parts of the body. The nutrients from digestion are extracted by the combination of the stomach, pancreas, gallbladder and small intestine, the last transferring them into the blood stream (p.63). The hormonal content is secreted from cells everywhere in the body[*]. The oxygen is transferred into the blood by the lungs (p.123), and the carbon dioxide, as a waste product of respiration, is produced at every cell in the body. The red and white blood cells are manufactured in the bone marrow.[47]

If considering only the nutritional aspect of blood, then the *Nei Jing* notion was partly correct. The blood *does* provide nourishment, only it is not restricted to *some* aspects of it (such as only the *yin* aspect) but provides all nourishment. The *Nei Jing* mistakenly thought the *yang* aspect of nourishment was provided separately (by the "constructive influence"[†]), but that both these aspects flowed together in the "meridians". The fact that both these aspects flowed together (the *yin*

[*] Page 91 provides an example of how hormones function.

[†] —Though the picture was complicated by the *Nan Jing*, which started referring to blood as "constructive influence", rather than this being the *yang* aspect of food influence, as stated in the *Nei Jing*; see p.185.

and *yang* aspects of nourishment) was true; they do. But they are, in fact, both part of the same substance, the blood, which flows in the blood circulatory system, whose true nature the *Nei Jing* was unaware of.

The blood is also the transport medium for our immunity, in the white blood cells and antibodies. The *Nei Jing* imagined the blood to have no defensive function but instead attributed this to a completely imaginary system that was transported in the "meridians" (the defensive influence, covered below).

The red blood cells transport oxygen. The *Nei Jing* did imagine a purpose for oxygen, but had no notion that it was needed by every cell in the body, nor that it was transported in the blood.

The hormonal content of blood serves as one of the major communication mediums in the body (p.91). The *Nei Jing* had no notion that the blood served any such purpose; and, indeed, the notion of bodily communication (in the sense of hormones and the nervous system) does not appear to have been considered by the *Nei Jing* authors. It could be argued that the various "influences" constitute communication between the organs and bodily tissues, but I do not believe the *Nei Jing* authors imagined it in this way. This is a modern conception, born from the knowledge of the nervous and hormonal systems.

The substance the *Nei Jing* authors had in mind when they described blood was certainly the same substance that we call "blood" today.[48] But because of their various misconceptions about metabolism, physiology, immunity and anatomy, they simply got the above mentioned details wrong. However, the *Nei Jing* statements about the nutritional aspects of blood can, in spirit, be taken literally, as long as the above caveats are born in mind.

Blood may also be called "constructive influence"

To add further confusion to *Nei Jing* metabolism, in the *Nan Jing* the idea was introduced that blood and constructive influence could sometimes be regarded as the same thing. This idea is discussed on page 185.

The notion of defence against pathogens

The *Nei Jing* authors deduced that something along the lines of an "immune system" was present in the body, which was impressive. But again, because they were working from pure logic (having made no practical observations of the internal workings of the body that could reveal how an "immune system" might work), they got the details wrong.

They imagined that another vapour-like substance, which they called "defensive influence" (*wei chi*), flowed in the spaces between the skin and muscles and thus provided the warmth to the skin and muscles, which warmth was what protected us from attack by external pathogens.

Today, we think of the immune system as consisting of various tiny components that aggressively attack and kill any foreign bodies that enter us (p.212). Because this concept is so well known today, when we interpret the *Nei Jing* notion of defensive influence it is tempting to imagine that they thought it produced its effect by "doing battle with" or "combating" the evil influence (*xie chi*), or "harmful wind", which was thought to enter us through the skin. But no such notion was in the minds of the *Nei Jing* authors. Instead, it is clear that the general thinking was that defensive influence (*wei chi*) provided the warmth to the skin and muscles and that it was this warmth that protected us from attack by external pathogens. The following *Su Wen* extract even clearly states that the defensive influence "does not merge with" the pathogens.

Extract from *Su Wen*, Chapter 43

Huang Di: The [constructive and defensive influence], do they also let a person have a block? [i.e. an obstruction]

Qi Bo: ...The [defensive influence], that is the violent [influence] of water and grain. This [influence] is fast and unrestrained and cannot enter the vessels. Hence, it moves inside the skin and in the partings of the flesh.... The [defensive influence] does not merge with the [influence] of wind, cold, and dampness. Hence, it does not cause a block.[49]

Hence, when a person was healthy, it was the warmth of their skin and muscles that protected them, but when a person was "deficient", so that their skin and muscles were not properly warmed, this enabled pathogens (such as harmful wind) to penetrate their skin.

Extract from *Ling Shu*, Chapter 66

When wind, rain, cold and heat cannot avail themselves of a depletion, their [harmful influences] alone are unable to harm man. When someone suddenly encounters a swift wind and heavy rain and does not fall ill, the reason is that he did not have a depletion.[50]

Hence, with a "deficient" person, the pathogen enters their skin. At this stage, the pathogen could be released from the body through various "holes" (acupoints) in the "meridians", or by inducing sweating, which also enabled (or compelled) the pathogens to escape.

Extract from *Su Wen*, Chapter 19

The wind is the chief cause of the one hundred diseases. Now, when wind and cold settle in a person, they let this person's entire finest body hair stand up straight. The skin closes and develops heat. At this time, the wind and the cold can be effused through induced sweating. In some cases block, numbness, swelling, and pain result. At this time, it can be removed through hot water and poultices, as well as through fire cauterization and piercing. If no cure is achieved, the disease enters the lung and lodges there. It is now called "lung block". It develops cough and rising [influences].[51]

Extract from *Su Wen*, Chapter 60

Huang Di asked: I have heard, the wind is the origin of the one hundred diseases. To treat it with needles, how to proceed?

Qi Bo responded: When wind enters the body from the outside, it lets a person shake from cold. Sweat leaves the body and the head aches. The body feels heavy and has an aversion to cold. Treat this at [Du-16 (*Fengfu*)].[52]

It was theorized that if this was not done, the pathogen lodged there, and then gradually made its way through the "meridian" network until it reached the internal organs, first the *yang* organs (*fu*), then the *yin* organs (*zang*). Once it reached a *yin* organ, a serious disease resulted, which was difficult to treat.

Extract from *Ling Shu*, Chapter 66

When a [harmful influence] strikes a person, in the beginning it is in the skin. When the skin is relaxed, then the skin structures are open. When they are open, the [harmful influences] enter via the body hair. Once they have entered, they proceed into the depth. When they are in the depth, the body hair will rise. When the body hair has risen, then that person shivers. Hence the skin aches. When the [harmful influences] remain there for some time and are not removed, then they are transmitted further and they will settle in the [meridians]. While they are in the [meridians] the muscles and the flesh are in pain... [This passage then goes on to describe the progress of the pathogen through the various sections of the body, with the symptoms produced at each].[53]

Every detail of this whole scenario is simply untrue; our protection from attack by external pathogens is performed by various elements of the immune system, where the "combat" takes place either in the lungs (p.123) or in the blood; and no part of the immune system is responsible for warming the skin.

However, the notion of defensive influence (*wei chi*) *could* be thought of as being analogous to the active components of the immune system, the lymphocytes and antibodies (p.212), since these perform the same function that defensive influence was thought to. But the notable differences are that in the immune system, a genuine combat *does* take place, but this happens in the lungs (when defending against airborne pathogens—p.123), whereas in *Nei Jing* physiology, no combat takes place but instead the warmth of the skin and muscles was thought to protect us from invasion by pathogens. And in contemporary physiology, once pathogens enter us, the combat then takes place in the blood generally, whereas in the *Nei Jing*, there was no concept of any such "immune" function taking place *within* the body.

The *Nei Jing* authors were aware that pathogens could either enter us from outside or be created within us.

Extract from *Ling Shu*, Chapter 28

As for the very first origin of all diseases, they all originate from wind, rain, cold and summer heat, from *yin* and *yang* [influences], joy and anger, from beverages and food and from living conditions, from being severely scared and from sudden fear.[54]

Hence, if illness was caused by mental or emotional factors (which could be considered internal pathogens), then it was thought that there was no protection against such pathogens, so they entered the *yin* organs (*zang*) directly and caused serious illness which was difficult to treat.

Interestingly, the same situation exists in contemporary physiology—as described in the sections of this book's organ chapters that deal with mental functions. Our thoughts and emotions directly induce organ malfunction; and once this becomes habitual, it is difficult to treat. In contemporary physiology, such "pathogens" (thoughts and emotions) are invisible to the immune system, and the induced organ malfunctions cannot usually be satisfactorily treated—such as IBS (p.67), all stress-related signs and symptoms (p.113), and so on.

The *Nei Jing* position on "defence" against such mental and emotional "pathogens" was to avoid excessive anger, etc., and you would not then become ill.

Extract from *Ling Shu*, Chapter 66

When joy and rage are immoderate, then that will harm the [*yin* organs (*zang*)]. When the [*yin* organs] are harmed, then a disease emerges in the *yin* realm.... Grief and pondering harm the heart. Repeated cold harms the lung. Rage harms the liver. To be drunk when entering the women's chamber and to sweat during sexual intercourse and then to be met by wind, will harm the [pancreas]. When someone overexerts himself, and then enters the chamber [i.e. has sex] and sweats, that will harm the kidneys. This way ... diseases are generated.[55]

Extract from *Su Wen*, Chapter 3

The fact is, the wind is the origin of the one hundred diseases. In case a person is clear and calm, the flesh and the interstice structures are firmly closed up and resist. Even though there is a strong wind which is a violent poison, it will be unable to harm that person. This is so because one follows the sequence of the seasons.[56]

However, once such illnesses have developed, it should be noted that Chinese acupuncture is usually adept at remedying the signs and symptoms, and also at helping the person to adjust the harmful mental and emotional habits—as described in the "mental functions" sections of the organ chapters.

Does *any* vapour-like substance flow in the "meridians"?

If there is no defensive influence (*wei chi*), nor constructive influence (*ying chi*), nor chest influence (*zong chi*) flowing in the "meridians" (which are imaginary anyway—p.29), does *anything* similar flow within the body?

From the point of view of today's Chinese medicine, this is a philosophical question. The *Nei Jing* notion of what equates to the term *chi*, is quite different to the notion adopted in the 1970's, and both these notions play no part in this book's scientific explanation of how acupuncture works (the intelligent tissue model). Chapter 3 (p.49) clarifies all these issues.

The notion of "original influence"

There are clear correlations between the ancient Chinese notion of original influence (*yuan chi*) and certain hormonal activity in the body—as described in the chapters on the kidneys and the lymphatic system (p.177 and 217). This means that, in effect, the ancient Chinese correctly worked out that a hormonal-like substance, which originated in the three kidney-related structures, circulated the body and controlled all its vital functions. To have worked this out over two thousand years ago was an impressive achievement (pp.177-179 and p.217).

The role of the kidneys, bladder and intestines

In the *Nei Jing* theories, the small intestine played no part in the extraction of nutrients from food. This was a further mistake; the small intestine plays a vital role in absorbing the digested food into the blood (p.205). And urine was theorized to originate from the digested food; it was thought to be extracted by the large intestine, which then passed it to the bladder (p.179). All these details are also untrue; urine is produced by the kidneys, during its filtering of the blood, and the kidneys then pass the urine to the bladder; whereas the *Nei Jing* contained no notion that the blood was filtered at all, nor that it served as a *transport* for digested nutrients and other vital substances (p.180).

Hence (considering the entire content of this *Conclusions* section) many details in the *Nei Jing* theories on metabolism and physiology are simply untrue. Their study, though, does provide a fascinating insight into the minds of physicians over two thousand years ago.

Does it matter that Chinese medicine uses metaphor?

The theoretical side of Chinese medicine is often metaphorical, and other aspects of the theories contain substantial factual errors, such as those highlighted in this chapter. However, the most significant elements of this healing system were discovered through practical observation, and those elements are fact based—and remain impressively accurate in clinic today, over two thousand years later. The key facts are the signs and symptoms related to each organ's pathology, the locations of the meridians (the *pathways on the skin*) and acupoints, and the causes of disease, including mental and emotional factors.

Even though much of the theoretical side of Chinese medicine is metaphorical, or relies on facts that are largely untrue, the overall system (perhaps *because* it is metaphorical) still works beautifully. The untrue theories and facts may be viewed as largely academic, since they do not affect treatment outcome. And the metaphorical aspects of the system can often help to produce a diagnosis and select the acupoints to use. Such a diagnosis is also usually metaphorical (such as "Stomach heat", "Excess liver yang", "Deficient kidney yin" and so on), yet the treatment still works.

This book helps students to identify whether a *Nei Jing* passage is either fact based, metaphorical, or simply untrue. But beyond this, the book also describes the key aspects of Chinese acupuncture (such as the organ functions) in relation to contemporary physiology. This enables Chinese medicine to be explained to patients using terms they can understand—while, within the practitioner's mind, any aspect of the *Nei Jing* may still be used to assist in forming a diagnosis and planning a treatment.

See also Chapter 14 (p.261), which analyses numerous passages from the *Nei Jing* to demonstrate how some of the untrue theories may have been formed.

Chapter 3. Today's notion of "chi"

When the term 氣 "chi" is used today, what is meant by this? There is certainly much mystique around the subject, but does the notion refer to something real or is it simply a misunderstood myth?

The term was first used in the medical context in the *Nei Jing*, which is a collection of separate scripts written by different authors around the 2nd century BC (p.14). The scripts describe every aspect of Chinese acupuncture. But there are two aspects to these scripts which need to be differentiated. There are the practical observations related to acupuncture, and there are the theoretical deductions.

The practical observations include the signs and symptoms that result when a particular organ is stressed in some way, including mental and emotional factors; and also the layout on the body of each organ's meridian, the key acupoints along those meridians, and the general results of stimulating those acupoints. This was the practical knowledge related to providing acupuncture treatments. As well as this, there was the patients' experiences related to the treatments, which must have been the same then as they are today. These include the following sensations.

- When an acupoint is needled, the patient usually feels a sensation at that acupoint, whose strength is usually proportional to the degree of stress in the related organ.
- On some patients, when an acupoint is needled, they sometimes feel a tingling sensation propagating a short distance along the meridian near to the needled acupoint; or they sometimes feel a tingling at another related acupoint.
- When an organ's function is poor, the skin at its key acupoints, or sometimes along sections of its related meridian, can feel cold to the touch in relation to the surrounding skin; and this coldness tends to clear immediately the organ is treated with acupuncture.
- A similar experience is that patients will sometimes feel a warmth flowing along a particular meridian during the treatment.

All these (and similar) experiences, and also the above knowledge of each organ's related signs and symptoms, are fact based. That is, they are real. This is confirmed in clinic today, where this ancient knowledge of an organ's related signs and symptoms is repeatedly encountered, and remains impressively accurate.

All well and good. But then the problems began. The *Nei Jing* intellectuals (be they practitioners or pure theorists) then attempted to explain what was happening inside the body to account for all these observations.

The *Nei Jing* model of how acupuncture works

Over 2,000 years ago, there was no useful knowledge of the body's internal anatomy (p.16), and no knowledge at all of the microscopic detail of the body tissue, of its chemistry, nor of the body's communication systems, such as the nervous and hormonal systems. In the absence of all this knowledge, how on earth could the internal workings of the body and the organs be explained? Their solution was to invent a metaphorical system, based on what they saw around them in the outside world.

When food was cooked in a pot, this produced steam which appeared to contain some essence of the food (it smelt like the food being cooked). Therefore it was theorized that the stomach perhaps worked in the same way. Food entered the stomach and was "cooked", so that a vapour rose from the food, containing its essence, and this vapour was imagined to travel around the body, delivering the food's nourishment to every part of the body. This vapour is the substance that was named *chi*. But how was it transported?

Bloodletting was then a common practice, and the superficial veins that blood was let from, the *Nei Jing* referred to as the *luo mai* 絡脈, or collaterals (p.31). From the rudimentary dissection of corpses, it would have been discovered that these superficial veins (and arterioles) flowed into deeper and larger vessels (what are known today as the arteries and deep veins). It is also clear that the *Nei Jing* practitioners would have been aware of the presence of *pathways on the skin* (what we today call the meridians), and it appears that they assumed that the arteries and deep veins followed these same pathways. It was these *imaginary*, deep vessels that they referred to as the *jing mai* 經脈, or "meridians" (p.29).

Hence, an imaginary system of deep, artery-like tubes was assumed to exist, which lay deep to the *pathways on the skin*. These tubes were thought to flow into one another, and also into the abdominal organs. And the blood, together with those imaginary vapours (*chi*), were thought to circulate within these deep, artery-like tubes.*

This highlights the root of a significant misunderstanding. In the *Nei Jing*, it was further theorized that when a person was cold, these deep artery-like tubes (the "meridians") could shrink, and thus obstruct the flow of the blood and vapours. And it was also theorized that by piercing acupoints on the *pathways on the skin*, the needle would go deep and penetrate these underlying tubes (the "meridians") and thereby release blood from the system; or even that the vapours could be affected by manipulating the needle in certain ways.

These notions were perhaps born from other assumptions—that when certain signs or symptoms existed in the patient, this was thought to be due to the blood and these vapours being excessive or deficient.

---

* As said on page 24, when this book places "meridian" in quotes, this is referring to the *Nei Jing* definition (i.e. deep, artery-like tubes). But when the term is used without quotes, this is referring to today's definition (i.e. to those *pathways on the skin*).

A practical (and therefore factual) observation was that when a person experienced certain signs or symptoms, and a needle was inserted into a certain acupoint, this would clear the condition. This was factual, but the intellectuals then appeared to have theorized that this therapeutic effect was achieved by enhancing the amount or flow of these vapours. This notion was convincing but entirely fictional, because there were no such vapours circulating the body and there was no network of artery-like tubes that lay deep to the *pathways on the skin*, and since these did not even exist, nothing, including vapours extracted from food (*chi*), could flow through them. Hence, this system could not possibly account for how the body works, nor for the effects of acupuncture. However, it is clear from the *Nei Jing* and its later commentaries that this model was understood to be literally true. Over a thousand years later, practitioners cited aspects of this model, clearly understanding it to be as true as any mathematics equation today (p.37 and 267).

The 1970's model of how acupuncture works

In the 1970's, there was a revived interest in Chinese acupuncture in the West. The therapy clearly worked and was extremely powerful, yet there was no explanation in today's physiology that could explain how it worked.

The *Nei Jing* was the earliest written account of acupuncture, and it also described their model of how acupuncture worked. In the 1970's, this was the only model available and the practitioners simply wanted to know how acupuncture worked, therefore this model may have initially been understood to be factual.

It may have been assumed that the ancient Chinese invented acupuncture, therefore they ought to know how it worked. This is still a common misconception today. The ancient Chinese did not invent acupuncture. By this, I mean that the mechanism that enables certain points on the body to be stimulated to correct health issues, such as stress in any of the main organs, this mechanism had always been present in the body. The ancient Chinese did not invent this system, they only discovered how to utilize it (p.18). Therefore, the *Nei Jing* model of how acupuncture (and the body) works, does not have any authority. It is merely a fictional model created by the *Nei Jing* authors to try to account for acupuncture-related phenomena. It was the best they could imagine, without any useful insights into how the body works to base their model on.

Consequently, when the *Nei Jing* model was closely read in the 1970's, many aspects of it would have seemed clearly fictional. There were no food vapours circulating in deep artery-like tubes (which the *Nei Jing* referred to as "meridians"), which followed those *pathways on the skin* (which are what we today call the meridians). And since these fictional tubes did not exist, they could not be shrunk when exposed to cold, so that the flow of blood and vapours would be blocked. And clearly when an acupoint was needled, the needle did not penetrate into these deep artery-like tubes—to free up such blockages of food vapours and blood and thereby effect a treatment; or to let out excess blood or to strengthen the deficient vapours, to also effect a treatment.

If the *Nei Jing* was read closely, such a model would have seemed fictional. However, the *Nei Jing* model was the only one available to explain how acupuncture worked, so all these ideas were taken to be factual, but modified using insights from today's anatomy and physiology.

It was decided that the reference to food vapours (*chi*) was really referring to some type of energy, and that it did not flow through deep, artery-like tubes (because it was now known that arteries did not generally align with the *pathways on the skin*), but instead it was assumed to somehow flow through those *pathways on the skin*, which it was also decided was what the *Nei Jing* authors were really referring to when they used the term *jing mai* (or "meridian"). Hence *chi* was regarded as being some vague type of energy that today's physics had not yet discovered.[1]

Another key concept that was adopted from the *Nei Jing* model was that of those fictional artery-like tubes (the "meridians") being shrunk by cold and hence causing the flow of blood and food vapours to be blocked within them. But this concept was reapplied to the *pathways on the skin* (what we today call the meridians), and it was assumed that the flow of this vague energy (what *chi* is now generally regarded to be) could be blocked within those *pathways on the skin*, and that acupuncture appeared to work by unblocking this flow, or, on other occasions, by somehow strengthening this vague energy, so that the function of the organ related to that meridian was improved.

Hence, in the absence of any scientific explanation, this was the general model that was adopted to explain acupuncture. This was done, despite the fact that no-one knew what this newly imagined energy really was, and no-one therefore had any idea of how such an imagined substance could flow through these *pathways on the skin*, which did not seem to have a dedicated anatomical structure. In this way, parts of the *Nei Jing* model were dismissed as being clearly untrue, and instead those parts were reinterpreted, based on the assumption that the overall model was still largely correct (even though it was based on fictional assumptions, such as vapours circulating the body in artery-like tubes). Hence, the 1970's model was derived, which is still widely adhered to today.

Common experiences that seem to support the 1970's model

In the absence of any scientific explanation for acupuncture, the 1970's practitioners used the above pick-and-mix approach to reinterpret the *Nei Jing*; and as well as their approach being guided by today's anatomy and physiology, it was doubtlessly also guided by their own experiences of practising and receiving acupuncture. The following common experiences are all apparently consistent with the 1970's model of how acupuncture works.

- When an acupoint is needled, and a sensation is felt at the needled acupoint by the patient, this could be interpreted as being a rush of this energy (*chi*) to that acupoint, whose conduction was previously blocked. And it might be thought that the "removal of this block" somehow allowed this energy to now flow along the meridian, which somehow "restored the meridian system to good health", which then accounted for the patient's overall health being restored. Though this is the usual perception, there is no specific notion of *how* this "energy flow" might interact with the patient's health (i.e. no idea of the specific physiological mechanisms involved), except perhaps the vague idea that when this energy is "flowing around the meridians", this somehow establishes the patient's good health.

- On some patients, when an acupoint is needled, they sometimes feel a tingling sensation propagating a short distance along the meridian near to the needled acupoint; or they sometimes feel a tingling at another related acupoint. These sensations are usually interpreted to be produced by the freshly unblocked flow of this energy, and hence interpreted to be direct evidence of the existence of this energy.
- When an organ's function is poor, the skin at its key acupoints, or sometimes along sections of its related meridian, can feel cold to the touch in relation to the surrounding skin; and this coldness tends to clear immediately the organ is treated with acupuncture. This returning warmth would also usually be interpreted as being due to the returning flow of this energy, which was previously not flowing in those locations. Again, this would be perceived as being direct evidence of the existence of this energy.
- A similar experience is that patients will sometimes feel a warmth flowing along a particular meridian during the treatment. Again, this would be interpreted as the effect of the return of this energy to those locations.

All these (and similar) experiences help to reinforce the 1970's model. They appear to be evidence of energy (of an unspecified type, which is unknown to today's physics or biology) "flowing along" the meridians and producing effects as a direct result of the acupuncture.

But the model does not stand up to scrutiny. For example, when an organ's function is corrected by acupuncture, the model cannot account for the communication between the acupoint and its related organ. The tingling feeling that some patients sometimes feel propagating along a meridian has been measured to travel at 18 centimetres per minute.[2] However, by taking a patient's pulses before and after needling an acupoint to correct an organ's function, it is clear that needling one of an organ's key acupoints usually corrects that organ's function in around one second. This is a common observation that most experienced acupuncturists must have made. And there are similar tests that can demonstrate this rapid communication rate between an organ and its related acupoints (p.369). Yet, when considering the tingling feeling propagating along a meridian and assuming this is *chi* (the supposed energy that accounts for acupuncture's effects), it would be impossible for a substance travelling at such a slow speed to account for the communication. When this supposed energy is thought to travel at 18 centimetres per minute, if it were manipulated at an acupoint, it would take several minutes for any change in that energy to reach the related organ, and several minutes for that change to then propagate out from the organ back to all its other related acupoints. (In the *Nan Jing*, a faster, theoretical speed of *chi* was given, of around 152 centimetres per minute[3], but even this is still far too slow to account for the communication).

Using today's anatomy and physiology, attempts have been made to explain acupuncture's effects. In 2010 it was hypothesized that sensory nerves may be responsible for communicating the needling sensation to the brain, but this idea also does not stand up to scrutiny for many reasons (p.401), and clearly cannot account for acupuncture's rapid effects on organ function. And the same is true of the primo vascular system (p.315). These structures are thought to coincide with the main meridian paths, yet the primo fluid that flows within this system, flows at the even slower rate of 0.3 millimetres per second (or 18 millimetres per minute, which is ten times slower than the propagation rate of "needle sensation" along a meridian—p.316). So, there is also no explanation in contemporary anatomy and physiology to account for the rapid effect of acupuncture treatment.

The fact that science (up until 2018) had no explanation for acupuncture's effect or for what meridians are, was perhaps a good reason for the 1970's model to be adopted by Chinese medicine. They had to have some explanation; science could offer none, so it must have seemed there was no choice but to invent a new model, loosely based on the *Nei Jing* model.

But until such myths (that form the basis of the 1970's model) are dispelled, Chinese acupuncture can never be taken seriously by other disciplines. It was in this context that, over many years, I developed the "intelligent tissue" hypothesis which explains what the meridians are, how acupuncture works; and accounts for every acupuncture-related phenomenon familiar to Chinese medicine. And in 2018, I started publishing objective experimental data that validated the key aspect of the hypothesis (pp.322-333). Hence there is now a simple model that can explain every aspect of acupuncture.

The intelligent tissue model of how acupuncture works

Central to the model is the notion that all bodily tissue interprets organ information conveyed on electromagnetic waves (p.333).

This ability in the tissue was probably present throughout the body's evolution. Assuming that (just as it does today) all bodily tissue always possessed the ability to interpret organ information conveyed on electromagnetic waves, then as soon as the first rudimentary digestive organs evolved, the body shape and the sense organs may have gradually evolved in response to organ information. In other words, an animal's body may have evolved to serve its abdominal organs. There is much evidence in Chinese medicine to support this notion—in each of the sense organs being associated with a particular abdominal organ (p.88) and also in the paths of the meridians. Each path tends to reflect the function of the associated organ (pp.351-353), and the layout of the meridians on the limbs exactly corresponds with the functional relationships between the organs (pp.345-351).

This suggests that throughout evolution, all bodily tissue was able to interpret organ information, and this caused the shape of the limbs, head and torso to form in response to this information. If this was the case, this would mean that the tissue that now correlates with the path of a particular meridian (say, the heart meridian), formed in that particular position to reflect the function of the related organ (the heart) and also its relationships with the other organs. This would mean that today, this bodily tissue that is situated along that meridian (in this case, the heart meridian), evolved to "listen to" and respond to the heart (its normal function, its physical condition, and its particular types of stress), so that this situation has now resulted in a body-shaped filtering system for organ information, as follows.

The information from all the organs is combined into a single, complex wave; but along each meridian, only the information from a particular organ is now responded to by the local tissue along that meridian. And it is this (in effect) filtering system that now produces the meridians. The tissue along a particular meridian, emphasizes the organ information from the related organ, so that when the organ is stressed in any way, this produces anomalies at various locations along its related meridian. At the key acupoints, the tissue would become tender when pressed; or if the organ function were weak, the skin at its key acupoints may feel cold to the touch; if the organ had "heat" (in Chinese medicine terms), the skin at its key acupoints may become reddened, or even feel warm to the touch. Also boils (acne), stiff or painful joints, or even shooting pains along a meridian may be produced by this same mechanism.

When the tissue at any of these key acupoints is needled, this appears to relax the tissue (i.e. causes it to shed its borrowed stress and hence return to normal function), and this pattern of the tissue returning to normal function, is also communicated body-wide on the same electromagnetic waves. The wave pattern of this transformation would be specific to a particular organ (the organ that caused the anomaly at the needled acupoint), and when this pattern (of the tissue shedding the stress that was borrowed from that particular organ) reaches that organ, this appears to persuade the organ to follow this same pattern and it also returns to normal function.

Hence, the meridians, rather than consisting of dedicated anatomical structures, are simply distal tracts of normal tissue that are affected by organ function (p.355).

This explains all acupuncture-related phenomena

In this way, this simple fact of bodily tissue interpreting organ information conveyed on electromagnetic waves, is able to explain every acupuncture-related phenomena familiar to Chinese medicine. Not only does it explain what meridians are, how they are produced, and how acupuncture works, but it is also able to explain how Chinese medicine organ pulses are produced (p.302), how organ information is able to radiate between people, so that we can feel when other people are upset, or even sometimes pick up their symptoms (pp.363-369). And the common phenomena listed on pages 52-53 are now explained as follows.

When an acupoint is needled successfully, the sensation felt at the acupoint by the patient (the so called "de chi" sensation) occurs when the related organ starts to correct its function and, in effect, release its stress. This process of the organ function transforming back to normal is reflected at the needled acupoint (due to the local tissue interpreting this new organ information), and this is what produces the sensation felt by the patient. This explains why, when the needle is first inserted, there is sometimes no sensation. But then, when the needle is stimulated, there reaches a point when the appropriate local tissue relaxes, and this state is reflected back to the related organ, causing it to release its stress, which process is then interpreted by the tissue at the acupoint, producing the sensation. And this also explains why the degree of the sensation is proportional to the degree of stress in the organ. When that stress is high (and consequently the acupoint was tender when pressed), the needle sensation often occurs the moment the needle is inserted, with no stimulation. On the other hand, when an organ's function is already normal, or near to normal, and one of its key acupoints is needled, it can be very difficult to obtain a needle sensation. This is because there is no great change of function to be induced in the organ, therefore a needling sensation (which is the reflection of a change in organ function) cannot be obtained.

After an acupoint is needled, the patient may sometimes feel a tingling sensation propagating along the meridian, or at other key acupoints related to the same organ. Again, this sensation simply represents the changing state of the organ function. After it is stimulated by acupuncture, the organ would begin to return to normal function; in other words, it would gradually shed its stress. When this process is reflected in the tissue near the needled acupoint (due to the local tissue interpreting this new organ information), this produces a tingling sensation that moves a little way further along the meridian, in a *yin*-to-*yang* direction. That is, the stress moves to a more superficial level of the organ's function (i.e. a more *yang* level), which movement is reflected at a gradually more and more *yang* location along the meridian (on a limb meridian, this means that it moves towards the tip of the limb). The sensation is usually only felt moving along a short section of the meridian, which reflects the fact that the majority of the stress only has a short "distance" to move to be completely shed by the organ.

In this same situation, a tingling is sometimes felt at a related acupoint. For example, if one of the *back shu* acupoints for the kidneys is needled (Bladder-23 *Shenshu*), then the patient may feel a tingling at Kidney-3 (*Taixi*), near their heel. Such a key acupoint for that organ (Kidney-3) would reflect any major functional improvement in the organ. Therefore, when such an improvement is induced (in this case, by needling Bladder-23), a sensitive patient may feel a tingling at this related acupoint, Kidney-3, which is simply reflecting the fact that the organ's function is improving. This situation is reflected at the distal acupoint, even though that acupoint was not needled, which confirms that the tingling sensation was not produced directly by the needling, but by the local tissue at the acupoint interpreting the organ's new information (which is instantly transmitted bodywide on electromagnetic waves—p.366).

When the skin at an acupoint or meridian is colder than the surrounding skin, this coolness (or absence of normal warmth) can also be explained by the local tissue interpreting organ information. Because an organ's function is poor, the reflection of this state in the local tissue at its key acupoints and meridian may cause the temperature of the skin in those locations to be correspondingly reduced. And when the organ's function is corrected by acupuncture, the skin's temperature at its related acupoints and meridian would also return to normal, which can even cause the patient to be aware of that returning warmth along the meridian.

The "electric shock" sensation

There is another occasional sensation, not mentioned above, which feels akin to an electric shock shooting along a meridian. This cannot be accounted for by any notion of *chi*, whose theoretical speed is far too slow for it to be able to cause such a sensation. However, the sensation can be accounted for by the intelligent tissue model.

When an acupoint is strongly stimulated and the patient feels a sensation akin to an electric shock shooting along an entire meridian, this may reflect the fact that the organ was shocked into suddenly changing its function in a significant way, rather than this happening gradually. This state would be "instantly" reflected at every location along its related meridian (theoretically, an electromagnetic wave propagates through human connective tissue 670 times faster than nerve impulses travel—p.366). But it would seem to the patient that an "electric shock" had rapidly travelled *along* the meridian, which could be accounted for as follows.

Even though the local tissue (including the sensory nerves) at every location along the meridian had simultaneously reflected the organ's suddenly changed function, the activation of each sensory nerve still needed to be communicated back to the brain for the patient to become aware of the sensation. And the further from the brain each nerve was, the longer this communication would take, which would give the impression that the nerves were firing in a long sequence, starting with those nearest to the brain and progressing along the meridian. In fact, such a sensation would seem to travel along the meridian at the rate that nerve impulses travel in the body (at around 100 metres per second). But this does not mean that a substance of any sort (including electricity) had travelled along the meridian, even though this is the impression the patient would be left with.

Experimental validation of the intelligent tissue model

Though the intelligent tissue model is still regarded as an hypothesis, its key aspect has now been validated experimentally. My own published experiments have demonstrated that the tissue at key acupoints physically changes to reflect states in the related organ, and does this in real time, with no discernible delay (pp.322-333).

How can practitioners who've learnt the 1970's model, accept the intelligent tissue model?

The 1970's model regards *chi* as being a vague form of energy which has not been discovered by today's physics and which is assumed to flow through "vessels" which have no dedicated anatomical structure.* Whereas the intelligent tissue model accounts for every phenomena related to Chinese acupuncture, but without the need for any substance or dedicated energy to flow in the meridians at all. Does this mean that *chi* does not exist?

To practitioners of Chinese acupuncture, this very suggestion may provoke outrage. In the 1970's model, the phenomena and experi-

* It is clear that primo vessels are not an integral part of the meridian system—p.322.

ences listed on pages 52-53 are convincingly accounted for by the notion of energy flowing along meridians. And indeed, once the 1970's model is accepted, the very existence of these phenomena, such as the needling sensation; the tingling sensation that occasionally propagates along a short section of a meridian; the coldness of the skin at key acupoints and along a meridian when the associated organ is functioning poorly; the apparent "blockages" to the flow of this energy that occur at meridian locations, which are then apparently "cleared" with treatment; all such experiences seem to constitute evidence of the existence of this vital energy that is thought to produce such phenomena.

Once a practitioner has experienced these phenomena for many years and always accounted for them by using the 1970's model of *chi* and its flow around the body, it is understandably difficult for them to then dismiss the 1970's model. There is no doubt that all these phenomena and experiences are real. However, the 1970's definition of *chi* is not a direct reference to a real phenomenon; it is only an abstract model designed to account for these real experiences. But the intelligent tissue model does not call for a complete revolution in the minds of existing practitioners. If practitioners want to hold on to their existing 1970's notions of *chi*, then the intelligent tissue model *could* be regarded as simply providing a scientific definition of *chi*. In this case *chi* would be defined as organ information conveyed on electromagnetic waves (or alternatively, *chi* could be regarded as the process of an organ's health being reflected at its related meridian), so that rather than consisting of some vague form of energy of a type unknown to today's science, it is simply organ information (or the reflection of that information). Does this interpretation of the intelligent tissue model work? And how would this new definition of *chi* fit into the 1970's model?

A scientific definition of *chi*

It might be helpful to first realize just how close the intelligent tissue model is to the *Nei Jing* model. In the *Nei Jing* model, *chi* is defined as a vapour released from ingested food, which then travels the body, along the paths of the meridians (even though this vapour was thought to travel through deep, artery-like tubes, it was still imagined to travel the exact paths that the meridians take, as we think of them today). This vapour was thought to also contain the essence of each organ (p.26); and it was thought that by manipulating this vapour at acupoints, this could effect changes in the related organ. Whereas, the same effects are achieved in the intelligent tissue model by organ information being conveyed to every part of the body on electromagnetic waves, with the information from each organ being emphasized at its related meridian. By stimulating key acupoints, changes can be effected in this organ information, which changes are then able to persuade the related organ to revert to normal function. Not only is the mechanism very similar, but (as said on page 28 above) organ information conveyed on an electromagnetic wave could certainly be regarded as being as ethereal as vapours rising from cooked food.

But to marry the intelligent tissue model to the 1970's model, we must now think of *chi* as existing of, not some type of energy, but as organ information conveyed on electromagnetic waves. It might be thought that organ information conveyed in such a way is energy anyway, so what's the problem? Isn't this just another way of saying the same thing?

Well, no, not really. In the 1970's model, it is this mysterious energy that is thought to produce the effects; perhaps in the same way that when electricity flows into a light bulb, it is the electricity that produces the light (or is converted into light). But in the intelligent tissue model, the organ information (which we are imagining to be a new definition of *chi*), does not carry some substance that is vital to life, and which, when delivered to any bodily location, is then able to nourish the tissue, so as to enable it to function normally. Instead, it is purely information. And when this information is changed (due to the related organ not functioning properly) this change is reflected in the tissue local to the organ's related meridian, to produce the tenderness when pressed, or the cold or red skin, etc. And when the information is then changed again at a key acupoint (by the location being stimulated, which returns the local tissue to *its* normal function), this change is then reflected at the related organ, persuading the organ to also return to normal function.

There is no life-giving substance that "flows along the meridians". Instead, the meridians are merely bodily locations where organ information is emphasized. Hence to marry the 1970's model to the intelligent tissue model, practitioners just need to appreciate that *chi* is not a substance in its own right, but instead it could simply be regarded as the expression of an organ's health (good or bad) at locations along that organ's related meridian. Followers of the 1970's model may still then continue to use all their other thoughts related to that model, so that only a slight adjustment (in the definition of *chi*) is required.

In truth, there is very little difference between the two models; and this whole discussion could be regarded as a merely philosophical exercise, or even as an academic distinction. There are many similarities between *all* the models, and all the same experiences and phenomena occur and are explained, and the therapy works today as well as it always has done, whatever thoughts are in the minds of the practitioner.

However, when looked at from a scientific point of view, the 1970's model of how acupuncture works, and the 1970's notion of *chi*, are pure fiction. Therefore, when talking to patients, healthcare workers, scientists, or the media, if Chinese acupuncture is going to have any credibility, it is necessary to use explanations that directly refer to reality (rather than using a metaphorical model). Here, the intelligent tissue hypothesis provides a credible explanation for all the phenomena related to acupuncture, including its ability to immediately correct organ malfunction; and its central concept (that bodily tissue interprets organ information) has now been validated experimentally (pp.322-333).

At the simplest level, rather than referring to *chi*, acupuncture might be described as achieving its effects by manipulating organ information. If curious patients then wonder what mechanism it uses to manipulate organ information, the overall process could be summarized as above. That is, due to the resonance between an organ and its related acupoints, the organ's health is reflected at those acupoints, which become tender when the organ is stressed; and by stimulating one of these acupoints, the local tissue returns to normal function, which persuades the related organ to also return to normal function.

Chapter 4. Pancreas and stomach

Attribution of Chinese medicine organs

As demonstrated in Chapter 2 (p.23) , many of the notions in *Nei Jing* metabolism and physiology are simply untrue, including some aspects of organ function (such as the stomach "steaming" vapour up to the lungs; the large intestine producing urine and passing this to the bladder; and so on). Due to these issues, this resulted in there being only a loose relationship between the theoretical *Nei Jing* organ functions and the actual anatomical organs (which I explain in more detail below). Unfortunately, this loose relationship led to one of the key *Nei Jing* organs being attributed to the wrong anatomical organ. And this misattribution continues to be used today in Chinese medicine, which causes confusion.

The main digestive organ in Chinese medicine is called *pi* 脾. In terms of the anatomical organs, this was associated with the spleen. However, when comparing this organ's main functions with those of the organs described in contemporary physiology, it is clear that the organ *should* have been associated with the pancreas.

The main functions of the Chinese organ *pi* are that it plays a key role in digestion and the production of energy; and is also responsible for the appetite (p.64). Whereas the pancreas produces juices and enzymes that digest carbohydrates, proteins and fats[1]; secretes the hormones *insulin* and *glucagon* to control the uptake of glucose, which is the body's main fuel[2]; and also secretes the hormone *pancreatic polypeptide*, which is thought to produce the appetite.[3] Hence this organ's main functions are also digestive and the production of energy and the appetite. It seems obvious that these two descriptions are referring to the same organ and that the Chinese medicine organ *pi* should therefore have been attributed to the pancreas.

The spleen (in contemporary physiology) is a part of the lymphatic system (it may be regarded as a large lymph node) and its main functions are therefore related to immunity[4]; but it also helps to maintain an appropriate amount of fluid in the tissues and purifies the body fluids, destroying debris such as dead cells[5]; so it is difficult to see why the Chinese medicine organ *pi*, the key digestive organ, is still equated to the spleen.[6]

Section 42 of the *Nan Jing* states, "The spleen weighs.... Its flat width is three inches. Its length is five inches,"[7] whereas the spleen (in contemporary physiology) is a rectangular structure with a thickness of about one inch, length of about 4.7 inches and width of about 2.7 inches.[8] Clearly this *Nan Jing* description is describing the spleen (of contemporary physiology), rather than the pancreas.

How was this mistake made?

Such dimensions could only have been obtained by dissecting a body, which raises the question: how was each anatomical organ associated with the theoretical organ functions then known?

Even though the knowledge of basic organ anatomy was known to *some Nei Jing* authors, [9] this knowledge could not have amounted to much more than an awareness of the organ masses in the torso. This would not have enabled the functions of those organ masses to be correctly worked out, since this would have required a knowledge of the chemistry and microscopic anatomy of the organ tissue, which knowledge simply did not then exist. So, even though there was basic knowledge of internal anatomy, this would have provided little assistance in working out the organ functions.

To some degree, it might be supposed that the physical "plumbing" between the organs may have provided a clue to each organ's main function, but due to the misguided notions of *Nei Jing* physiology, the presence or absence of physical links or "tubes" between the organs was not necessarily a guide or a limitation. For example, it was theorized that nutrients passed around the body in the form of vapour. All *Nei Jing* authors shared this belief. They imagined that the essence of food, rose from the food, much like steam from a cooking pot, and this steam, or vapour, then circulated in the "meridians" to every location in the body (p.23). Hence, it was imagined that the stomach extracted this vapour by "cooking" the food, so that the vapour rose from it, much as happens in real life. And some *Nei Jing* authors theorized that this "steam" rose from the stomach and passed to the lungs, which then circulated it in the "meridians" (p.41). The fact that there is no physical link between the stomach and lungs was not a limitation, since their model of physiology did not require a physical link. Instead, since they believed that nutrients travelled in the body in the form of vapour, there was no reason to think that this vapour was not capable of steaming between one organ and another, so that a physical link between such organs would not be found during dissection. And the same is true of their misguided theory that the large intestine produces urine, then passes this to the bladder (p.47). There is no anatomical link between the intestines and bladder, but this (if known about) would not necessarily have been a limitation, since they could have imaged the exchange also taking place in the form of vapour. This is what I mean by there being only a loose relationship between the physical organ masses and the theoretical *Nei Jing* organ functions.

If the "plumbing" between the organs was not a guiding factor, and it was not possible to work out an organ's function from its tissue, how did they manage to attribute the other organs correctly?

Generally, the discomfort produced when an organ is stressed may have been the guiding factor. With the liver, kidneys, stomach, heart, lungs or intestines, the discomfort would have helped identify which anatomical organ produced the symptoms. With the

Chinese medicine organ *pi*, any such discomfort would have been in the region of the stomach organ, and perhaps mistaken for being produced by the stomach. So to find which anatomical organ to associate with the Chinese organ *pi*, its theoretical function was perhaps the only clue.

The requirement was to locate *an* organ near to the stomach, since this was suggested by the organ *pi's* digestive function. The spleen is a relatively large organ mass adjacent to the top part of the stomach, and when viewed from the front during dissection is much more visible than the pancreas (which would be hidden from view, behind the stomach),[10] which may explain why the spleen was selected rather than the pancreas. The fact that there is no physical link between the spleen and stomach would not have been a limitation, since the *Nei Jing* notions of physiology did not require there to be a physical link. Any substances that passed between the organs could have flowed as vapours (as they were thought to do between the stomach and lungs). Understandably, due to their mistaken notions of metabolism and physiology, they had no idea that the spleen, even though it was a large organ adjacent to the stomach, played no role in digestion.

Unfortunately, due to this original misattribution, the term "spleen" is now used in Chinese medicine to refer to this organ, *pi* (the pancreas), and also used in clinic, in discussions with patients. But in order to clear up this confusion and enable contemporary minds to understand discussions of Chinese medicine, I believe it is important to correct this misattribution, and throughout this book I therefore refer to this organ as the pancreas. But when reading other Chinese medicine texts, you should be aware that this same organ would usually be referred to as the spleen.

The functions of the pancreas

As stated above, in contemporary physiology, the main functions of the pancreas are that it

- produces pancreatic juice, which contains enzymes that digest carbohydrates, proteins and fats[1] (these enable the small intestine to absorb the nutrients into the blood stream—p.205);
- secretes the hormones *insulin* and *glucagon* to control the uptake of glucose,[3] which is the body's main fuel[2]; and
- secrets the hormone *pancreatic polypeptide*, which is thought to produce the appetite.[3]

The Chinese medicine approach

In contemporary physiology, the notions of the organ functions were formed by dissecting the body, examining the organs and systems at the microscopic level, and attempting to work *backwards* from those observations. But in ancient China they used a different approach. At that time, the contemporary knowledge of the chemistry and microscopic anatomy of the body did not yet exist, so could play no part in their reasoning. Instead they relied purely on practical observation. They observed the signs and symptoms that were produced when an organ was stressed, and which cleared once that organ was treated. And this was all they needed to know. The concept of organ functions, as we think of them today, did not then exist. Later though, Chinese intellectuals did work out many theories to attempt to explain *how* the various symptoms were produced, which theories are described throughout the *Nei Jing*. However, many of these are simply untrue, such as most of their notions of metabolism (pp.40-48); and also see my analysis of five phase theory and its misapplication to attempt to explain signs and symptoms (pp.263-277).

Today's Chinese medicine avoids this issue by using an approach reminiscent of that used by the ancestors of the *Nei Jing* authors. Rather than describing organ functions in terms of *how* the signs and symptoms (and normal functions) are produced, general phrases are instead used to summarize an organ's main functions and also the *effects* of those functions.

The difference between functions and effects

For example, in the following list the pancreas is described as "providing strength and substance to the muscles". This phrase does not describe a function but an indirect effect. The effect is fact based, but this could not be described as a literal function of the pancreas, since the pancreas (in contemporary physiology) only enables the completion of digestion and then regulates the uptake of glucose. It is the presence, or absence, of the digested resources that then produces the *effect*, which is to provide the muscles with strength and substance. Hence this is an effect rather than a function.

These descriptions have the advantage of being true—since they avoid repeating *Nei Jing* theories and focus on practical observations.

It is important to make the distinction between such functions and effects, so as to facilitate communication with healthcare practitioners outside of Chinese medicine—and also with your own patients. If an effect such as the pancreas *providing strength and substance to the muscles* were referred to as a pancreas function, this notion could only be rejected by anyone familiar with contemporary physiology, since there is no direct functional link between the pancreas and the muscles. Whereas if these qualities in the muscles were described as an indirect *effect* of the pancreas function, this would enable contemporary physiology to at least consider the phenomenon.

Hence, in today's Chinese medicine, the functions and effects of the pancreas are described as follows.

The Chinese medicine functions and effects

The pancreas

1. completes digestion, enabling the digested resources to be transported around the body;
2. provides strength and substance to the muscles;
3. produces the sense of taste and the colour in the lips;
4. prevents haemorrhage;
5. counters the effect of gravity on the organs; and
6. has mental and emotional functions.

Below I explain each of these functions and effects in turn and relate them to contemporary physiology.

1. Completes digestion, enabling the digested resources to be transported around the body

The first part of this description ("completes digestion") is a direct function rather than an effect.

The *Nei Jing* authors noticed that when the pancreas function was poor, the patient often experienced some or all of the following signs and symptoms:

- general weakness,[11]
- emaciation and malnutrition,[12]
- poor appetite,[13]
- abdominal bloating and discomfort[14] with excess gas,[15] and
- loose stools.[16,17]

From this, it was deduced that the pancreas *completes digestion*—since, when the pancreas function is poor, the resources from ingested food are unavailable, rendering us weak and malnourished. And it was also deduced that the pancreas *enables the digested resources to be transported around the body*—since, when its function is poor, no digested resources are transported to any part of the body, including the muscles (making us generally weak) and internal organs (producing the signs and symptoms of abdominal discomfort, bloating, excess gas and loose stools[18]).

The second part of this description is an effect rather than a function. In contemporary physiology, the pancreas does not literally transport resources around the body; instead it enables the small intestine to absorb the resources into the blood stream, and the blood then transports the resources. Therefore, this description does not refer to a literal function of the pancreas but to an indirect *effect*—which is that the resources are *able* to be circulated, simply because the pancreas produced them.

It is possible that this *effect* may seem a mere play on words, since it may not seem to be stating anything beyond the obvious. But it is describing an observation made by the *Nei Jing* authors, which clearly seemed clinically significant. And also, it cannot be denied that it is literally true. But in Chinese medicine, descriptions of such effects only tend to remain true as long as *Nei Jing* theories are not offered to explain them.

Extract from *Su Wen*, Chapter 29

All the four limbs are supplied with [influence (*chi*)] by the stomach, but the stomach [influence] is unable to reach the [meridians] directly. It is only because of the [pancreas] that the four limbs get their supplies. Now, when the [pancreas] has a disease and is unable to move the body liquids on behalf of the stomach, the four limbs are not supplied with the [influence] of water and grain. Their [influence] weakens day by day; the vessel paths are no longer passable. The sinews and the bones, the muscles and the flesh, none of them has [influence] to live. Hence, they do not function.[19]

In the above extract, the author offers his theory to explain this pancreas function and effect. Curiously, on first reading, the essence of this extract's description *seems* to correlate with the main pancreas function of contemporary physiology. The pancreas completes the digestion begun by the stomach, so that if the pancreas did not do this properly, the nutritive resources (including glucose, proteins, vitamins and minerals) would not be properly absorbed by the small intestine into the blood, therefore malnutrition would occur, resulting in the signs and symptoms mentioned.

It is the theoretical passages in the *Nei Jing* that tend to be either metaphorical or untrue (p.261); whereas its passages based on practical observation are usually fact based and have stood the test of time—such as its descriptions of the signs and symptoms associated with a particular organ's malfunction. Therefore the above *Su Wen* extract, which expresses a theory, seems remarkably accurate.

But this is only the case if the Chinese medicine notions of metabolism are ignored. These were described on pages 33 to 48. Their general notions were that some type of vapour-like essence is extracted from ingested food (akin to steam rising from a cooking pot) which is modified and split into separate parts, all of which are transported through the "meridians", along with the blood, to every part of the body, with the separate parts of the vapour performing different roles. There was no notion that oxygen (clear influence) was required to enable glucose (food influence, or constructive influence) to be made use of by the body tissue; no notion that the small intestine played any part in absorbing nutrients; and the details of the roles played by the other organs also varied between different authors within the *Nei Jing*, leaving a tangled web of contradictions.

This is only to be expected when none of this knowledge was based on practical observation of the body's inner workings; but instead on the speculations of intellectuals, using the analogy of their state's administration. The upshot is that all their above notions of metabolism are untrue.

When the above *Su Wen* extract is considered in this light, the statement that the pancreas "moves the body fluids on the part of the stomach" is now understood to mean something quite different to the notion in contemporary physiology—that the pancreas completes the digestion begun by the stomach. The flow of substances in contemporary metabolism is entirely different from that in *this* version of *Nei Jing* metabolism, or in any other version of it. It is only when considering this *Su Wen* extract in isolation of the other passages in the *Nei Jing* that it *appears* to resemble the pancreas function of contemporary physiology.

In today's Chinese medicine, the descriptions of an organ's effects, such as the pancreas "enabling the digested resources to be transported around the body" only remain true as long as the *Nei Jing* theories of metabolism are not cited to attempt to explain *why* the organ has this effect. In other words, such descriptions are only useful clinically, and in discussions with patients, as long as they are left as a general overview.

It should also be born in mind that the general inaccuracy of such *Nei Jing* theories does not in any way diminish the power of acupuncture or Chinese medicine. Acupuncture was not invented by the Chinese; it is a natural phenomenon in the body that has always existed (p.18); therefore the *Nei Jing* theories on *how* acupuncture (and the body) works, even though not factual, do not in any way affect the outcome of acupuncture treatments.

The advantage of Chinese medicine

In some areas (*because* of its approach) Chinese medicine achieves results that are yet to be matched by contemporary medicine.

The signs and symptoms related to each organ's malfunction were identified through practical observation, and this was done *before* any theories were developed to attempt to explain those signs and symptoms and how the body produces them—the theories came later (p.261). This means that, no matter how inaccurate the later theories are, the associations of the signs and symptoms with a particular organ's malfunction are fact based; and when acupuncture corrects an organ's malfunction, the signs and symptoms are cleared and the person's health improves.

In contrast to this, contemporary medicine is often unable to account for the signs and symptoms that Chinese acupuncture routinely treats. For example, when trying to account for the intestinal symptoms of abdominal bloating, discomfort, excess gas and loose stools, there is no knowledge in contemporary physiology that is able to properly explain them. Therefore such symptoms are usually regarded as being without explanation and the condition is labelled a *syndrome*, which means a collection of symptoms with no known cause. And in this case the term "irritable bowel syndrome" (IBS) is used to describe the condition. However, the fact remains that through practical observation in ancient China, these symptoms were all observed to occur when the pancreas function was poor, and once the pancreas function is successfully treated with acupuncture, the symptoms clear.

Patient example
Male, aged 56. This patient had poor energy, a poor appetite, poor sense of taste, soft stools, and felt tired after eating, all of which cleared with treatment. See the full case history on page 246.

Patient example
Male, aged 49. This patient had a long history of IBS, which responded well to treatment. See the full case history on page 253.

It could be said that labelling this condition a syndrome (of "unknown cause") is inappropriate, since there *is* an indirect link between the pancreas and these symptoms—in contemporary physiology. The small intestine is about five metres long in an adult and is the main site in the digestive system where nutrients are absorbed into the blood stream. The process of absorption is heavily dependent on the enzymes secreted by the pancreas. It is therefore not difficult to imagine that when the pancreas function is poor, the workings of the small intestine would be heavily affected, which may account for the intestinal symptoms of a bloated and tender abdomen, excess gas and loose stools. And the weakness and emaciation in the person would be the obvious result of this poor digestion.

However, it should be acknowledged that the Chinese acupuncture treatment of the pancreas (which clears this condition—and is described later) probably could not currently be explained in biochemical terms. Chinese acupuncture has no idea how the body works at the chemical level—and does not *need* to know this—so it can provide no assistance in this matter. Therefore, in contemporary medicine, the condition will probably continue to be regarded as being of "unknown cause".

Explanation of Chinese medicine terms

In today's Chinese medicine, to describe the main pancreas function and effect it is usually said that the pancreas "governs transportation and transformation".[20] The term "transformation" is usually understood to mean the transformation of food into the resources the body needs, which, in *Nei Jing* terms, are the various influences (*chi*), blood and liquids. And the term "transportation" is usually understood to mean the transmission of these substances around the body. The pancreas is also understood to be the main digestive organ, in that it "governs" these processes. To translate this description into something more meaningful to today's readers, I describe the function and effect as "completes digestion, enabling the digested resources to be transported around the body". But is this a valid translation of today's Chinese medicine phrase?

When textbooks and practitioners use this phrase (that the pancreas "governs transportation and transformation"), the meaning they have in mind is usually a literal belief in selected aspects of *Nei Jing* metabolism. They understand "transformation" to mean that the pancreas enables and oversees the transformation of ingested food and liquids into the various influences (*chi*), blood and body liquids; and they understand "transportation" to mean that the pancreas enables, or directly produces, the circulation of such resources around the meridian network. These are *selected* ideas from *Nei Jing* metabolism (there is no definitive version of *Nei Jing* metabolism, due to the contradictions from different authors—p.125), but, even though selective, every detail is still untrue. Influences do not really exist, and neither these nor blood really flow in the meridians (pp.40-47), and the circulation of these (in effect) "imaginary" substances is not effected by the pancreas (in contemporary physiology). Even any analogous substances within contemporary physiology—such as glucose, fats, vitamins and minerals, blood, or oxygen—are not circulated by the pancreas.

The Chinese medicine organ functions and effects only remain true, as long as *Nei Jing* metabolism is not cited to attempt to explain *how* they are produced. In recognising this, my translation of this description is expressed in a way that is both meaningful to today's readers, and also avoids any mention of *how* the effects are produced. Thus this main pancreas function and effect remains fact based.

Note that there is nothing wrong with students or practitioners referring in their own mind to the *Nei Jing* theories of metabolism and physiology, as long as it is realized that the Chinese medicine described by such theories is conceptual only, and is certainly not literally true, so that a practitioner should not expect to be able to mention such theories to patients or to anyone outside of Chinese medicine and remain credible.

2. Provides strength and substance to the muscles

The *Nei Jing* authors noticed that when a person's pancreas function was poor, the muscles of their limbs may became weak and soft.[21]

As said on page 64, this is an effect rather than a direct function. The pancreas (in contemporary physiology) enables the completion of digestion and then regulates the uptake of glucose. It is the presence, or absence, of the digested resources that then produces the effect. When these resources are not present, malnourishment results. In this situation, the initial poor pancreas function would have resulted in us becoming weak and having wasted muscles.

In today's Chinese medicine, to explain this effect it is usually said that the pancreas "dominates the muscles and the four limbs".[22] When the "four limbs" are referred to in the *Nei Jing*, this usually means their functioning, which, in other words, means the ability to move about. And this could also be understood as meaning the general strength and stamina.

3. Produces the sense of taste and lip colour

It was noticed that when the pancreas function was poor, the patient experienced a weak sense of taste or even no sense of taste at all,[23] and also had pale lips;[24] and that after the pancreas was successfully treated, the patient's sense of taste returned and their lips regained their normal redness.

The production of lip colour is certainly an effect rather than a function. And the production of the sense of taste is probably also an effect, though this is uncertain. There is the possibility that this could be a direct function of the pancreas, in the same way that the production of the appetite is recognised as a pancreas function in contemporary physiology. However, this pancreas effect (or possible function) has not been fully explored in contemporary physiology, so it is not possible to determine whether it is a direct function or an indirect effect. Physiologically, nerves from the taste buds activate parasympathetic nerves that enter the pancreas, providing a direct neuronal link between the taste buds and pancreas.[25] This does provide a direct informational link between the two, so that there is at least the possibility that the pancreas may directly produce (or contribute to) the sense of taste—in contemporary physiology.

The only thing that can be said for certain is that both these effects (or the function and effect) are fact based, since they were based on practical observation by the *Nei Jing* authors and are still routinely encountered in clinic today.

In today's Chinese medicine, these effects are usually expressed by saying the pancreas "opens into the mouth and manifests on the lips",[26] the term *opens into the mouth* meaning there is a strong association between the pancreas and the sense of taste.

4. Prevents haemorrhage

It was noticed that when the pancreas function was poor for an extended period, some patients suffered various kinds of haemorrhage, such as

- blood in the stools,[27]
- uterine bleeding,[27]
- purplish spots or patches on the skin, and
- the tendency to bruise easily.

And after the pancreas was successfully treated, these signs tended to clear, which led to the observation that the pancreas prevents haemorrhage.

This is certainly an effect rather than a function. In contemporary physiology, the pancreas has no direct control over the blood vessels, nor over whether the blood maintains its proper place in the vessels or tissue. Its main function is focused on enabling the small intestine to complete digestion. But nonetheless, this effect is still a fact-based observation—that when the pancreas function has been poor for some time, haemorrhages tend to occur.

In contemporary physiology, haemorrhaging is most often associated with either a reduced platelet count or with vitamin K deficiency. Reduced platelet production would usually be due to bone marrow deficiencies; and vitamin K is usually synthesised in the intestine by bacterial action.[28] However, contemporary physiology does not currently associate these factors with poor pancreas function, which does not, of course, mean there is no link. Contemporary physiology also does not associate poor pancreas function with the symptoms of IBS, yet within Chinese medicine this association has been known for over two thousand years—and was discovered through practical observation, in the same way that the association between poor pancreas function and haemorrhaging was.

In the same way that poor pancreas function affects the function of the intestine (to produce the symptoms of IBS), it is possible that it may also affect the synthesis of vitamin K within the intestines, which would account for the signs of haemorrhaging. It is also possible that the malnutrition that would result from poor pancreas function could lead to a deficiency in the bone marrow, reducing platelet production, which could also account for haemorrhaging. These points are speculation. However, even though contemporary physiology is currently not able to explain some of the common disease mechanisms known in Chinese medicine (such as the association of the pancreas with IBS, the "kidneys" with asthma and hay fever, and the liver with many stress-related signs and symptoms) this may change in the future. For now, all that can be said is the these *Nei Jing* symptomatic observations are clearly fact based—since they are still routinely encountered in clinic today.

In today's Chinese medicine, this effect is usually expressed by saying the pancreas is responsible for "controlling the blood".[29] I have translated this to "prevents haemorrhage", since it implies an indirect effect rather than the direct function of "controlling" the blood, which the pancreas does not literally do.

5. Counters the effect of gravity on the organs

It was noticed that when the pancreas function was poor for some time, signs and symptoms could occur featuring an unnatural downward movement in the body (which signs and symptoms cleared once the pancreas was successfully treated), such as

- a bearing-down sensation in the abdomen;
- prolapse of the anus; and
- prolapse of organs such as the uterus, stomach, kidneys or bladder.

This is clearly an effect rather than a direct function. And one way to account for this effect using contemporary notions of physiology is as follows. The pancreas enables the body to obtain energy and nutrition from the food we eat, which then nourishes the muscles and also the tissue of each organ. And in the same way that the muscles lose volume and become flaccid when we are malnourished, the internal organs may also suffer similar effects—becoming weak and possibly flaccid and (to some degree) losing their proper form. In this state, they would tend to no longer retain their proper place in the abdomen.

6. Has mental and emotional functions

From the time of the *Nei Jing*, a connection was noticed between the mental and emotional activity and the functioning of the organs—such that it appeared that each of the main organs produced certain thoughts or emotions.

> **Extract from *Ling Shu*, Chapter 8**
> The liver stores the blood. The blood hosts the *hun* soul. The liver [influence (*chi*)]... if replete, then rage results. The [pancreas] stores the [constructive influence (*ying chi*)]. The [constructive influence] hosts the intentions.... The heart stores the vessels. The vessels host the spirit. The heart [influence]: if depleted, then the patient will be grieved. If replete, then he will laugh without end. The lung stores the [influences]. The influences host the *po* soul.... The kidneys store the essence. The essence hosts the mind."[30]

In this passage, the theories expressed as to how each organ produces its mental or emotional activity are not significant. These, like many of the theories in the *Nei Jing*, tend to be either metaphorical and not intended to be interpreted literally, or simply untrue (p.261).

To take the "heart" theory as an example—the passage states that the heart is associated with the "vessels" (which, at that time, meant only the "meridians", which the blood was considered to be transported through—p.42), and that these "meridians" host the "spirit" (which was considered to be the portion of the heart that produces its particular mental and emotional traits). Then, the passage states that when the heart influence (heart *chi*—which would have been understood as some kind of vapour that contained some essence of the heart's current state), when this vapour becomes either depleted or replete (as it flows through the "meridians"), then it is this changed state that somehow produces the mental traits of the patient being either "grieved" or "laugh[ing] without end". The quality of being "grieved" is open to interpretation, but the trait of laughing "inappropriately" is certainly one that in clinic is still clearly associated with heart problems (p.234). But as to the theory about *how* these states are produced by the heart, if this is interpreted literally then it is clearly untrue, since the influences do not really exist anyway (pp.40-47), so that their state within the "meridians" also does not exist and could not therefore produce these emotions. But further, the idea of our thoughts and emotions being produced within the "meridians" does not seem credible. This thinking was perhaps a product of the *Nei Jing* notion that all states in the body are the result of the movement of influences through the "meridians".

However, if we choose to be generous for a moment and interpret the theory as being intended metaphorically, then I can see the validity of it. The state of the heart influence (heart *chi*) in the heart "meridian" was thought to directly reflect the state of the heart; and when the theory states that it is the heart influence in the "meridian" becoming either replete or depleted that produces the mental or emotional states, this could be understood as meaning that the function of the heart itself is changed, and that it is this changed function in the heart that produces the mental or emotional state. This I can accept as being true. But I do not believe the *Nei Jing* authors intended their theory to be metaphorical; I believe they understood it to be literally true—but each reader must decide this for themselves.

Likewise, the extract states that the pancreas stores the constructive influence (*ying chi*), and that the constructive influence hosts the "intentions".

Incidentally, when interpreting any passage from the *Nei Jing* that expresses a theory, it should be remembered that other *Nei Jing* authors (in separate chapters) will sometimes express a conflicting theory,* which should caution the reader about accepting any passage at face value.

This particular passage seems to be expressing the theory that the mental activity associated with the pancreas comes from something extracted from the food we eat (i.e. the constructive influence), rather than from the pancreas itself. At face value, this would have to be dismissed as nonsense. However, interpreting the passage metaphorically, I can see its validity. As expressed below and in the following chapter, the pancreas is responsible for digesting food, and this function appears to be used by the conscious mind to also digest our thoughts. The "constructive influence" is a theoretical vapour-like substance that the stomach and pancreas extract from the food we eat, and which contains some essence of the original food that can be used to nourish any part of the body. When the conscious mind uses the pancreas to digest a thought, the thought takes the place of the physical food the pancreas normally digests, and it is thought that the pancreas may process that thought in the same way it processes the food (p.93). In other words, the contents of our thoughts are equivalent to the contents of our food; i.e. the constructive influence. Therefore, to say that the constructive influence hosts the "intentions" (i.e. the pancreas's mental and emotional functions) is not too far from the truth—when viewed metaphorically. But again, I think it is more likely that the *Nei Jing* author understood their theory to be literally true.

However, the significant aspect of the above *Ling Shu* extract (and any other similar passage), is not the theories expressed about how or why the symptoms are produced, but simply the fact that the *Nei Jing* authors associated mental and emotional traits with the main organs. It is true that, to an outsider (someone not familiar with Chinese medicine), these untrue theories tend to devalue such passages. But putting the theories aside, the mental and emotional traits associated with the organs are still routinely seen in clinic today—and this book presents a somewhat different explanation for how they may be produced (see below).

A more impressive passage on this topic is Section 16 of the *Nan Jing*. This passage sticks entirely to the facts, without theorizing about them. It discusses how organ malfunction can be diagnosed. Once such an "illness" has been detected in the "pulses", it states that the illness can be confirmed by the presence of the

* See Chapter 2, on Chinese medicine metabolism, particularly pp.33-48.

main physical, mental or emotional signs and symptoms that were known to be present when any of the five main organs were "afflicted". On the pancreas, it states

> **Extract from *Nan Jing*, Section 16**
> Consider feeling a movement in the vessels that is associated with an illness in the [pancreas]. External evidence of such an illness includes a yellow face, a tendency to belch, a tendency to ponder, and a fondness of tasty food.... The illness, as perceived by the patient, consists of a swollen and full abdomen; his food is not digested; his body feels heavy and the joints ache. He is tired and weary, desires to lie down, and is unable to pull his four limbs together. If this evidence is present, the [pancreas] is afflicted. If it is not present, the [pancreas] is not afflicted.[31]

Note that "a tendency to ponder" is cited as the main mental trait associated with the pancreas, which, in my experience, is more clinically accurate, and useful, than the description of the pancreas as housing "intention". And this is supported by Chapter 5 of the *Su Wen*, which, when describing the traits associated with the pancreas, states "among the states of mind it is pensiveness".[32] Today, "pensive" is defined as "deeply or seriously thoughtful, often with a tinge of sadness".[33] This seems to perfectly describe the manner of a person whose conscious mind is dominated by this aspect of the pancreas function.

For contemporary readers, the notion of the abdominal organs playing any part in our mental and emotional activity may be hard to accept. But this ancient knowledge was based on practical observation; and the associations of certain thoughts and emotions with certain organs is still routinely seen in clinic today.

Since this subject is so clinically significant, the whole of Chapter 5 is devoted to exploring it. Using concepts from contemporary physiology, the chapter provides detailed explanations of how it may be possible for the main abdominal organs to produce many aspects of our mental activity—and conversely, for similar mental activity to be able to impede the functioning of the abdominal organs. But for now, the following introduces the topic.

It is clear that the pancreas provides us with the ability to mentally digest facts, just as it provides us with the ability to digest food. The following observations (amongst others), which are routinely encountered in clinic, support this notion.

Habitual thinkers tend to develop poor pancreas function. And when such people then indulge in a bout of intensive thinking, this usually weakens further their pancreas function, producing a flare up of the related signs and symptoms, such as feeling bloated and tired after eating, having a tender abdomen, poor energy, frequent loose stools, excess gas, and intolerances to certain foods. It is as though the pancreas's resources are drained by the activity of us mentally digesting facts.

Further (some time *after* the *Nei Jing*), it was recognised that the activity of the organs have a daily rhythm and each organ is most active in a particular two hour period (p.379). The pancreas function is known to be strongest between the hours of nine and eleven a.m., and to then gradually diminish until it reaches its weakest at nine p.m. And the habitual thinkers who develop poor pancreas function find they can think clearly only in the morning, until about midday, and if they try to mentally digest facts later in the day, they find this increasingly difficult. This suggests that the ability to mentally digest facts depends on the strength of the pancreas function. In other words, that it is the pancreas that is responsible for this ability. And also, if this mental ability were a function of the brain alone, unrelated to the pancreas function, it would not be time dependent.

Today, this is a common pattern amongst students or any person whose work involves heavy thinking. And when revising for exams or when the demands of their work are intensified, this can induce a flare up of the signs and symptoms of poor pancreas function (known as IBS in contemporary medicine).

And even our own recent ancestors appear to have had an awareness of the possible association between the organs and thoughts, since this awareness is fossilized in the very language. We still use phrases such as "food for thought" and "chewing over an idea" which suggest the knowledge that the digestive organs are associated with our ability to mentally digest facts; and phrases such as having a "gut feeling" or a "gut instinct", indicating that instinctive ideas seem to somehow come from within the abdomen.

A possible physiological explanation of how the pancreas could provide us with this mental ability is given in Chapter 5.

Improper function

When the pancreas function is poor, any of the above mentioned pancreas functions and effects could become defective, which could cause a *selection* of the following signs and symptoms to occur:

- poor appetite[13] (prefer to only eat small amounts);
- general weakness[11] (and hence the tendency to avoid speaking),[34] and feeling tired after eating;
- abdominal bloating and discomfort[14] (particularly after eating), excess gas,[15] frequent loose stools[16];
- intolerances for certain foods, such as dairy or wheat;
- poor sense of taste[23];
- cravings for sweet food (p.82);
- muscles of limbs are weak and soft (emaciated)[12];
- tendency to bruise easily or have mild haemorrhages or purple spots or patches on the skin, blood in the stools, excessive menstrual flow or bleeding of the uterus[27];
- feeling a bearing-down sensation in the abdomen, possibly with prolapse of the anus or of internal organs such as the stomach, kidneys, uterus or bladder; and
- pain or discomfort anywhere along the pancreas or stomach meridian.[35]

People with this condition would tend to be habitual thinkers or worriers,[36] and all the above signs and symptoms would tend to be made worse after extended periods of heavy thinking or studying.

Today's Chinese medicine term for this condition is analogous to "poor pancreas function". The condition would usually be called "Pancreas chi deficiency" (or, in other texts, "Spleen chi deficiency"). Using this book's convention, this would be written

"Pancreas influence deficiency". The phrase "pancreas influence" is analogous to pancreas function (p.27), therefore today's Chinese medicine term for the condition is analogous to poor pancreas function.

How a diagnosis is made

When a patient first comes for treatment, they often have problems with several of their main organs but have come to clinic to address a single issue which is often a complication of one of the main problems. I would usually begin by asking whether they had certain signs and symptoms related to each of the main organs. If the patient had around three of the signs and symptoms listed above, this would suggest they had poor pancreas function, and I would confirm this by examining their pulses and tongue (see the *Nan Jing* extract on page 73 above).

Facial colour and tone of voice

This initial questioning could also be guided by my impressions of the patient, including their general manner, complexion, and the sound of their voice. When poor pancreas function is pronounced, there may be a yellow hue visible on their face.

> **Extract from *Su Wen*, Chapter 10**
> If the complexion is generated by the [pancreas], it resembles a *gua-lou* fruit [which, when ripe, is a shining yellow colour] wrapped up in white silk.[37]

And Chapter 37 of the *Ling Shu* states "...when the [pancreas] has a disease, the lips are yellow...",[38] where the 'lips' refers to the skin around the lips, rather than the red part.

Chapter 5 of the *Su Wen* associates a "singing" tone of voice with the pancreas.[39] And in clinic today, when a patient's health is dominated by their pancreas function, they will often have a singing quality to their tone of voice and will also often hum or sing to themselves.

The pulses

The taking of pulses has been a part of Chinese medicine from its beginnings. Today, these are taken only at the patient's wrists, though at the time of the *Nei Jing*, the "pulses" (then known as the "movement in the vessels") were felt at certain acupoints on the meridian of each organ; it was the *Nan Jing* that introduced the novelty of taking all the pulses only at the wrists (p.299).

The pulse is felt in three different positions on each wrist, each position providing information about the functioning of a different organ. This is conveyed in the quality of the pulse, rather than merely its speed; and the possible qualities could involve the width of the pulse, the firmness, or tautness, the shape of the rising and falling, the strength, the depth, and so on—with each quality indicating a particular type of malfunction in the corresponding organ*.

A typical pulse with poor pancreas function

When there is poor pancreas function, the pulse would often be weak and deep at the second position on the patient's right wrist (which corresponds to the pancreas†), and the pulse would tend to have a quality known as "slippery". The sensation of feeling a "slip-

* For a detailed description of the mechanism that may enable pulses to contain this information, see page 302.

† The pulse positions are shown on page 301.

pery" pulse could be imagined as being akin to feeling treacle flowing beneath your fingers rather than water—as though the blood were thicker than it should be and moves more slowly, so that the rise and fall of the pulse may seem somewhat lazy.

The term "dampness"

"Dampness" is said to result in us when the digestion, particularly the pancreas function, is poor; or, to put it another way, when the digestive ability is unable to cope with a particular type of food we eat—in the quantities we eat it in. Hence, the state is related to the digestion.

When a person has just eaten a large meal, their pulses usually adopt a "slippery" quality. But after a short while, their digestion of the meal progresses and this quality usually clears from their pulses. However, if their pancreas function is poor, this "clearing" process may take longer, or may never completely finish, leaving the person with pulses that are permanently "slippery". This state is then known as *dampness*, which could be understood as meaning that the person's digestion is weak—and the not-properly-processed digestive substances constitute the *damp* within the person. In time, oedema may result (see below for an explanation).

The above are the facts in practical terms. But what could the presence of "dampness" be equated to in contemporary physiology? In other words, what effects might happen in the body due to poor pancreas function?

The "slippery" pulse after eating, represents a state in the functioning of the organs—as all Chinese medicine pulses do. In the blood (in contemporary physiology), the products of digestion are being circulated, and there is a sudden surplus of glucose (the body's main fuel) and also proteins and fats. All the organs would be exposed to this sudden surplus, therefore the "slippery" pulse quality usually appears in all pulse positions. But this excess of glucose, fats and proteins is usually regulated and returns to normal. This regulation is performed by

- the pancreas, by secreting *insulin* and *glucagon* to control the uptake of glucose—p.63;
- the liver, which stores much of the glucose for use later, and converts fats into *triglyceride* to store them in the fatty tissues of the body—p.99;
- the kidneys, which also store glucose for use later, just as the liver does—p.153; and
- the adrenal glands, which regulate the blood glucose level by counteracting insulin, and play a significant role in releasing the stored glucose from the liver, kidneys and muscle tissue, and also mobilize the energy stored in the body's fat reserves—p.154.

When this "slippery" quality remains in a person's pulses throughout the day, this suggests that some part of all the above regulation is not working properly.

From Chinese medicine observations, it is clear that this state usually begins with poor pancreas function, but any of the other organs mentioned above may also be involved. However, since the treatment focuses on the pancreas, this may be the main organ involved. In contemporary physiology, it is possible that this simply consists of a malfunction in the pancreas's ability to control the uptake of glucose, but to a lesser degree than exists in diabetes—to be, perhaps, the forerunner of diabetes.

Also in contemporary physiology, it is probably not possible to accurately define all the processes and organs involved in producing the state known as "dampness" in Chinese medicine. But it could perhaps be best visualized as follows. The products of digestion are not properly regulated, and due to this "fault" in the supply of nutrition to all the organs and processes, the organ functions become "sluggish", and in time oedema may develop, which may be explained as follows.

In Chinese medicine, the term "kidneys" includes the kidneys and adrenal glands (p.153), and both these structures work closely with the pancreas to regulate the processing, storage and supply of glucose. Once the poor pancreas function fails to properly regulate the uptake of glucose, this may impede the function of any other organ also involved in this process, including the "kidneys", and once the kidney function is impeded, this may produce the oedema (p.163).

The above explanations are speculation, which sometimes cannot be avoided when attempting to explain Chinese medicine using contemporary physiology.

Tongue examination

In Chinese medicine, it is recognised that the malfunction of the organs produces visible changes to various aspects of the tongue. On the body of the tongue, different areas are associated with particular organs and when an organ is stressed, its associated area may have a changed body colour (it may be unusually red or pale); or there may be a change in the tongue shape, such as a dip in that area; or the tongue coating may show a change in its thickness or colour (p.383).

The stomach and pancreas are associated with the central area of the tongue, and with poor pancreas function there may be a dip in this region. But more reliably the tongue's general body shape would tend to be noticeably swollen with teeth indentations along both sides.

In clinic, this type of tongue is a reliable indication of poor pancreas function. And I also find that people with such a tongue are, without fail, heavy thinkers or worriers. This has often caused me to wonder which came first. Was it that the person developed poor pancreas function, which then caused them to become habitual thinkers; or were they always prone to continuously thinking, which led to them developing poor pancreas function, which in turn tended to worsen their thinking habits (since the thinking became harder) and the more they indulged, the more this weakened their pancreas function, so worsening their digestive symptoms, until they arrived at an impasse where they suffered chronic digestive symptoms and could not think clearly. This, of course, is the worst case scenario, but many habitual thinkers or worriers may be able to relate to the description. As to which came first, it may not be possible to tell; the only certain thing is that poor pancreas function and heavy thinking seem to go hand-in-hand.

Treating poor pancreas function

Once diagnosed, an acupoint would be selected to strengthen the pancreas function. Some typical acupoints are Stomach-36

(*Zusanli*), Pancreas-6* (*Sanyinjiao*), Pancreas-3† (*Taibai*) and Bladder-20 (*Pishu*).

Note that usually only a single acupoint would be used. In acupuncture, there is often a choice of several different acupoints that could achieve the same effect, and the above are amongst the most commonly used acupoints to affect the pancreas function.

Due to the resonance between the pancreas and these acupoints, when poor pancreas function is present, the acupoints tend to become tender. When one of these acupoints is stimulated, this utilizes the same resonance but in reverse, which encourages the organ to cancel out the malfunction in itself that caused the tenderness (p.372), and the organ returns to normal function. The pancreas pulse would then become much stronger (where it was previously weak) and usually changes in quality.

Since the problem is corrected by the organ itself, is hormonal activity also normalized?

The monitoring of the body's hormonal activity (or of any similar factors in the blood considered in contemporary physiology) plays no part in Chinese medicine. However, since part of this book's purpose is to relate Chinese medicine to contemporary physiology, this issue needs to be commented on.

Acupuncture utilizes the associations between the organs and specific locations on the meridians to encourage the organs to cancel out any malfunctions themselves. And once a course of treatments is successful, the person feels good and any signs and symptoms they previously suffered in relation to the treated organ would have cleared—which is one of the measures of the treatment's success. Since hormones are simply an organ's communication medium, and other similar factors in the blood are merely a measure of that organ's activity, and the condition has been corrected by the organ itself, it is difficult to imagine why such factors would not also have returned to normal—assuming they were abnormal before the treatment.

For example, one key symptom experienced by people with poor pancreas function is a poor appetite. In contemporary physiology, it is considered that the secretion of the hormone *pancreatic polypeptide* (*by* the pancreas) may be responsible for producing the appetite (p.63). Once poor pancreas function is successfully treated with acupuncture, the patient's appetite usually dramatically improves. If our appetite *is* produced by the hormonal activity of the pancreas, this would suggest that the acupuncture treatment of the pancreas caused the organ to correct its hormonal activity.

Another common example is acupuncture's treatment of hay fever. In contemporary physiology, hay fever would usually be considered an immune-system issue. In Chinese medicine terms, the underlying cause of hay fever is usually poor "kidney" function. When the "kidneys" are mentioned in Chinese medicine, this also encompasses the adrenal glands (p.153) which, from evolution's point of view, are a part of the "kidneys" (p.153) and are therefore treated whenever acupuncture corrects the function of the "kidneys". The adrenal glands secrete the hormone *cortisol*. One of cortisol's many actions is the development and maintenance of normal im-

* Also called Spleen-6.

† Also called Spleen-3.

munity (p.154). In my clinical experience, acupuncture treatment of hay fever is usually extremely effective, often transforming the lives of life-long hay fever sufferers, who find that after successful treatment, when they are exposed to all the same allergens as before, they now experience no signs and symptoms. In contemporary physiology, the patient's immune system is now clearly working properly, whereas before the treatments, it was not, which suggests that the acupuncture treatment of the "kidneys" (which includes the adrenal glands) caused the adrenal glands to correct their hormonal activity.

The progress of treatment

In Western countries, acupuncture sessions tend to be given at weekly intervals initially, then the time between treatments is increased as the signs and symptoms improve. On the second visit, most patients report an improvement in some of their symptoms, which could include an improvement in their sense of taste, energy or digestion, with less bloating and tiredness after eating, or the absence of loose stools; and some even report an improvement in their ability to think, with their mind seeming more clear. After the first session, this improvement may only last for a day or two, particularly when the symptoms were present for many years. But after each successive treatment, the improvements usually last longer, until the patient remains symptom free between treatments. At this point, the interval between treatments is increased. Many patients then only return for a further treatment once they start to feel less well. This might be once a month or even just once a season, depending on how stressful their life is.

Patient example

Male, aged 56. This patient had a wide range of symptoms that had built up for years, including poor appetite, feeling tired after eating, having a poor sense of taste, sweet cravings, loose stools, and he found it hard to think after midday. All these symptoms cleared after a few treatments. See the full case history on page 246.

The value of regular maintenance treatments

Once a patient's health problem has been resolved, they usually appreciate the value of good health and realize that this can be maintained by regular treatments, with the frequency being determined by the degree of stress in their life.

> **Extract from the *Su Wen*, Chapter 2**
>
> The sages did not treat those already ill, but treated those not yet ill; they did not put in order what was already in disorder, but put in order what was not yet in disorder.... Now, when [treatment is sought] only after a disease has become fully developed—when attempts at restoring order are initiated only after disorder has fully developed—this is as if a well were dug when one is thirsty, and as if weapons were cast when the fight is on. Would this not be too late?[40]

Causes of poor pancreas function

This condition is widespread in developed countries, since they are "thinking" societies. Many jobs are mentally demanding, the education system itself demands intensive study over many years, and perhaps the situation of wealth itself tends to produce citizens who are prone to thinking and worrying—due to the pressures of consumerism.

Extract from *Su Wen*, Chapter 29

When one is invaded by a robber wind or depletion evil, the *yang* [meridians] receive it. When food and drinks are consumed without restraint, when rising and resting occur out of time, the *yin* [meridians] receive it.

When the *yang* [meridians] receive it, then it enters the six [*yang* organs (*fu*)]. When the *yin* [meridians] receive it, then it enters the five [*yin* organs (*zang*)].

When it enters the six [*yang* organs], then the body becomes hot and one lies down when it is not the proper time. In the upper part of the body this causes [shortness of breath].

When it enters the five [*yin* organs], then distension and obstruction result. In the lower part of the body this causes outflow of undigested food. If this lasts for long, it causes intestinal [gas].[41]

As usual with any *Nei Jing* passage, the important detail to focus on is the content the authors gained from practical observation. In the above extract, this is that when exposed to external pathogens, this tends to produce the signs and symptoms of a cold or flu; i.e. we become hot and weak (lying down when not the proper time) and have shortness of breath. But when "food and drinks are consumed without restraint" and when we do not keep to normal hours (rise and rest out of time), this affects the *yin* organs (*zang*), including the pancreas, which produces the symptoms of "distension and obstruction", loose stools (outflow of undigested food), and intestinal gas.

The untrue elements in the above extract, which resulted from theorizing, were that both external and internal pathogens affect us by entering the "meridians"; and the ideas on the nature of those pathogens (p.44). However, this aside, all the practical observations about the causes of illness and the resultant signs and symptoms are reliable and have certainly stood the test of time.

When considering the pancreas, an important point to realize is that "consuming food and drinks without restraint" also refers to mentally digesting information without constraint; i.e. always thinking, studying or worrying.

All this mental activity tends to impede the pancreas function. Chapter 5 uses concepts from contemporary physiology to provide a detailed description of how this relationship between our thoughts and pancreas function may be possible. But in summary—when the conscious mind needs to digest a thought, it uses the pancreas's digestive function, since that function existed for millions of years before such thoughts came along. But many of the ideas we try to digest are difficult to understand, and we may fail to properly digest them. And since this mental function mirrors the pancreas's physical function, a failure in the one produces a corresponding failure in the other. Therefore, when we fail to properly digest a thought, this impedes the pancreas's ability to extract nutrition from food. And the more we study difficult topics, or rack our brains to understand something that is beyond us, the more the pancreas function is impeded.

The body was designed to be used

Through most of evolution the body was physically active, which would have been relied on when nature designed the digestive system. Nature does things efficiently, and it would have been wasteful to create a digestive system that worked perfectly whilst we remained largely inactive. Therefore the body was designed to rely on normal usage to assist *all* its systems to work effectively. And gentle exercise after a meal aids the digestive process. But most of today's occupations demand lack of exercise, which only makes it harder for the digestive organs to work properly.

And finally, the very fact that we live in a developed society seems (paradoxically) to demand that we eat unhealthy food, making it even harder for the overworked digestive organs to extract the nourishment the body needs. The pancreas cannot cope with the demands we place on it, and many of the signs and symptoms listed on page 74 develop.

Acupuncture highlights unhealthy lifestyle factors

Acupuncture normalizes the functions of the main organs, and at the end of a treatment patients often comment on how relaxed they feel, and some even describe their state as euphoric. I usually tell them that what they are feeling is normal, but that normality only feels this good to them because they were so used to living in a stressed state.

This "normality" does begin to wear off in the days following the treatment, since the patient returns to their previous stresses, and responds to them in the same way. But after a few treatments, patients often make spontaneous changes to their lifestyle. It is as though the treatments make them aware of the factors in their life that detract from this "normality"—that is, the factors that encourage their organs to work in ways that do not feel right. And a patient with poor pancreas function might become less inclined to overthink, or to worry, since they can now so clearly feel how exhausting this is, or how unwell it makes them feel. Or they may restrict their thinking to mornings and avoid it for the remainder of the day, where possible; and perhaps start to introduce more light exercise, particularly after eating, and also changes to their diet.

Helpful changes to the diet

When a patient has poor pancreas function, it would be beneficial for them to avoid eating any of the following (since these foods are harder to digest, so they may lead to the build up of *dampness*):

- all heavy dairy produce, such as cheese and cream;
- pork and rich meat;
- roasted peanuts (such as in peanut butter);
- concentrated juices, especially orange and tomato;
- bananas, sugar and sweeteners; and
- if the poor pancreas function is pronounced, wheat could be avoided in the early stages of treatment.[42]

And in general all meals should be cooked and warm, and liquids should also be at body temperature or above. This is to aid the digestive process—since, when we eat raw or cold foods, the stomach and pancreas need to work harder to digest them; while if foods are cooked and warm, they can be digested more easily.

Sweet cravings

Chapter 10 of the *Su Wen* states that "the [pancreas] longs for sweet flavours".[43] And most patients I see in clinic who have poor pancreas function describe themselves as having sweet cravings. This is because food that is naturally sweet tends to benefit the pancreas. However, in developed countries, people often satisfy this craving by eating chocolate or other foods high in refined sugar, which may provide a short term boost in energy but ultimately only weakens the pancreas further. This is because the sweetness is far too high. The remedial flavours that we crave should be taken in small doses, which have a beneficial effect; but when taken in large doses, this tends to overwhelm the organ and have a negative effect.[44]

The following foods are naturally sweet and would all tend to have a beneficial effect (when adequately cooked):

- sweet root vegetables, such as carrot, parsnip, sweet potato, potato;
- rice, oats, millet;
- cauliflower, pumpkin, squash, string beans, broad beans, lentils, peas;
- blueberry, cherry, date, fig, grape, strawberry;
- salmon, herring, or any white fish; and
- chamomile and jasmine.[45]

Other terms used for pancreas conditions

When poor pancreas function has been present for many years, or is particularly pronounced, this could cause signs and symptoms beyond those mentioned above. However, since these signs and symptoms result from a worsening of the poor pancreas function, their treatment is very similar. These extra, less common signs and symptoms might involve

A. extreme lack of energy, with the body feeling heavy;
B. excessive feeling of coldness, particularly in the limbs, and an aversion to cold;
C. undigested food in watery stools; and
D. bright yellow face, eyes and skin, with scanty, yellow urine.

In today's Chinese medicine, items "A" to "C" are called "Pancreas yang deficiency".* There are a number of possible interpretations of this term. Here, *yang* could be referring to the function of the organ, so that "yang deficiency" means an absence of organ function (or barely detectible function), and this condition is understood to be a progression from the state of poor pancreas function. Or another interpretation of "yang deficiency" is that the condition has reached the stage where the *yang* aspects of the body have been affected. In this context *yang* refers to the quality of warming, animating, of adding colour and life. Due to the poetic and metaphorical nature of such terms, it is not always possible to clearly equate them to a single concept in contemporary physiology. And item "D" is called "Damp heat in the pancreas" (page 181 explains the term *damp heat*).

Such terms are relatively recent adoptions

It should be noted that the above terms were not used in the *Nei Jing* or *Nan Jing* and were

* Or "Spleen yang deficiency" in other books.

adopted more recently (p.449). However, in the *Nei Jing* there was no single way of referring to or describing an illness in an organ. Different authors used different approaches and different terms. The *Nan Jing* extract on page 73 above is a good example of a simple approach, where it was said that if a range of signs and symptoms were present, together with a "movement in the vessels" related to that organ (i.e. an organ pulse indicating the organ function was not normal), then the organ was said to be "afflicted", whereas if these signs were not present, then the organ was not afflicted. In other words, an organ was either ill or not ill (p.449). And this book follows this simple approach by using a single term to describe illness in an organ—usually "poor (organ) function", meaning that the organ is stressed in some way.

Effects on the quality of the blood

The *Nei Jing* notion of blood was that it provided nourishment, but only the *yin* aspect of nourishment (the validity of this notion is discussed on page 42). The blood was considered to be manufactured by the digestion. As regards the nutritional content of blood, this is also true in contemporary physiology (but see page 42). Therefore the quality of this aspect of the blood depends on the good function of the pancreas and stomach. And an exhausted pancreas would lead to a reduction in the quality of the blood, which could cause a range of signs and symptoms, including

- a pale complexion, pale lips and fingernails;
- dizziness, vertigo;
- dry stools, constipation; and
- dry skin or hair, with the skin being itchy.

And if the heart were affected by the poor quality blood, this could produce

- poor long-term memory;
- insomnia (where it was difficult to fall asleep, rather than waking during the night); and
- palpitations, anxiety.

And if the liver were affected, this could produce

- numbness[46] or weak tremors in the limbs;
- blurred vision, floaters (seeing dark specks in the field of vision); and
- scanty or delayed menses.[47]

In today's Chinese medicine, the above conditions would be termed "Blood deficiency", "Heart blood deficiency", or "Liver blood deficiency" respectively.

However, once the poor pancreas function was treated, all the complications would tend to clear, so it would seem unnecessary to regard all the above signs and symptoms as belonging to separate conditions, each requiring separate treatment. It is true that in acupuncture there are many ways of tackling the same problem, and there are certain acupoints that are recognised as being helpful in the above situations. For example, the acupoint Bladder-17 (*Geshu*) is often used to help nourish the blood. But essentially, the treatment aims to normalize the function of the pancreas and once this is done, all direct signs and symptoms, and also the complications, would tend to clear.

In contemporary medicine, this condition would usually be called anaemia.

Dietary assistance

The following foods are all able to nourish the blood, and selected items could be added to a patient's general diet:

- beetroot, dark leafy greens, spinach;
- date, fig, grape, apricot;
- liver, beef;
- kidney bean, aduki bean;
- chicken egg; and
- sardine, octopus, oyster.[48]

Stomach conditions

The stomach works closely with the pancreas. Of the two, the pancreas is the most important digestive organ, and problems with the pancreas are far more common in clinic than problems with the stomach. However problems with the stomach do occur, either along with the pancreas or separately.

The functions of the stomach

In contemporary physiology, the main function of the stomach is to begin the digestive process by mixing the food with gastric juices, including water, hydrochloric acid and enzymes which begin to break down the food and liquefy it, ready for it to be passed on to the small intestine where the pancreatic juices complete the digestive process.

In the way that we think of an organ's function today, such as in the above description, the *Nei Jing* did not really ascribe a function to the stomach. In combination with the pancreas it was ascribed a function, but when considered on its own, it was thought of more as a temporary store for food, which was then quickly passed on to other organs.

Chapter 8 of the *Su Wen* states "The [pancreas] and the stomach are the officials responsible for grain storage. The five flavours originate from them."[49]

Chapter 21 of the *Su Wen* states "The [influence] of food enters the stomach. The stomach spreads essence to the liver.... The [influence] of food enters the stomach. The turbid [part of the influence] turns to the heart.... Beverages enter the stomach. Overflowing essence [influence] is transported upward to the [pancreas]."[50] Here, the notion is portrayed of the stomach as a temporary store for food, which is then quickly moved on to other organs which then perform their functions; but there is no real notion portrayed of the stomach *doing* anything to the food.

Section 31 of the *Nan Jing* states "The [*san jiao**] encompasses the passageways of water and grain [in the body].... The central section of the [*san jiao*] is... responsible for the spoiling and processing of water and grain."[51] This passage ascribes a function, but this is to a section of the *san jiao*, not to the stomach. In this context, the *san jiao* may be considered as a summary of the functions of the organs located in the three separate regions of the torso, so that the passage is referring to the stomach and pancreas in combination (the "central" section of the *san jiao*).

Hence, the impression is that the stomach was generally thought of as a temporary storage for food, which was then quickly passed on to the other organs which then performed

* Also called the triple burner.

their function. The food influence (*gu chi*) that was passed on from the stomach, was then split into different components, such as constructive and defensive influence, but there was no mention of where this splitting took place, nor of what it involved; i.e. which organ performed the splitting and what the organ did to the food influence to divide it (p.37).

The authors of the later *Nan Jing* appear to have decided that a general "spoiling and processing of water and gain" must have taken place by a combination of the stomach and pancreas. Whereas the *Nei Jing* passages describing metabolism were contradictory and lacking sufficient detail to be able to ascribe any particular function to the stomach (pp.33-48).

In today's Chinese medicine, the *Nan Jing* description above has generally been assumed to be describing the stomach function alone. But it should be born in mind that this is a modern adoption, informed by today's knowledge of the stomach's function.[52] Does this matter? The description of "spoiling and processing the grain", which is also translated as "rotting and ripening the grain", is describing the stomach function as it is defined today, only using different terminology. The process of chemically breaking down and liquefying the food, is very much akin to that of rotting it. However, the exercise of properly understanding Chinese medicine does not simply consist of substituting the *Nei Jing's* perceived oversights with descriptions from contemporary anatomy and physiology. Instead, it is instructive to try to imagine Chinese medicine as the *Nei Jing* authors might have done.

Improper function

It was noticed that when the stomach function was weak, any of the following signs and symptoms could occur:

- nausea, vomiting,[53] belching;
- sour regurgitation, hiccup[54];
- feeling discomfort or heat or coldness in the *epigastrium* (heartburn);
- discomfort over the ribs on the front, left side of the body (beneath which the stomach is situated), usually called indigestion;
- bleeding gums or mouth ulcers;
- bad breath—either an unpleasant odour or a burnt odour; and
- pain or discomfort anywhere along the stomach meridian.[35]

With all the above signs and symptoms, the treatment would be very similar, and would involve the use of an acupoint that strengthens the stomach function. Some key acupoints are Stomach-36 (*Zusanli*), Ren-12 (*Zhongwan*), and Bladder-21 (*Weishu*).

When poor stomach function is present, these acupoints tend to be tender due to their association with the stomach. When one of these acupoints is stimulated, this encourages the organ to cancel out the malfunction in itself that caused the tenderness at the acupoint (p.372), and the organ returns to normal function.

The causes of stomach problems

Such problems often happen when a person has low energy in general, which is often due to them developing poor pancreas function; or occurs after a long illness. And once this situation is reached, the person's eating habits would then play a big part. Any of the following habits may lead to a weakening of the stomach function and the occurrence of signs and symptoms from the above list:

- eating too quickly and not chewing the food sufficiently;
- eating too much at one sitting, or not eating enough in general, such as when dieting;
- eating foods that are hard to digest, such as any cold or raw foods, or foods from the list on page 81; and
- being emotionally upset when eating.

Avoiding such habits would help the patient to avoid developing stomach problems. But more importantly, any weaknesses that make the patient prone to stomach problems should also be addressed, such as poor pancreas function.

Finally, as with all the organs, the stomach function can also be impeded due to mental and emotional factors. Any sustained situation in our life that we find hard to *stomach* could have this effect. In other words, when we are unable to *start* to mentally digest a fact or situation, this failure is duplicated in the stomach and impedes *its* ability to begin the process of digesting food.

Patient example
Male, aged 14. The patient's parents split up when he was aged ten, and a year later he developed stomach cramps. His elder brother then left home to attend university, which he also found hard to accept. This case was a clear example of the disruption of an organ's function due to emotional factors. He found it hard to stomach these circumstances, which then impeded his stomach function. See the full case history on page 250.

The knowledge of this particular cause-and-effect has become so clear to people over the centuries that it is now fossilized in the very language. It is possible that this is the origin of such expressions as: finding something *hard to stomach*, or *having no stomach* for something, or: something that *makes you sick*, where such emotions or ideas produce physical symptoms in the stomach, such as pain, nausea or indigestion. The following chapter provides a possible physiological explanation for how such mental factors can impede the function of the organs.

Chapter 5. The mental functions of the organs

Throughout the *Nei Jing* there are references to the mental and emotional causes of illness,[1] and to the specific thoughts and emotions produced when certain of the abdominal organs become stressed. For example, the following observations were made:

- that a stressed liver causes a person to become excessively tidy and prone to rage,[2] and that excessive rage harms the liver[3];
- that a stressed heart causes a person to be anxious, easily startled, to be introverted, to avoid contact with others, and also affects the person's speech[4];
- that a sense of loss or sadness harms the lungs[5];
- that an emotional shock, or the loss of status, harms the kidneys,[6] which then makes a person more fearful;[7] and
- that thinking excessively harms the pancreas,[8] which then only increases the tendency to ponder.[9]

To account for these mental (and emotional) functions, the *Nei Jing* authors merely stated that each of these organs possessed a "soul", the assumption being that it was this soul that performed the functions. Each of these souls was given a name. The *yi* 意 was the soul of the pancreas[*]; the *hun* 魂 the soul of the liver; the *po* 魄 the soul of the lungs; the *zhi* 志 the soul of the kidneys; and the *shen* 神 the soul of the heart.

In ancient China it was the custom to describe such phenomena in this way. But to the contemporary mind the notion of an organ having a "soul" is difficult to understand or accept, and the notion of the abdominal organs having anything to do with our thoughts is counter-intuitive and would be resisted by most Westerners. Our thinking appears to take place in the brain, so how could some (or most) of our thoughts be produced by the abdominal organs?

Yet, to any practitioner of Chinese acupuncture, it is clear that this is exactly what happens. These age-old observations are still routinely encountered in clinic today and are able to explain the mental causes of many common conditions.

This *Nei Jing* knowledge was gained from practical observation (by observing a symptom and being able to associate it with an organ—since, when the organ was treated,

[*] Also called the spleen in Chinese medicine (p.61).

the symptom cleared), rather than gained from theorizing. Therefore the observations are fact based, so it ought to be possible to account for them using contemporary physiology. And this is the challenge tackled by this chapter. It uses concepts from contemporary anatomy and physiology to provide one possible explanation of how the abdominal organs may be able to produce thoughts and emotions, and also how those same thoughts and emotions may be able to adversely affect the function of their associated organ.

The organs are self-governing

A surprising fact is that the abdominal organs are largely self-governing. That is, they mostly function independently of any input from the brain. The *enteric nervous system* (ENS) is a large mass of neurons situated near to the abdominal organs, which is dedicated to this purpose. It works independently of the brain and spinal cord and continues to function without any outside input.[10] For this reason, the ENS is often called the "brain of the gut" or the body's "second brain". The ENS is an immense system, containing almost as many neurons as exist in the spinal cord. It does receive some signals from the sympathetic and parasympathetic nervous systems to help regulate its functions, but it is still considered to be largely self-governing.[11]

This is why organs can be transplanted, without their nerves being re-connected, and yet the organs generally continue to function normally. For example, the autonomic nervous input to the liver appears to serve non-essential functions. It is known that when the autonomic nerves entering the liver are cut (as in a liver transplant), the auto-regulatory mechanisms inside the liver are fully able to control liver metabolism in non-stimulated conditions; but that the autonomic nervous input to the liver may play a part in helping to regulate metabolism during the fight-or-flight responses (when quicker communication is required between the organs).[12]

This makes sense in evolutionary terms

When we consider the early evolution of animal life, this situation is less surprising. In terms of the main structures in the body (the brain, sense organs, digestive organs, and the general form of the body as it is today—with limbs and a head) it seems probable that the digestive organs would have begun to evolve *before* all these other structures, for several reasons. Primarily, the first, primitive digestive organs would have been necessary to take in food and make available the vast amounts of energy needed to *enable* the evolution of other complex structures in the body—and then support those structures, once evolved. But also, within Chinese medicine itself there is evidence that supports the notion that the main abdominal organs existed (even if only in an early form) *before* the senses began to evolve—and therefore before large parts of the brain existed.

The associations between the organs and senses

Chinese medicine has identified functional associations between the main organs and senses, which can provide further evidence to support the above notion. But more importantly, these functional associations also provide a clue to the nature of the relationship between the organs and thoughts.

Each of the five main organs is associated with a sense; and for that sense to function well (or sometimes to function at all), the associated organ must also function well, as follows.

When the pancreas function is normal we have a strong sense of taste, but when its function is poor the sense of taste is also poor, or even absent (p.69).

When the liver function is unimpeded the sight is strong, with vivid colours and straight lines; but when the liver function is stagnated, this can produce visual disturbances, pains around the eyes, poor eyesight and dry and sore eyes (p.106).

When the lung function is normal, we have a strong sense of smell and can breathe easily through the nose; but when its function is poor, the sense of smell is also poor, or even absent, and we cannot breathe easily through the nose (p.130).

When the kidney function is normal, we have good hearing, but when it is poor, the hearing is also poor, sometimes with low pitch tinnitus, or we may even become deaf (p.166).

When the heart function is normal, we have a fluent faculty of speech, but when its function is poor, we quickly develop speech problems, such as stuttering, stammering and even indiscriminate verbalising (p.189).

The fact that each of these organs must function well to enable the related sense to also function well (or sometimes even at all) suggests that each organ must somehow enable its related sense to work. If this is the case, then the evolution of that sense must have been reliant on the existence of its related abdominal organ. This suggests that all these organs, including a complete digestive and circulatory system, began to evolve before the senses and brain even existed. And as described in the remainder of this chapter, this notion also sheds light on some aspects of the relationship between the organs and thoughts.

The organs have their own intentions

All the organs, and these five main organs in particular, have their own intentions, which are produced by their physical function. The following passages suggest how these intentions may have evolved, and then describe how they may produce our thoughts.

Each organ possesses a "will"

It is clear that each of the abdominal organs possesses a "will" of its own. But what do I mean by "will"? Every piece of living matter (whether animal or vegetable) must have the urge to be alive and to continue to live. At the microscopic level, this would include the many components of living matter that combine to make up even a single-cell creature. But beyond the existence of this fundamental urge, I mean "will" in a larger sense. I mean the *intention* to do something. In living matter, such an intention would be created by adding together many of these microscopic pieces of living matter until they create a larger form that *does* something. At the smallest level, this starts with a single cell. All such cells do something, and this activity could be considered the expression of that cell's intention.

When such cells are added together, a more complex structure is created. For example, if we imagine a small piece of our own skin—this is a collection of cells that behaves in a specific way. It could be viewed as a collection of living matter that is *determined* to form itself into skin (and do all the things that skin does). And when that skin is damaged in some way, the living matter repairs itself, so determined is it to be skin. All this type of activity requires intention. This is the difference between living matter and non-living matter. If a pebble is chipped, it does not repair the chip in itself; it is entirely passive and no matter what is done to it, it will not respond. Whereas, if any living matter is damaged, it will attempt to repair itself. And if stimulated in other ways, it usually has a particular response, such as its response to light, heat, cold or pressure (even though that response is biologically programmed into it and happens automatically). And these such responses, together with its determination to be a piece of skin (or the stem of a plant, and so on), are what make up its intention.

Beyond single-cell creatures, evolution then progressed to the first creatures with a digestive system, but before the stage when they had limbs or a recognisable head. Such creatures may have possessed a primitive stomach, pancreas, intestine, liver, heart, lung, kidney (or at least, an embryonic form of these organs), which were probably the key organs needed to efficiently take in complex food from the outside, break it down, convert it to various types of useable nourishment and transport this to every part of the creature, including the internal organs themselves.

Each of these organs was by now a complex structure in its own right. It had a role to play within the creature's body; it acted within a team of organs, responded to what the other organs were doing and performed its own role when called upon to do it.

The organs were the "brain" of the early creatures

This hypothetical creature at an early stage of evolution would not yet have limbs, a head, or even a brain—since there was not yet any senses. So, where was the driving force within the creature?

The only centres of major activity within it were its organs, each of which was driven by its own intention. When considering the organs in this way, particularly at the stage of evolution before the creature had a head or brain, it is possible to accept that each of the creature's organs could be considered a complex creature in its own right. Admittedly, these creatures might seem somewhat alien-like to us, and they were each bound in servitude to the other creatures around them and to the overall body that contained them, but they could, nonetheless, be considered creatures in their own right.

For example (as still happens today), this embryonic stomach took in food from outside and broke it down to begin the digestive process. Here, the stomach acted in response to the other "creatures" around it; *something* told it when to act. It then transported the food to the embryonic pancreas, which added the particular mix of enzymes necessary to complete the food's digestion (that is, assuming these embryonic organs acted as they do today). And again, here, the pancreas could be considered as a separate creature, performing a very specialized role in response to the other creatures around it.

This team of creatures *drove* the overall creature. They were its only major centres of activity, of intention. In the way we think of the brain today, this team of organs was the brain of this early creature.

What was the nature of this "thinking"?

Each of these digestive organs had a particular role to play within the overall team of organs and this required cooperation and communication between them.

At the same time that these embryonic organs were forming, we can assume that a network of nerves must have developed between the organs, and also *chemical messengers* were probably circulated through the blood (clearly an embryonic blood circulatory system would have also needed to develop simultaneously). The chemical messengers were unique chemicals (such as hormones) that acted as a signal. Just as happens today, it is reasonable to assume that one of these chemicals was secreted by an organ when it wanted to communicate a particular state; and when other organs detected the chemical, they responded in a certain way. This is the system of communication that still exists in most creatures today and there is no reason to think it, or a similar system, was not present from the start.

For example, when food leaves the stomach and enters the *duodenum* (which is the tube through which food exits the stomach, and is the start of the small intestine), cells in the walls of the duodenum sense the presence of acid material from the stomach and release the hormones *secretin* and *cholecystokinin* (CCK), and when the pancreas detects these hormones, it secretes pancreatic juices which then continue the process of digesting the food, enabling the small intestine to absorb the nutrients into the blood stream.[13] And nerves work in a similar way.

Nerves as a communication system

The nerves within the body form a communication system. They are used by the organs to sense various states in the other organs, and to also communicate various states *to* those other organs.

For example, in the wall of the stomach and gut, there are many neurons (nerve cells) that only react to specific chemicals. The nerve cells act like sensors. They are exposed to the material passing through the stomach and gut and when a specific chemical comes into contact with each neuron, this causes that neuron to fire (its sodium channels are *chemical gated*—p.389). The presence of this particular chemical causes the nerve cell to open its sodium channels, which causes the electrical potential on its membrane to suddenly rise; and this triggers a chain reaction along the nerve connected to the neuron. At the other end this signal causes something to happen. Many of these nerves enter the pancreas, and the signals cause the pancreas to secrete various enzymes to assist in the digestion of food. The amount, type, and speed of the secretions are timed to coordinate with the particular type and amount of food being digested.[13]

These particular nerves (along with the chemical messengers) could be considered analogous to antennae extending from the pancreas (and all other organs), enabling the pancreas to sense the type and amount of food that needs to be digested and exactly *when* the digestion needs to take place.

The logic of the organ network

This network of nerves and chemical messengers are the communication medium between the twelve organs, which enables each organ to sense when its own functions are needed, to what degree, and to communicate to others what that organ itself needs—which decision-making process must contain knowledge of each organ's own functions, so as to make the decisions. The network consists of (in effect) a mass of on/off switches which determine the actions of each organ, and the network acts very much like the logic of computer software—which itself is just a mass of on/off switches connected so as to enable particular tasks to be performed. As such, this network of nerves and chemical messengers that travels to and from each organ (the antennae of that organ) is a representation of the decision-making processes of that organ—which contains the logic of the organ (its decision-making "software") and also has knowledge of the functions of the organ.

How might this organ logic be used to process our thoughts?

It seems that each organ's logic is also used to process our thoughts. That is, the same processing the organs do on the physical substances in the body, they appear to also perform on our thoughts. But how do we know this is happening, when did it begin, and how might it be possible?

Our thoughts mimic the functions of the organs

There are similarities between each of the main organ functions and particular thought patterns, and there are also clear signs that each organ is involved in the production of that particular thinking.

For example, the pancreas digests food; and the process of us mentally digesting facts seems to be linked to this pancreas function—in that, when this function is weak, we are less able to digest facts. And this ability is also time-dependent; it is at its strongest when the pancreas function peaks, and people with poor pancreas function find it much harder to digest facts at other times of day (p.73). If this task of digesting facts were purely a mental one, unrelated to the abdominal organ functions, it would not be time dependent, which also seems to support the notion that it is the pancreas that performs this type of thinking.

The liver plays a largely organizational role in the body, organizing the supply and flow of the energy and other nutrition; and it seems to perform the same role on our thoughts by organizing every aspect of our life and the tasks we perform—and when such thoughts are blocked, this blocks the liver's physical function (p.107).

The lungs extract precious oxygen from the air we breathe, and they seem to perform this same role on our thoughts by looking for quality in intangible things, which enables us to appreciate quality (p.133).

The kidneys are concerned with our survival, both immediate and long-term; and it seems this function is also applied to our thoughts—to enable us to identify situations that are immediately dangerous to us or that threaten our long-term survival, or to spot beneficial opportunities (p.168).

The heart circulates nourishment to all the other organs, and it seems that this function also produces our concern for other people and our desire to share our good fortune with them. And when our social connections are mentally impeded, this weakens our heart's physical function (p.190).

When might this have begun?

To return to the hypothetical primitive creature at the stage of evolution when the digestive organs first began to evolve—it is most likely that the creature did not yet possess a head, nor any senses. And since such a creature did not yet have a brain, it could have had no thoughts—as we think of them. Or could it? It had a team of organs, all of which had their own intentions. In other words, they processed physical substances. Therefore, these same thoughts (or intentions) did exist in this early creature—even though it had no head or brain.

The whereabouts of our conscious mind

The beginnings of the brain (as we know it today) may have consisted of the neuronal matter related to the sense organs. And our conscious mind seems to simply consist of the activity of monitoring the senses. That is, the fact that this sense information exists, seems to have created the role of "monitoring that information", and it may be the necessity of having this role that created our conscious mind.

Such a scenario (if correct) provides another possible explanation for how the organs may interact with our thoughts. The main organs are closely associated with the senses, whose processing takes place in the brain, therefore this provides a possible route that could enable the organs to interact with the brain, and hence our thoughts.

The processing of complex thoughts

Once the senses evolved, the information from these needed to be responded to, but initially only simple, life or death decisions had to be made, such as deciding what was food, how to get to it, and what was dangerous to the creature itself and how to avoid it.

It was not until we ventured onto land—millions of years later—and started living in societies, using tools and shaping the environment to ourselves that much more complex thoughts would have occurred to us. At this stage, there was a mass of logic related to the abdominal organs that had already been present for millions of years (the so called brain of the gut), and whenever one of these new ideas needed to be processed, if it were possible that some of this pre-existing gut logic *could* process that thought, then this would probably have happened—in place of the creature waiting for a considerable amount of time until new brain matter evolved to do the same job. After all (apart from the urgency of the situation), why create new brain matter to perform a task when some logic already exists that could do the job?

The key point here is that the thoughts needed to be *capable* of being processed in the same way that an organ processes other substances.

How could an organ's logic process a thought?

Looking at this conceptually, and taking the pancreas as an example, how might the organ's intention act on our thoughts?

The physical function of the pancreas could be summarized as: *to further break down food* (which process the stomach began) *to find any inherent nutrition and to control the body's uptake of the main nutrition.** And these words also serve as a summary of the pancreas's intention, since its function and inten-

* This is a summary of the functions in contemporary physiology, which are described on page 63.

tion are one and the same (its intention being to act in a certain way, and those *actions* are then the pancreas *functions*).

Originally this intention acted on food alone, but once our conscious mind evolved to the point where complex ideas presented themselves to us, this pancreas intention may also have been capable of acting on those ideas—to *further break them down to find any inherent nutrition.* Here, the *nutrition* would be any new ideas that were somehow embedded within the original ideas.[14]

For example, suppose a thought entered our conscious mind—something we saw or heard, or words we heard or read, or some memory we recalled. Initially, our thought may not make sense to us. But there may be *nutrition* within it somewhere, and the pancreas logic may then process this thought, to *break it down so that any nutrition within it could be found.* And in this way the idea may be broken down and transformed, usually into a different idea, and that (the *nutrition* obtained from the original thought) stored in the memory—just as nutrition is extracted from food and utilized in the body, sent to where it is needed or stored for later use.

Another way to look at the above concept is this. Our thought processes appear to mimic the functioning of the abdominal organs. One simple explanation for this is that our thought processes came into existence *because* of this already-existing logic, and it was therefore the particular way the abdominal organs function that *created* the particular way we now think.

Is this processing done in the organs or brain?

The symptomatic observations made by Chinese medicine suggest that it is the digestive organs themselves that perform any unconscious thinking, rather than the brain.

For example, the ability to mentally digest facts depends on the strength of the pancreas function. Once this becomes poor, we find it harder to digest facts and can only do this effectively when the pancreas function peaks (in effect, between seven and eleven a.m., which includes the time when the stomach function peaks). And when the pancreas function is poor and we indulge in heavy thinking for a few days, this usually causes a flare up of the physical signs and symptoms related to poor pancreas function (p.71). These facts suggest it is the pancreas itself that performs the thinking, rather than the brain.

The alternative scenario

However, another possibility is that the organ logic was duplicated in the brain matter that processes the senses, which could have happened as some facet of the association between the main organs and senses. But another requirement of this scenario is that there would still need to be immediate, two-way communication between these brain-matter copies of the organ functions and the organs themselves, so that what happens in the one is immediately duplicated in the other, in both directions (though the communication would need to take place via some medium other than nerves). This scenario would then account for every related phenomena identified in Chinese medicine.

To take the above pancreas example—the organ's brain-matter copy could process our thoughts—taking them from our conscious mind, processing them, then handing back the results. And since there would be immediate, two-way communication between this brain-matter copy and the pancreas itself (via some unknown method), when the brain-matter copy was working hard on our thoughts, this would have the same effect on the pancreas that attempting to digest an endless banquet of food would have. Consequently, the pancreas would become tired. And this process would work in both directions. Due to this two-way communication, when the pancreas function was poor, our mind's ability to digest thoughts would also be poor, since the brain-matter copy would reflect any state in the organ. And these effects would be made worse in people who frequently attempt to digest challenging thoughts, since, when our mind fails to digest a thought, this *failure to digest* would also be duplicated in the pancreas (as well as the situation of being worked hard), which would then fail to digest physical food.

Comparing the two scenarios

As another example—in my experience, when a patient has their gallbladder removed, from that moment onwards they usually find it almost impossible to make decisions (which is a mental function of the gallbladder—p.121). But their brain has not changed, so how come they can no longer make decisions? This seems to suggest it was the abdominal organ itself that made the decisions. Or does it? Perhaps the brain *is* no longer the same. In the alternative scenario, there is a two-way connection between the brain-matter copy of the organ's logic (its function) and the organ itself, so that what happens in the one is duplicated in the other. Therefore it would not be surprising that when the organ were removed, the brain-matter copy of its function no longer worked—so the evidence could be interpreted to support either scenario.

As another example—when we have been thinking for a while and become tired of trying to digest new facts, we may feel a mild pain across the forehead, which seems to imply that this thinking takes place in the brain, rather than in the stomach. But another common experience that sheds light on this situation is ice-cream headaches. Typically, with people who already have poor stomach function, when they eat an ice-cream, they feel a sharp pain across their forehead. This is produced by the chilling effect of the ice-cream on their stomach, and is communicated to their forehead via the stomach meridian (or, more correctly, by utilizing the same process that creates the stomach meridian—see p.355), which rises to either side of the forehead. This mechanism could also explain the forehead pain experienced by people who have become tired of digesting new facts. The stress could be felt by their stomach—which *begins* the process of digesting new facts, just as the physical stomach *begins* the process of digesting food, which is then completed by the pancreas. And this stomach stress would be communicated to their forehead via the stomach meridian, which could be taken to indicate that the act of us *beginning* to digest facts takes place in the stomach, rather than the brain. But then again, this digestion could also be happening in the brain-matter copy of the stomach function; and due to the two-way connection between this and the stomach itself, the process of us starting to digest any new fact would be communicated to the abdominal organ, where any stress would be felt, and this would then be communicated to the forehead via the stomach meridian. So again, the evidence could be interpreted to support either argument.

However, a common phenomenon related to heart transplant patients suggests that the processing takes place in the organs. The mental (and emotional) function of the heart is to form social connections with people and to also form bonds with the things we love, such as certain activities or food (p.190). And on page 195, I describe the experiences of some heart transplant patients, who, after the surgery, inexplicably retained some of the memories of the things the donor loved, or details of some of their social interactions. This not only serves to support the Chinese medicine notion of the heart's mental function, but also suggests that the memories of that function may be stored in the heart itself, which supports the notion that the heart's mental function is performed in the heart, rather than the brain. But this raises the following question.

How might thoughts be communicated between the organs and mind?

What a thought might consist of is unknown. Does it possess some sort of molecular (or similar) structure? This is difficult to visualize, but since thoughts are a product of the physical body, and clearly interact with the body, then there must be a structure of some sort that represents each thought.

Since this is unknown, then a medium (or mechanism) that may be capable of communicating thoughts around the body can only be speculated on. What *is* known is that since our thoughts are usually about the world around us, they must have all originally begun with the senses, primarily sights and sounds (including words).

The senses present our conscious mind with information, which information is obviously located in the brain, since that is where our conscious mind is. But the senses rely on the good function of the abdominal organs (p.88), which implies that the abdominal organs may play some part in processing (or producing) the sense information.

It might be argued that the organs only *enable* the brain tissue to work, which then processes the information itself. But this presupposes that the key neuronal masses that perform each separate function in the brain each require a separate type of nutrition for that collective mass of neurons to work.

For example, there is a mass of neurons associated with sight, and for these to work properly they would require a particular blood-born nutrient that was only made available when the liver function was normal. And the same would need to be true of the neuronal masses associated with taste, hearing, smell, and the faculty of speech. For each of these separate masses of neurons to work properly, they would require a specific type of nutrient that was only made available when their associated organ was functioning normally.

This scenario is not credible. But further, with the heart at least, it is clear that the link between the improper function of speech and the impeding of the heart function happens almost instantly (p.192), therefore this hypothetical nutrient could not be supplied through the blood, which only seems to leave the possibility that each of these organs somehow utilizes either nerves or a signal carried on an electrical wave to enable the particular neuronal mass in the brain—which processes their associated sense—to function properly. This requirement seems to make the scenario even less credible—since, why would some immediate signal from each organ be necessary to enable the brain's processing of the organ's associated sense to take place? It is difficult to imagine a purpose for such an arrangement (accidental or otherwise). This only leaves the possibility that the organs play some direct role in processing the sense information, which suggests that the sense information must be somehow communicated between the brain and abdominal organs.

The medium of communication

If the sense information is communicated between the brain and organs, the speed required would rule out any *conventional* medium other than nerves. But since there is no *direct* nervous input from the brain or spinal cord to the organs (p.88) this would also seem to rule out nerves. This only seems to leave the possibility of communication via electrical waves—or similar.

As regards the sense information, this does not immediately seem credible. Though it should be noted that the entire primo vascular system (p.316) was unknown to contemporary science around twelve years ago; and this book's intelligent tissue hypothesis and its notion of communication of organ information over electrical waves (p.372) is unknown to contemporary science today (it may be years before every aspect of it is proved), so on this scientific frontier, nothing can yet be entirely ruled out.

The information from the senses (sights and sounds—including words) are very close to being thoughts, so that a biological mechanism that *could* communicate such information between the senses and abdominal organs, could just as well communicate thoughts between the brain and organs, in both directions.

However, the difficulties of imagining (and finding) such a communication system would not exist if the alternative scenario turns out to be correct—that the organ logic is duplicated in the brain, probably associated with the areas that process the senses, so that all communication between the senses and organs, and communication of thoughts between our conscious mind and organs, is able to take place within the brain. But this would still leave the problem of accounting for the evident two-way communication between the organs and brain, despite there being no direct neuronal link.

Chapter 17 describes new evidence of communication between the organs and their related acupoints via information conveyed on an electromagnetic wave, and also evidence that bodily tissue is constantly interpreting this information and reacting to it (pp.322-328). These discoveries shed light on how such communication between the organs and brain may be achieved.

A scientific frontier

Elements of the above arguments are, by necessity, speculative. This whole area is scientifically unexplored—a true scientific frontier.

What *is* known is that all these close associations exist between the main abdominal organs and the senses, and between the functioning of those organs and our thoughts and emotions. What I have presented here is one possible way to explain and account for these facts.

It has to be said that the notions in this chapter would be resisted by many of the scientists who currently regard the body as being very much brain-centric; that is, that everything within us starts and ends with the brain, which is akin to an all-powerful computer that drives the body which is regarded as merely a machine. But once the scientific exploration of these areas begins in earnest and makes progress, the view may become more widely held that the body is far more viscera-centric than brain-centric. Chinese medicine has known this for thousands of years; it is hoped that contemporary anatomy and physiology may one day also "discover" this same knowledge.

Chapter 6. Liver and gallbladder

The functions of the liver

In contemporary physiology, the main function of the liver is to regulate the supply of energy to every part of the body, including the other organs, which it does as follows.

The main fuel source in the body is glucose, which is extracted from the food we eat. The stomach, pancreas and small intestine perform a large part of the digestive process (p.387), but this is very much regulated by the liver. Immediately after eating, a large amount of glucose is extracted from the carbohydrates in our food, but the liver stores much of this and gradually releases it back into the blood supply between meals, so as to keep the level of glucose in the blood at a stable level throughout the day. It does this by converting the glucose into *glycogen* (which is a form that can be more readily stored in the liver and also in the muscles) and then converts this back into glucose when needed.[1]

The liver also breaks down the fats in our diet by producing bile; the fats can then be used as energy, but fats that are beyond our immediate needs are converted to *triglyceride* and stored in the fatty tissues of the body (triglyceride is made by combining free fatty acids and glycerol, and is the molecule used to store fats).[2]

After eating, if we have taken in carbohydrates or proteins beyond our immediate needs, the liver also converts these into triglycerides, which are then stored in the fatty tissues of the body. Between meals, when the level of glucose in the blood starts to fall, the liver stops synthesizing fats in this way; and the triglyceride molecules stored in the fatty tissues begin to be broken down into free fatty acids and glycerol, which are released into the blood. The liver then converts the glycerol molecules into glucose, which helps to maintain the correct level of glucose (the process is known as *gluconeogenesis*).[3]

The liver also completes the process of digesting proteins. These are broken down into amino acids by the digestive system; and then the liver breaks these down into another form of energy, known as ATP (p.387), which is used to supplement the ATP that powers every cell in the body (most cells produce a certain amount of ATP within themselves, and this is supplemented by the ATP that the liver produces); or the liver can also convert these amino acids into new glucose molecules to also be used as fuel in the body; and it can also synthesize extra glucose from some carbohydrates.[4]

As well as storing and producing energy, the liver also stores many essential nutrients, vitamins and minerals, such as vitamins A, D, E, K, and B12, and the minerals iron and copper; and by doing this it ensures a constant supply of these essential substances for use in the body.[5]

The liver also cleanses the blood to remove toxins such as bacteria, fungi, parasites, drugs, alcohol, and worn out blood cells, and also generates many essential components of the blood, such as clotting factors (*prothrombin* and *fibrinogen*) and essential proteins (*albumins*).[6]

It also transforms and removes from circulation hormones produced by the body's own glands for messaging purposes, such as insulin, glucagon, cortisol, aldosterone, thyroid and sex hormones (which is yet another way in which it regulates the activities of the other organs—as well as regulating the energy that drives them).[7]

Overall, the liver regulates the production and supply of energy (and other nutrition) to every tissue in the body, including those of the other organs, thereby enabling the proper function of the muscles and organs.[8]

The Chinese medicine functions and effects

As with all the organs, the *Nei Jing* authors used a practical approach to work out the functions and effects* of the liver.[9] When the liver function was not normal, a range of accompanying signs and symptoms were identified which cleared once the liver was successfully treated. This enabled the physical functions and effects, as well as the mental and emotional ones, to be identified, as summarized below. The liver

1. stores the blood,
2. maintains the smooth function of the organs,
3. maintains the smooth movement of the muscles,
4. influences the quality of the nails,
5. has a close association with the eyes, and
6. has mental and emotional functions.

1. Stores the blood

This is a direct function rather than an effect.

Through practical observation alone, the *Nei Jing* authors managed to deduce that the liver stores the blood and hence regulates the volume in circulation.[10] It was also noticed that when the liver function was not normal, patients sometimes suffered

- muscle cramps or twitches[11];
- numbness of the limbs[12];
- blurred vision;[13] and (in women)
- irregularities of menstruation, such as infrequent or even absent menstruation.[14]

These symptoms, which cleared once the liver was treated, were understood to be the result of an inadequate supply of blood to the tissues and other organs, or a reduction in the quality of the blood (which amounts to the same thing), and these observations may have

* See page 64 for an explanation of the term "effects" in this context.

contributed to their deduction that the liver stores the blood.

In contemporary physiology, the liver is also recognised as a major reservoir of blood.[15] During physical activity, blood is normally released from the liver, increasing the amount in circulation; and during rest, a proportion of the blood returns to the liver, reducing the amount in circulation.

2. Maintains the smooth function of the organs

This is a direct function rather than an effect.

The *Nei Jing* authors observed that when the liver function was not normal, patients could suffer a range of symptoms due to this and also the other organs (particularly the digestive ones) failing to function properly. The symptoms could include

- nausea, vomiting, belching—due to the stomach function being impeded (p.85);
- abdominal distension, diarrhoea—due to impeded pancreas function (p.74);
- a feeling of tightness or a distending pain in the region of the liver (the *hypochondriac* region), a general feeling of "stuffiness" and pressure in the chest,[16] period pains (*dysmenorrhoea*),[14] due to the liver's own function being impeded; and
- emotional symptoms such as depression, weeping,[17] irritability, anger, paranoia,[18] also due to impeded liver function (p.107 onwards).

Once the liver was successfully treated, these symptoms tended to clear, which suggested that one of the liver's functions was to "maintain the smooth function of the organs". In today's Chinese medicine, this function is usually expressed as "maintaining the free flow of influences (*chi*)".[19] But in the *Nei Jing*, the function was often expressed indirectly.

Extract from *Su Wen*, Chapter 9

The liver is the basis of exhaustion to the utmost. It is the location of the *hun*-soul. Its effulgence is in the nails. Its fullness manifests itself in the sinews. It serves to generate blood and influences.[20]

Interpreting *Nei Jing* passages is often difficult. The expression "exhaustion to the utmost" is unclear, and the *Su Wen* commentaries offer at least four different interpretations of the first sentence from the above quote:

- Man's movement originates from his sinews. The sinews are generated and ruled by the liver; they are closely related to the liver. When the sinews become tired, the liver [influence (*chi*)] stops this (Duan Yucai, 1988).
- The liver is the basis of the endurance of taxation and of the shouldering of hardships (Gao Shishi, 1980).
- The liver is the basis of the relaxed or tight status of the sinews and membranes (Cheng Zhaozhi, 1988).
- The liver stores the blood and rules over the sinews. All the movements of the human body depend on a taxation of the liver's sinews and on the function of the liver's blood (the *Kuang ya* 廣雅).[21]

All these interpretations offer similar meanings, which might be summarized as "the liver empowers the sinews, muscles and the other organs to function, no matter how much or how little they are worked." And the last line of the above extract "[the liver] serves to generate blood and influences" supports this interpretation. In other *Nei Jing* chapters, it is said that the blood is either manufactured in the stomach or in the vessels (pp.33-44); and that the various influences (*chi*) are produced either by the stomach, the pancreas, the lungs and heart, or by different combinations of these (pp.33-47). Here, in Chapter 9 of the *Su Wen* it is now said that the liver generates both. One possible meaning of this, in the light of the first line of the above extract ("The liver is the basis of exhaustion to the utmost"), is that the liver appears to enable the generation of these substances by the other organs—in varying circumstances, of high and low taxation. In other words, it "regulates" the production of these vital substances, so that their smooth supply and flow can be maintained.

In contemporary physiology, the liver is responsible for regulating the level of glucose in the blood (glucose being the body's main fuel source), and the liver also synthesizes extra glucose itself, and also ATP (another form of energy, which is used directly by the cells in the body—p.387), and also regulates the smooth flow of other vital substances to every tissue in the body (by storing vitamins, minerals, and producing other vital substances). All this activity ensures the smooth function of the organs and tissues. Therefore, the Chinese medicine liver function (*maintaining the free flow of influences*) can be understood as referring to the role the liver plays in regulating and supplementing the supply of vital resources to every part of the body, including the organs.

This is the most important liver function, and the impairment of this function is one of the commonest problems seen in clinic. Its effects are mainly in two areas: the digestion and the emotions.

The effects on digestion

The liver clearly has a large involvement in the digestive process, not only due to its own production and excretion of bile (which is essential for the digestion of fats), but also due to its regulation of the supply of vital resources to the other organs, including the stomach and pancreas.

In contemporary physiology, there is close cooperation between the liver and pancreas in the regulation of the level of glucose in the blood. Chemical messages are circulated in the blood which control this (the hormones *insulin* and *glucagon*). These are secreted by the pancreas, but the trigger for the pancreas to do this comes from outside the pancreas. The liver senses the level of glucose in the blood and these sensors may use the brain as an intermediary to control the pancreas's secretion of these hormones. This area has been the subject of much research, though there is still more unknown than is known.[22,23] However, this provides one example of the close cooperation between the liver and pancreas, which helps to explain (in contemporary physiology) how the liver regulates the supply of vital resources to the other organs, including the pancreas; and may also provide another explanation for the liver's direct influence on the function of the pancreas.

In Chinese medicine terms, when this liver function (*maintaining the free flow of influences*) is impaired, this may cause the stomach function to be impeded, producing such symptoms as belching, nausea, or vomiting (p.85); or it may impede the pancreas function, producing such symptoms as abdominal distension, diarrhoea, or any of the pancreas-related signs and symptoms listed on page 74.

The Nei Jing theory of movement contrary to the norm

These were the symptoms referred to by the *Nei Jing* authors, which would have been first discovered through practical observation by their ancestors (p.261). But the *Nei Jing* authors then produced theories to try to explain the symptoms. At that time, most theorizing about how the body works was done in relation to the movement of influences (*chi*), since (at the time) this was the (imaginary) system in the body that *appeared* to have the biggest effect on the body's ability to function normally.

Chapter 60 of the *Ling Shu* states that "All diseases are either movements contrary to or movements in accordance with the norms," and gives many examples of signs and symptoms that represent a movement contrary to the norms, such as a bloated abdomen, noises in the abdomen associated with a feeling of fullness, unending nosebleed, cough, discharges of blood in the urine.[24]

The stomach and pancreas symptoms of belching, nausea, abdominal distension and diarrhoea were understood in this way; they were movements contrary to the norms.

The stomach function is normally associated with movement in a downward direction. Food is taken in by the stomach and travels in a downward direction through the body. But when the stomach function is disrupted, this direction is reversed, producing symptoms such as belching, acid regurgitation, vomiting and heartburn (a feeling of heat rising), which are all symptoms involving an unusual upward movement.

Likewise, the normal pancreas functions feature an upward movement; it was seen as the main organ responsible for producing the body's influences, which enable us to counter gravity, give us muscular strength, and also enable the organs to counter gravity. But when the pancreas function is disrupted, this direction is reversed, producing such signs and symptoms as low energy, loose stools or diarrhoea, and the possible prolapse of the organs—which all feature a *downward* movement.

But this still did not explain *why* the symptoms developed; that is, when the liver had a disease, why would this also sometimes cause the stomach and pancreas to have a disease?

This was accounted for using the five phase doctrine, another cornerstone of *Nei Jing* theorizing.

The five phase "domination" cycle

Military analogies were frequently used in *Nei Jing* medical thinking. When a person was weak, outside forces would take advantage of this weakness and invade them (p.44), and the same thinking was applied to the organs. When an organ was weak, any other organ in a position to do so may take advantage of that weakness and "invade".

In five phase theory, there is such a relationship between the phases of Wood and

Earth (or "soil", as it was usually referred to in the *Nei Jing*), where liver belongs to the Wood phase, and the pancreas and stomach both belong to the Earth (or soil) phase. And between these particular phases, there was said to be a "domination" relationship, whereby the liver (Wood phase) would be capable of "dominating" the pancreas and stomach (Earth phase), but only if there was an imbalance between the two phases. That is, when the liver became excessive, or the pancreas and stomach became deficient.

Extract from *Su Wen*, Chapter 69

If in a year associated with wood, there is great excess of the [influence] of wood, wind [influence] prevails everywhere. The [pancreas], which is soil, receives [harm]. People suffer from outflow of undigested food and they eat less. Their bodies are heavy. They suffer from vexation and grievance, intestinal sounds, and propping fullness in the abdomen.[25]

Wang Bing (in 762 AD) commented on the above extract: "When the [influence] of wood is present in surplus, the [influence] of the soil yields." And Zhang Jiebin (in 1957) commented: "The transformation of wood is wind. When wood dominates, then it overcomes the soil. Hence the [pancreas organ] receives [harm]."[26]

This is the "domination" cycle of five phase theory (p.263). As well as the term "domination", other militaristic terms are also used, such as "subdue", "attack", "invade", "control", where one organ is said to "invade" another. Hence, when stagnated liver function affects the stomach, this is often termed "Liver invading stomach", and when the pancreas is affected: "Liver invading pancreas*", or sometimes "Disharmony of the liver and pancreas".

For example, Chapter 5 of the *Su Wen* states "If he is harmed in the Spring by wind, he will develop outflow of undigested food in summer."[27] Commenting on this line, Wang Bing (in 762 AD) stated: "When wind strikes the exterior, then the liver corresponds to this internally. The liver [influence] invades the [pancreas] and this results in outflow of undigested food."[28]

Though there are sometimes practical situations where this "domination cycle", and other aspects of five phase theory, seem to fit, in the majority of situations, the theory does not stand up to scrutiny (pages 263-277 analyse the theory in detail and demonstrate that many of its correspondences and relationships are arbitrary).

There is no doubt that this particular relationship between the liver and pancreas exists—so that when the liver is stressed, this often affects the pancreas and stomach, producing the symptoms the *Nei Jing* authors observed. We know those observations are fact based, since the same circumstances are routinely seen in clinic today. But these organ symptoms do not occur *because* of the supposed correspondences and relationships of five phase theory (since the theory does not stand up to scrutiny). Therefore, there must be some other explanation.

In contemporary physiology, such conditions are probably best understood by imagining what might be physically happening in

* It should be noted that the term "spleen" is used throughout Chinese medicine to refer to the pancreas—see page 61.

the body. The liver regulates the flow of energy and other resources to the stomach and pancreas (as well as to the other organs), and when the liver function is disrupted, this would therefore disturb the flow of energy to the stomach and pancreas, causing them to no longer function properly and they may produce the symptoms described above.

Hence a translation of the term "Liver invading stomach" using the concepts of contemporary physiology, could be "the liver fails to properly regulate the flow of resources to the stomach, so the stomach no longer functions properly".

The effects on the emotions

The *Nei Jing* authors noticed that when this liver function (*maintaining the free flow of influences*—in other words, regulating the generation and supply of energy in the body) was impaired, it also often impacted on the emotions, producing such symptoms as depression, weeping, irritability, anger and paranoia.

The topic starting on page 107 below describes how the mental functions of the liver are produced, and also provides explanations for the above emotional symptoms.

3. Maintains the smooth movement of the muscles

This is an indirect effect rather than a function, since the liver has no direct functional control over the muscles. Instead, as an indirect consequence of the liver function, the smooth movement of the muscles is affected.

The *Nei Jing* authors noticed that when the liver was stressed, patients could suffer such symptoms as: stiffness of the "joints" (meaning the muscles*), cramps, spasms, tremors, or twitches in the muscles,[29] all of which cleared once the liver was successfully treated. In today's Chinese medicine, these signs and symptoms are accounted for by stating that one effect of the liver is to maintain the smooth movement of the muscles.

In contemporary physiology, the liver completes parts of the digestive process so as to manufacture blood and also acts as a reservoir so as to regulate the amount of blood in circulation; and it also regulates the amount of energy in circulation (the supply of glucose and ATP). Both these functions, when defective, may play a part in accounting for the above symptoms, since the poor quality and inadequate supply of blood, together with the inadequate and irregular supply of energy may contribute to the improper function of the muscles—and hence the stiffness of the "joints", and the tremors, spasms, or twitches in the muscles.

4. Influences the quality of the nails

This is an indirect effect rather than a function.

The *Nei Jing* authors noticed that when the liver function was normal, the nails were strong and had a smooth surface, while when the liver function was not normal the nails often bore ridges and could be soft, thin, withered, or even deformed or chipped.

In Chapter 10 of the *Su Wen*, this idea was expressed by saying "The correlate of the liver

* The joints are moved by the muscles and tendons, so in this context "stiffness of the joints" refers to a joint's inability to move smoothly due to the inability of the muscles and tendons to contract and relax properly—rather than due to physical anomalies, such as arthritis.

are the sinews; its splendour appears in the nails."[30] And commenting on this line, Wang Bing (in 762 AD) commented: "Nails are outgrowths of the sinews. Hence they are where the splendour of the liver appears externally."[31]

This explanation, of course, is not literally true. The nails are not "outgrowths" of the "sinews". But because of the symptomatic associations between the liver, the muscles (which were called the "sinews" by *Nei Jing* authors) and the nails, it was theorized that the nails were somehow an extension of the muscles. The reasoning must have gone something like this. When the liver is stressed, this produces signs and symptoms in the muscles, and sometimes also in the nails. The muscles run along the limbs, and the nails appear at the end of the limbs. And since signs and symptoms appear in both, in response to stress in the same organ, then there must be some physical association between the muscles and the nails. Considering the lack of knowledge of the body's internal anatomy (p.16), this conclusion seems reasonable.

In contemporary physiology, the same explanation for the poor movement of the muscles may be seen as also accounting for the poor quality of the nails. In particular, the poor quality and inadequate supply of blood to the extremities may be understood as accounting for the nails not being properly nourished.

5. Has a close association with the eyes

This is an indirect effect rather than a function, since the liver has no functional link with the eyes. Instead, as an indirect consequence of the liver function, the eyes and eyesight are affected.

The *Nei Jing* authors noticed that when the liver function was not normal, any of the following symptoms could occur:

A. dryness or redness of the eyes, blurred vision, night blindness, floaters (light or dark specks seen by the patient in their field of vision)[32]; and
B. pain associated with the eyes (either behind the eyes, around the eye sockets, or on the temples),[33] and visual disturbances.

In today's Chinese medicine, the symptoms in list "A" are said to be due to the effects on the liver of poor quality blood. This disrupts the liver function in a certain way, and one of the effects of this is the production of these signs and symptoms associated with the eyes. This is therefore known as "Liver blood deficiency". And the symptoms in list "B" are all associated with migraines and are produced by a particular malfunction in the liver—which is described in detail on page 118 below.

After successfully treating the liver, all the above symptoms tend to clear, which not only confirms the association between the eyes and liver, but also suggests that proper function of the liver is necessary to enable the eyes to work well. This is also observed by patients in clinic today; after treating the liver of patients who tend to experience the above symptoms, they often report that their vision is clearer and the colours brighter.

There is also said to be an internal liver meridian that ascends to the eyes,[34] and the gallbladder meridian begins beside the eyes, which suggests a possible mechanism that could enable the liver to affect the eyes and eyesight. A similar effect is produced at acupoints, and also anywhere along an organ's meridian, when that organ malfunctions—and the effect can be instant. The organ malfunction appears to cause the local tissue at certain of its acupoints to also malfunction, hence they become tender when pressed; or redness, heat, coldness, itching, pimples, or even shooting pains may result. And when the organ's malfunction is corrected, the malfunction at those distal locations immediately clears (pp.369-370). There is no reason why this same mechanism could not also explain the disruption in the sense organ associated with each of the main organs, in this case the eyes and eyesight.

6. Has mental and emotional functions

Over millions of years, each organ evolved logic to enable it to carry out its functions and coordinate these with the other organs (p.91). And once our conscious mind started having complex thoughts about the world around us, it is possible that this pre-existing organ logic may have been used to process such thoughts. Today, this notion is supported by the clear two-way associations between the liver function and certain of our mental processes, as described in the remainder of this chapter.

The thoughts produced by the liver function

In contemporary physiology, the liver's physical functions could be summarized as regulatory. It monitors the organs and tissues of the body and regulates the production and supply of energy and also the circulation of blood—and the resources it transports (p.99). The liver's physical function could be summarized in words as follows. *To monitor the flow of substances to the organs and tissues, and when this does not seem right, to regulate the flow.*

When the liver's logic associated with this function is used to process thoughts, what thought patterns might result?

In the body, the liver regulates the flow of physical substances, but when this function is applied mentally, our thoughts become the equivalent of those substances. This includes all our thoughts about the world around us: the things we see, how they appear (how tidy, disorganized, pleasing or displeasing), how tasks are done; other people's general appearance, their clothes, the way they speak or conduct themselves (including these same ideas about our own conduct), or our thoughts about any other aspect of the world around us. The liver acts when something *does not seem right* in the flow of substances*. In this case, this means: whenever the flow of our thoughts is obstructed—which would happen whenever we were troubled by a thought, or when another person or object obstructed our thoughts. But how are our thoughts able to interact with the liver?

It is not certain where the logic of the liver is located. It may be contained in the biological matter that makes up the liver itself; in the network of nerves and chemical messengers that communicate between the liver and the other organs (p.91); in brain matter perhaps related to the processing of sight, where the

* Page 232 describes *how* the liver knows when *something does not seem right* in the flow of our thoughts.

liver's logic may be copied in neurons (p.94); or in a combination of all these separate elements working together. But the significant point is that the physical liver and its logic are dependent on one another, and there is two-way communication between the two. Therefore, what happens in the one is duplicated in the other—in both directions. Both therefore perform in the same way; they regulate the flow of substances. And when an obstruction to the flow of substances occurs in this logic (whether the logic is located in the brain, the liver, somewhere between the two, or in both), the obstruction is duplicated in the liver. Hence, an obstruction to the flow of our thoughts, tends to cause the liver to act as though there were an obstruction to the flow of the *physical* substances in the body.

Creative thinking

In the body, when the flow of substances is obstructed, the liver solves the problem by finding a creative solution. It regulates the flow of substances by (creatively) interchanging them when necessary, calling on reserves to solve a shortfall, creating new energy—such as ATP—and so on (p.99). When this same function is applied mentally, the liver can just as well perform similar actions on our thoughts to remove any obstacles to *their* flow—where the "reserves" it calls on are our memories or newly-created ideas, which may be interchanged with the original ideas, or *parts* of those ideas, until the obstruction is removed.

The following are common examples of the type of creative thinking the liver performs:

- At work you were asked to perform a task, but with the tools you had and the time available, it was not possible to perform this task to your standards. Here, the *obstruction* to the flow of your thoughts was the fact that you were obliged to perform a task that was not possible.
    - Your solution was to make a complaint to the company about your unrealistic workload; or to think of a way to divide the task between you and someone else; or to decide that since the company did not care about the standard of work, it was okay to lower your own standards and do poor quality work to get the task done; or to devise a scheme to get your manager into trouble, so that he would be removed.
- Something someone said to you did not make sense. The *obstruction* here was that a rule was being broken—they did not make sense and we expect people to make sense.
    - Your solution was to think of a question to ask to clear up what they meant, so that their comment *did* make sense; or to decide they were using words in an unconventional way, which caused you to misunderstand what they meant; or to perhaps decide they had a "feeble mind" and the things they said could not be relied on, so you simply dismissed their comment as meaningless nonsense.
- A new acquaintance was suddenly being favoured over you by an old friend of yours, which deeply offended you.

The *obstruction* here was that you wanted to be valued more by your old friend, just as he used to, and you felt your old friend's change of allegiance was wrong—it broke your rules about how people should behave.

- Your solution was to think up something to restore you in his affection, such as acquiring an item you knew he admired (in an attempt to make yourself more desirable to him), or changing your appearance, or beginning a campaign of misinformation to turn him against the new acquaintance.

In all these situations (or any similar situation), where do these *solutions* come from? If you think back to when you were last in any such situation, this type of creative thinking—this suddenly coming up with an idea that solves a problem—is something that appears to just happen by itself. You were aware of the problem, then the solution appeared in your conscious mind, as if it had come from elsewhere. This type of creative thinking is the task the liver performs.

Does the liver produce our dreams?

The liver function peaks between the hours of one and three a.m. (p.379), and a typical person's first dreams of each night tend to occur around one a.m. and then at around two-thirty a.m., after the two deepest portions of sleep.[35] And dreams are certainly creative; and their content is often a clear creative response to things that were on our mind during the day. The obvious inference is that it is the liver's creative ability that produces our dreams. But further, most people find that problems that foxed them during the previous day, tend to be solved while they sleep, so that on waking the solution appears in their mind—hence the phrase "sleep on it". It is notable that this unconscious creative thinking is performed most effectively at the time of day when the liver function is strongest (between one and three a.m.), reinforcing the notion that it is the liver that may perform this unconscious creative thinking.

This creative ability produces countless "rules"

Throughout our life, the liver's creative ability works out how best to do each task. These solutions are, in effect, our own liver's "rules". And there are other, general rules—such as the rule that we must join a queue at the back, rather than pushing in; or speak politely to other people; or not drive through a red traffic light, and so on. These rules have all been worked out by either someone else's or our own liver's creative ability.

From the liver's point of view, such rules serve as a short cut, enabling it to avoid *again* working out how best to do a particular task (which is hard work); instead, it simply applies its prearranged rule. And when our conscious mind is aware that such a rule is being broken, this obstructs the flow of our thoughts, but the liver's normal response of working out a creative solution is bypassed (since this has already been done) so instead the liver moves directly to its "emergency" response.

The liver's emergency response to obstructions

From the liver's point of view, this situation is a serious threat to the body's health and is almost an emergency situation, so the liver produces a powerful force to attempt to remove the obstruction. It produces the emotion of anger, irritation or frustration; which is often accompanied by a feeling of tightness or congestion at the physical location of the liver—indicating that the emotion originates from this location.

If the obstruction were purely physical, the person would be likely to stand up and perhaps jump around, panting or shouting, and this physical activity would be likely to do the trick, since such an obstruction in the physical body would most often only occur after many hours of stagnation. And when the obstruction is in the mental context and the person feels this same emotion, their instinct would be to react in a similar way and perhaps jump up and down, shouting angrily. But due to social constraints, most people would try to control their reaction. However, most people manage to express this frustration or anger to one degree or another (some, of course, appear to exercise little constraint and would simply start shouting at the slightest cause). Sometimes their display would do the trick and the other person may submit, comply with the "rule", and the obstruction would be removed.

But in many situations such obstructions cannot be removed. For example, when the other person objects to being controlled or has alternative ideas about how something should be done, so refuses to change their behaviour. Or sometimes this scenario may not directly involve another person. For example, your work situation might constantly prevent you from doing your work in the way *you* think it should be done. This might include you being given tasks to do in too short a time, or tasks which you do not have sufficient resources to do "properly" (as *you* see it). All these situations produce a similar obstruction to the flow of our thoughts—and expressing our frustration would often have no effect on removing the obstruction. Or sometimes such an obstruction might be caused by an inanimate object, such as computer software, or machinery of some sort; and in all *these* instances, no amount of shouting at the software or machinery or work process, is going to have the slightest effect on removing the obstruction.

Alternatively, for whatever reason, some people may choose to suppress their anger or frustration, in which case such obstructions would certainly not be removed. When a person suppresses anger or frustration, that suppressed powerful force only then adds to the stagnation, which produces a feeling of melancholy.

This situation causes a considerable problem for the liver. The flow of substances has been obstructed in the mental context, which then causes the liver to act as though the flow of physical substances had been obstructed in the body. And its "emergency" measure of producing the emotion of anger has failed to restore the flow, has been suppressed by ourselves, which only increases the stagnation, producing melancholy or even depression, which then only increases the stagnation everywhere in the body.

Patient example
Female, aged 29. This patient had a history of depression and panic attacks, and also a wide range of other symptoms. After a few treatments, all her symptoms improved markedly. See the full case history on page 245.

When the liver function is stagnated in this way, the body's digestive processes and hence the production of the resources our energy is made from are affected, as is the circulation of those resources, which then also affects the function of *all* the organs. If the situation continues for any length of time, the symptoms listed on page 113 start to appear; and the longer this stagnation is in place, the more the symptoms are likely to increase, both in number and severity.

I have noticed that when I recall an unresolved injustice, this can produce *heat* in the region of my own liver within a few seconds, indicating that such thoughts can affect the liver function almost instantly. The same observation can be made on the effects of certain thoughts on the heart function, which also appears to be almost instant (p.193). Such observations indicate how quickly and powerfully our thoughts can affect the function of the main organs.

The melancholy state and creativity

It is common for us to suppress our irritability and anger, due to it being socially unacceptable, which only causes this strong force to "turn inwards" and produce the emotion of melancholy. However, in some instances this state can be productive. As a creative person, I have found that the melancholy state is almost a prerequisite for creativity (in writing, musical composition and any other form). The creative process is very similar to the process described above. You encounter a problem—something you want to express—which you cannot solve, which then sends you into a melancholy state. And while the liver is producing this emotion of melancholy, it appears to be working creatively; its powerful energy has "turned inwards" and appears to be working flat out to find a solution to the creative problem (how to remove the obstruction), and then the solution starts to pour out—whether it is in the form of words, music or some other form which suddenly appears in your conscious mind. And once the problem has been solved, the melancholy lifts.

Each person's general nature

With most people, the interaction between their organs is often unbalanced, so that one becomes predominant, which then tends to influence the person's general nature. Such an imbalance is often inherited, in which case it can even affect such things as the general shape of the person's body and the sound of their voice. These features can be uncannily revealing, sometimes making it possible to diagnose a patient merely by listening to their voice (see below, p.114).

Traits of a liver-dominated person

When the liver dominates us, our mental activity would also tend to be dominated by the "concerns" of the liver, causing the following traits to become excessive.

We would tend to *over* regulate our environment. At the simplest level, we may find ourselves frequently (almost unconsciously) adjusting the position of objects: straightening a picture on the wall or an object on our desk. This is due to the liver function monitoring the flow of our "thoughts" (in this case, visual images), finding that something *does not seem right*, and creatively transforming the image into something that *does* seem right, which then causes us to straighten the picture (or other object) to make it match this more pleasing image in our mind.

> **Extract from *Nan Jing*, Section 16**
> External evidence of [an illness in the liver] includes a tendency towards tidy appearance, a [green] face, and an inclination to become angry.... The illness, as perceived by the patient, consists of swollen and stiff limbs, dripping urine and difficult stools, as well as twisted muscles. If [some of] this evidence is present, the liver is afflicted. If it is not present, the liver is not afflicted.[36]

Our vision is the only sense in which we routinely do this (adjust objects to make them tidy), which probably reflects the fact that the liver is closely associated with eyesight, and *may* also be directly involved in producing our sight—by rearranging (or "regulating") the visual field into "sensible" shapes, patterns and lines, so that the flood of light particles the eyes receive, becomes a meaningful picture in our mind. And the liver involvement is also indicated by the visual disturbances that are sometimes produced when the liver is stressed, such as straight lines and edges appearing wavy, and also all migraine-related visual disturbances (p.118).

As well as constantly adjusting objects, we would tend to minutely organize every other aspect of our life. We may spend much time planning—writing lists, organizing our own and other's schedules and itineraries, organizing things such as filing systems or inventing other such systems to minutely organize the activities of everyday life, both our own and other people's. And since the liver function peaks between one and three a.m., we may often find ourselves waking at that time with our mind busily planning and organizing any and every aspect of our life.

Over-applying the liver's creative ability would also cause us to create an excessive amount of "rules" which we would expect all people (including ourselves) to obey. We would be constantly telling people how to do each task, or rebuking them for doing a task the "wrong way". In this context, since it is *ourselves* doing the looking, the "right way" would mean obeying the rules *we* consider important or doing things the way *we* think they should be done. Or, often in the workplace, we may design intricate routines to perform tasks and expect other people to follow our routines; or may simply insist that each task, once *we* had decided how to do it, must be performed by other people in the particular way *we* worked out. Other people would certainly regard us as being a controlling person. And in a parent-child relationship, this control might extend to every aspect of the child's life. Of course, in many situations a certain amount of control is appropriate, but it is when that control becomes too much and too often that problems occur.

For a person who is dominated by their liver's concerns, a major health problem is caused in them when the people (or objects) around them decline to obey their "rules". This routinely blocks their liver function, producing the following condition.

Improper function

The liver plays a major role in the regulation, production and circulation of the resources that *all* our energy is created from. Consequently, when the liver ceases to function normally, this tends to produce powerful physical symptoms. In Chinese medicine terms, the following is the commonest liver condition.

Stagnated liver function

It was observed that when the liver function stagnated, this usually led to the patient experiencing *some* of the following symptoms:

- discomfort at the front or back of the torso at the level of the liver (the *hypochondrium*),[16] frequent sighing or hiccupping;
- feeling of irritability, with outbursts of angry shouting[18];
- muscular spasms, cramps, twitching,[29] stiff neck[37];
- a feeling as though something were stuck in your throat[38];
- fluctuations of mood, melancholy or depression, paranoia[18];
- migraines or headaches with pain on the top or sides of the head or associated with the eyes,[43] visual disturbances[32];
- dizziness, vertigo, hearing high pitch ringing sounds (tinnitus), insomnia;
- strong pain, stiffness or discomfort anywhere along the liver or gallbladder meridian, particularly on the head, neck, hips, outside of the legs[37];
- (in women) irregular periods with cramps, tender breasts, either scanty or absent menses or, alternatively, heavy flow with clots, and emotional fluctuations and irritability in the pre-menstrual phase (PMS)[14]; and (in all patients)
- effects on other organs, producing constipation,[39] or the alternation of constipation with loose stools and other digestive signs (p.104).

Causes of stagnated liver function

Stagnated liver function[40] (also called "Liver chi stagnation") is extremely common in developed countries, since the condition is primarily caused by mental and emotional stresses of the kind that are rife in such societies. As described starting on page 109 above, the liver's creative ability produces countless "rules" about how things should be done or people should behave or life should be organized, and when our rules are disobeyed, this obstructs the flow of our thoughts, which causes the liver to act as though the flow of *physical* substances in the body were obstructed. As an emergency measure, the liver generates anger or irritability to try to remove the obstruction, but if this fails or we suppress our anger, the liver function remains stagnated. And when this is present, any of the above (often powerful) symptoms occur.

> **Patient example**
> Female, aged 32. This patient sought treatment for issues related to her menstrual cycle, primarily acne but also PMS and painful periods. All these issues were addressed by the treatment, which focused on alleviating her stagnated liver function. See the full case history on page 252.

Diagnosis and treatment

When a patient has stagnated liver function they would usually have a selection of the symptoms listed above (p.113), which the practitioner would determine by questioning. And the diagnosis would be confirmed by examining the patient's tongue and pulses (p.383 and 299). To the practitioner, the liver pulse would resemble the feel of a taut wire under the fingers—and is called "wiry" in Chinese medicine. Some of the other organ pulses may also have this same "wiry" quality, since the stagnation often extends to the other organs as well. And the body of the patient's tongue would often have "stagnation dots" and also red sides, to one degree or another—the more pronounced the stagnation, the more this redness would be obvious. In tongue diagnosis, the left side of the tongue relates to the liver and the right to the gallbladder (p.383).

Facial colour and tone of voice

When the stagnated function is pronounced or chronic, the patient would tend to have a green facial hue which other people can often see.

> **Extract from *Su Wen*, Chapter 10**
> If the complexion is generated by the liver, it resembles [a light blue-green colour] wrapped up in white silk.[41]

The patient example on page 252 provides a striking example of this, where a boy's problems were caused by stagnated liver function, and his family reported that his complexion was notably green when his condition was at its worst.

This is also doubtless the origin of the expression "green with envy". When a person is prone to stagnated liver function, this would tend to create within them states such as envy and paranoia (page 231 describes the process whereby the liver creates paranoid thoughts). The enviable situation would be seen as the breaking of rules (it is unfair that the other person has this desirable advantage, rather than me; it is an injustice), and the more this "injustice" were focused on, the more the person's liver function would stagnate, heightening their green hue.

Chapter 5 of the *Su Wen* associates the liver with a "shouting" voice.[42] When a person is prone to stagnated liver function, they would usually have a loud voice and when in normal conversation would sound as though shouting. This is a reliable diagnostic sign, and easy to recognise.

Treatment

When stagnated liver function is present, one or more of the key acupoints related to the liver tend to feel tender when pressed. The key acupoints on the front of the body are Liver-3 (*Taichong*), Gallbladder-41 (*Zulingqi*), Gallbladder-34 (*Yanglingquan*), Pericardium-6 (*Neiguan*), and Liver-14 (*Qimen*). And the key acupoints on the back of the body are Bladder-18 (*Ganshu*) and Bladder-14 (*Jueyinshu*).

These acupoints become tender due to their association with this particular liver malfunction. When one of these acupoints is stimulated, this encourages the organ to cancel out the malfunction in itself that caused the tenderness (p.372), and the organ returns to normal function.

The effect is often immediate, or could sometimes take a few minutes, when the "wiry" quality in the patient's pulses would clear, indicating the organ function was now modified. I have also noticed that any red areas on the patient's tongue also tend to clear within seconds of the liver acupoints being needled. And, of course, patient's often feel considerably less stressed at the end of the treatment, since their liver function is now more normal.

In this way, as with all acupuncture treatments, the problem is corrected by the organ itself (p.78).

The progress of treatment

As when treating all conditions, after the first treatment the positive effects of the treatment may wear off after a day or two. But with each successive treatment, the positive effects tend to last longer. This phenomenon is partly due to resistive factors in the patient's lifestyle.

Acupuncture can "get under the radar" to address mental and emotional issues

Each person may have adopted patterns in their thinking and emotional behaviour that tend to encourage their main organs to malfunction. This is particularly so with the liver (as summarized on page 113 above), but it is also true with the other four main organs.

Their habits might include being too controlling of other people (and themselves), resulting in constant obstructed thoughts, irritability and (almost inevitably) stagnated liver function. And any difficulties might be compounded by a tendency to *not* express their frustrations or anger.

With all these patterns, there may be particular key incidents in a person's life which marked the start of the pattern, such as traumatic events; and the memory of these experiences can make it harder for the person to break the pattern. Ordinarily, mental and emotional patterns of these types would need to be changed in order for the patient's organs to return to functioning normally, and for their symptoms to thus clear—since, if these mental and emotional patterns remain the same, after every acupuncture treatment, the organs would soon re-adopt the same malfunction.

The process of us gradually changing such habits is normally a long and slow one, and with some people it may be beyond them. But acupuncture seems to "get under the radar" of our conscious mind and directly regulates the function of the main organs, which in turn tends to encourage us to spontaneously change our mental and emotional habits. I often find patients return after a few treatments and tell me about such changes; they find themselves suddenly becoming more assertive (when it is appropriate), or expressing their frustrations appropriately, or being more relaxed about which "rules" they like to see obeyed; and, in general, being more able to spot what elements in their life are bad or good for them.

However, it is still possible for a particularly strong-willed patient, who may be stuck in a mode of thinking or feeling, to doggedly cling to their familiar mental and emotional habits and thus reverse the treatments (see page 238). With such patients, their journey in life towards good health would tend to be an extended one.

> **Patient example**
> Female, aged 28. This patient sought treatment for a neck pain. Initially her symptoms improved, but the pain returned. She continued with treatment, which gave her the clarity and courage to resolve a relationship problem, and her neck pain was then able to clear. See the full case history on page 247.

Changes to lifestyle

When receiving acupuncture treatment, patients also often spontaneously change their physical lifestyle—since the treatments seem to make them more aware of which of their habits are unhealthy. But as a general rule, long periods of inactivity are detrimental to the liver, since this encourages physical stagnation in the body, which the liver abhors. And long periods sat at a desk under stressful conditions would be particularly damaging, since the mental and emotional stresses tend to worsen the stagnation. The body is designed to be used, to be physically active during daylight hours, so incorporating a variety of physical activities into our day is key to maintaining the health of the liver—and is a great way to dissipate the effects of mental and emotional stresses. However, routine *excessive* exercise would tend to have a depleting effect on the body's key resources and in the long term could be just as damaging to our health. One of the key principles advocated by Chinese medicine is balance, in every area and aspect of life.

Other liver conditions

The following terms are also used in today's Chinese medicine in relation to liver conditions, though it should be noted that such terms were not used in the *Nei Jing* and have been adopted more recently (p.449).

Once stagnated liver function is present, this tends to affect the function of the other organs and hence the production of blood. When this situation is present, this may lead to signs and symptoms such as

- blurred vision,[13] night blindness, dryness of the eyes, seeing either light specks or dark patches in the field of vision[32];
- poor quality nails, including soft, thin, withered, or deformed nails;
- numbness of the limbs,[12] weak muscles;
- pale complexion, pale lips; and
- increased tendency to experience muscular cramps and spasms.[11]

These signs and symptoms are thought to be produced by a combination of the stagnated liver function and the effects of poor quality blood, which itself came about due to the long-term stagnated liver function. In today's Chinese medicine, the condition is known as "Liver blood deficiency" (p.106).

If the stagnated liver function eventually affects the function of the stomach, this may produce

- a feeling of indigestion (discomfort around the lower, front ribs on the left side—the location of the stomach);
- belching, nausea or vomiting, acid regurgitation (p.85); and
- a rising sensation of heat in the centre of the chest (heartburn).

In today's Chinese medicine, this condition is known as "Liver invading stomach" (p.104).

> **Patient example**
> Male, aged 14. The patient's parents split up when he was ten, and a year later he developed stomach cramps. This case provides a textbook example of "Liver invading stomach". See the full case history on page 250.

> **Patient example**
> Female, aged 32. This patient sought treatment for acne. The case includes a clear example of "Liver invading stomach", which produced *heat* in the stomach, manifesting as acne. See the full case history on page 252.

And if the function of the pancreas were affected, this could produce

- a bloated and tender abdomen,
- loose stools alternating with constipation, and
- intestinal noises (p.74).

In today's Chinese medicine, this condition is known as "Liver invading pancreas" (p.104).

As stated on page 113, once the liver function is stagnant, this is likely to produce such symptoms as: constant feelings of dissatisfaction, frustration, resentment, repressed anger, possibly leading to depression. And over time, the following symptoms could also occur:

- frequent bouts of angry shouting[18],
- violent rages,
- migraines and headaches with severe pain,[43] and
- dizziness, vertigo, tinnitus.[44]

In Chinese medicine terms, the influences (*chi*) are considered *yang* in comparison with the blood, which is *yin*. Theoretically, it is thought that the above symptoms are due to the influences stagnating within the liver, becoming excessive and therefore "consuming" the blood (the *yin*), so that the *yin* can no longer restrain the *yang*, which then surges up into the patient's head (the influences moving contrary to their regular course), causing the powerful symptoms. Therefore in today's Chinese medicine, the condition is known as "Liver yang rising".[45]

As with many such Chinese medicine theories, the theory is not literally true. The notion of the influences (*chi*) "moving contrary to the norm" is a common *Nei Jing* conception used to explain symptoms (p.103), as is the notion of the interaction of the influences (either with the blood, or with pathogens or other substances, such as "wine influence" or "cold influence"—p.28). But in reality the influences themselves do not exist (pp.41-47), therefore any theory based on their movement (or their interaction with the blood) can only be untrue. However, as also is usually the case, the symptoms and the syndrome are fact based, since they were discovered through practical observation. Therefore it ought to be possible to account for them using contemporary physiology, which is done in the section *The causes of migraine* below.

Treatment of these conditions

All the above syndromes simply describe conditions that are either complications of stagnated liver function (and can therefore be successfully treated by treating that condition) or are due to problems with one of the other main organs and would be addressed by treating that organ (as well as treating the stagnated liver function), so that in the above examples, the stomach and pancreas could also be treated, as described on pages 77 and 85.

The causes of migraine

When any organ malfunctions, this tends to disrupt the function of some aspect of the local tissue at its associated acupoints, which is what produces the tenderness at those acupoints, with the degree of tenderness being proportional to the degree of the malfunction (p.370). Once the liver function stagnates, this same mechanism may produce "tenderness" at any location along the liver or gallbladder meridians. Initially the patient may not be aware of the tenderness. But as the stagnation increases, so does the intensity of the sensation, which may gradually build to produce the usual migraine symptoms. These typically occur along the path of the gallbladder meridian (over the temples and on the sides of the head), and are usually also associated with the eyes (an internal meridian is said to ascend from the liver directly to the eyes—p.106).

Stagnated liver function is most commonly produced, and then exacerbated, by stress, which is very much a mental factor, resulting from our own thoughts about the injustices in our life, the breaking of our "rules", and so on (p.113). The fact that the condition is brought on by mental factors may explain why the most intense pains are experienced in relation to the liver-related meridians on our head.

The liver may also play a part in processing vision and producing the images we see (p.112). However, this notion is not much more than informed speculation on my part. But what is much more certain is that, whichever way you look at it, the health of our eyes and vision do appear to be dependent on the good function of the liver (p.107). And this may explain the visual disturbances that are common.

In summary, the symptoms of a migraine are simply the pain felt by the liver when its function is impeded, which pain is reflected at various locations on our head due to the association between the liver and those locations.

The kidney-related cause

As stated above, it is mental stresses that tend to produce stagnated liver function, which can sometimes then go on to produce migraine symptoms. But this does not happen in all people. Some people are more prone to migraines, and these people often also have poor kidney function (p.174), which could be viewed as a common underlying factor.

In today's Chinese medicine, the particular kidney condition is known as "Kidney yin deficiency". The theory is that the syndrome occurs in people who have a constitutional deficiency of *yin* and excess of *yang*.[46] In other words, their kidney function is poor, producing a deficiency of *yin* (since the kidney is the most *yin* of the organs—p.348) and their liver function is frequently stagnated, which produces an excess of *yang*. In this case these *yang* qualities may be anger, irritability, rage, heat (the red face and sensation of heat in the body), trembling, twitching, tremors (when a person "trembles with rage"). And all these signs and symptoms are known as "liver wind" because they have been produced in the liver; they are the result of the "stirring up of liver wind". In this scenario, the insufficient *yin* is unable to restrain the *yang*, which then surges up into our head (moving contrary to its usual course) and produces the symptoms.

As with most such *Nei Jing* based thinking, the theory is not literally true. In clinic today, the theory may be a useful diagnostic tool but it is not literally true. However, the syndrome is fact based, since it was discovered through practical observation. It is true that people whose thoughts are dominated by "liver-related concerns" and who also have poor kidney function, are prone to migraines; and that when the poor kidney function is successfully treated, the migraines reduce in frequency, or clear completely. So, it ought to be possible to account for the syndrome using contemporary physiology. The following is one possible explanation.

When a patient has poor "kidney" function, this would also include possible malfunction of the adrenal glands (one of the three kidney-related structures—p.153); and since a key function of the adrenal glands is to help regulate the body's usage and storage of the resources that create our energy (p.154), this could impede the liver's ability to regulate those resources, resulting in stagnated liver function. Hence, the intense stagnated liver function associated with a migraine is being produced by two factors, the usual mental stresses and also this intra-organ factor from the kidneys, which could only amplify the degree of any stagnation in the liver function.

Together, these two factors may produce a malfunction in the liver that is significantly worse than would otherwise occur. And when this increased, or aggravated, malfunction is then reflected at the liver-related locations on the head (as any organ malfunction is reflected at the local tissue along its related meridians) this may account for the intensity of the symptoms.

The above is one possible scenario to account for the syndrome. Even though the scenario is speculative, what the above *has* demonstrated is a functional relationship between the kidneys and liver.

Patient example
Male, aged 24. This patient had a ten-year history of migraines. He was born with poor kidney function. This was the underlying cause of his migraines, which were triggered by stress at work. See the full case history on page 249.

Patient example
Male, aged 49. This patient had a long history of migraines and IBS, which all responded well to treatment. See the full case history on page 253.

Migraine usually responds well to acupuncture treatment. The function of the liver is treated directly, and any underlying causes are treated at the same time, such as poor kidney function. Key acupoints on the head, such as Gallbladder-20 (*Fengchi*), are also usually used, which tends to begin to relieve the symptoms immediately.

Treating any underlying weakness in the functions of the other organs (such as the kidneys), tends to reduce the frequency of migraines. But often, there are persistent factors in the patient's lifestyle which tend to exacerbate or bring about these weaknesses, which means that in the long term the migraines can only be kept to a minimum with regular treatments, or with the patient making lifestyle changes, which could include not driving themselves to work excessively (which weakens the kidney function) or, where possible, avoiding stresses of the type that cause stagnated liver function (p.110).

Gallbladder conditions

In contemporary physiology, the gallbladder is attached to the back of the liver by connective tissue[47] and has the following functions.

- It acts as a reservoir for bile, which is excreted by the liver and stored in the gallbladder, ready for use in digestion.
- It concentrates the bile by extracting water from it.
- When fats are present in the duodenum (the tube through which food exits the stomach), it releases bile into the duodenum to break down the fats to aid in their digestion.[48]

In the *Nei Jing*, the gallbladder's main function was considered to be mental—that of making decisions (see below). Throughout the *Su Wen*, the gallbladder was only mentioned in this capacity. The gallbladder was considered to contain "gall liquid" but this was not thought of as having the digestive function known today, and was thought of more as an extension of the liver's function.

Extract from *Su Wen*, Chapter 44

When the liver [influence] is hot, then the gall flows away. The mouth has a bitter taste; sinews and membranes turn dry. When sinews and membranes are dry, then the sinews become tense and are cramped...[49]

Commenting on this passage, Wang Bing (in 762 AD) wrote

The gallbladder is tied to the lobes of the liver and the flavour of its juice is extremely bitter. Hence, when the liver is hot, then the gall liquid overflows. When the gallbladder has a disease, then the mouth has a bitter taste. In the present case, the gall liquid overflows. Hence, the mouth has a bitter taste.[50]

Extract from *Nan Jing*, Section 42

The gall is located between the short lobes of the liver. It weighs three ounces and three *chu*. It is filled with three *ko* of essential sap.[51]

Commenting on this passage, Chang Shih-hsien (in 1510), wrote

The gall is the [*yang* organ (*fu*)] of clarity and purity; it does not accept anything dirty. It contains only three *ko* of essential sap.[52]

And Liao Ping (in 1913) wrote

The essential sap of the liver is stored in the gall. Both liver and gall master the blood. The two [*yin* organs] liver and gall are tied to each other; they constitute one entity. In this they resemble the heart and lung.[53]

It is clear that at the time of the *Nei Jing*, and even as recently as 1913, the gallbladder was not considered to have the digestive function known today. And yet in a contemporary Chinese medicine textbook, the main gallbladder function is stated as "The Gall Bladder receives bile from the Liver which it stores ready to excrete when needed during digestion. From this point of view, the function of the Gall Bladder is identical with that of Western Medicine."[54] This notion is clearly a modern invention, perhaps born from the desire to "update" the *Nei Jing* in the light of today's knowledge of physiology.

Improper function

Due to the close functional link between the liver and gallbladder (bile is produced by the liver), in an acupuncture clinic it would often be impossible to determine whether certain signs and symptoms were due to malfunction of the liver or gallbladder. For example, the following signs and symptoms could be due to malfunction of either: pain in the liver region, jaundice, nausea, and a bitter taste in the mouth. However—also due to this close functional link—treating the liver with acupuncture would also treat the gallbladder, and for this reason there is not usually the need to separately consider conditions of the gallbladder.

Also due to this close relationship, acupoints on the gallbladder meridian are often used to treat liver conditions. For example, the acupoints Gallbladder-34 (*Yanglingquan*) and Gallbladder-41 (*Zulingqi*) are often used to treat stagnated liver function, since (also due to this close relationship) these acupoints often become tender when the liver function stagnates.

The mental functions of the gallbladder

Through observation of mental and emotional symptoms and responses to treatment, the *Nei Jing* authors (or their ancestors) were able to observe that the gallbladder was responsible for the ability to make decisions, and having the courage to act on them.

Chapter 8 of the *Su Wen* states "The gallbladder is the official functioning as rectifier. Decisions and judgments originate in it" (a "rectifier" being the title of an official responsible for assessing the moral standing of certain people).[55] And Chapter 9 of the *Su Wen* states that there are "Altogether eleven [organs]. They receive decisions from the gallbladder."[56]

When the gallbladder is not functioning well, patients are usually indecisive and timid, which symptoms tend to clear once the gallbladder function has returned to normal. This mental function can be graphically observed in contemporary patients whose gallbladder has been surgically removed. The ones I have questioned, state that they are now unable to make the simplest of decisions, which they clearly associate with the removal of their gallbladder. Unfortunately this condition cannot be treated with acupuncture, since the treatment relies on the presence of the organ.

The logic of the gallbladder

The physical function of the gallbladder (in contemporary physiology) could be summarized in words as follows: *to distinguish between digestive substances, and when a particular type is detected, to take action to break it down to aid its digestion.* And this function (this decision-making process) would also constitute the logic of the gallbladder (p.91).

As with all other organs, the gallbladder logic can be used to process our thoughts. In this case, the function enables us to make decisions. That is, to *distinguish between digestive substances* (which, in the context of our conscious mind are any "thoughts" we have), and *when a particular type is detected* (that is, something where a decision is required—do I choose this way or that, this option or that), it then *takes action to break it down to aid its digestion* (that is, to pick one or other of the choices so that the result can be settled on—can be digested by our mind).

I have noticed that in patients whose job involves much decision making, the gallbladder meridian on their legs is often tender when pressed; and when I test this and the patient finds it particularly tender they will often say they had a hard week at work and feel "decision fatigued". This is also noticeable in a patient who comes for treatment after having made some hard decisions recently.

The path of the gallbladder meridian reflects its function

It is notable that the path of the gallbladder meridian reflects this mental function. The gallbladder meridian is the only one that zigzags; all the other meridians travel in straight lines, or follow the contours of the limb they travel along. The gallbladder meridian begins at the eye, then zigzags over the head—travelling back and forth over the side of the head four times—then zigzags down the side of the body and down to the foot. Its path seems to imitate this decision-making action: shall I go this way or that?

As said on page 351, this may be one further sign that during evolution a mechanism such as "resonance filtering" positioned the meridians by taking account of the symmetry between the organ functions and the geometry of the body, which would explain why the path of the gallbladder meridian reflects its physical (and mental) function. And it is notable that the location of the most intense zigzagging is on the sides of the head, which is the location of the thoughts which the decisions are made in connection with. (Or in another interpretation, it could be said that the most intense zigzagging happens on the head simply because this is the most *yang* part of the body.)

Chapter 7. Lungs and large intestine

The lung functions

In contemporary physiology, the primary function of the lungs is to take in oxygen. This is then transported to every cell in the body via the blood; and it is the "burning" (or *oxidizing*) of glucose within the cells, in the presence of oxygen, that enables the cells to create the energy they need (p.387). The lungs also expel carbon dioxide (CO_2) from the body, which is the waste product of this process.

Within the lungs the airways branch out in an inverted tree-like formation, but in place of each "leaf" is a structure called an *alveoli*, which is where the oxygen is transferred into the blood from the air we breathe, and the CO_2 is transferred *from* the blood back into the air which is then exhaled—through the "trunk" of the tree, which correlates with the throat.[1]

Defensive functions

The lungs also play a key role in protecting us from airborne pathogens (viruses, dust particles, pollen, and so on). This protection begins in the *upper airway*, which is the passage that extends from inside the nose, passes through the *larynx* (which contains the vocal cords), the windpipe (*trachea*) and down into the lungs. The inner surface of the nose is lined with mucus which begins to filter out small particles from the air we breathe, such as dust and *microbes* (viruses and bacteria); and the pharynx (the next part of the airway) contains lymphatic tissue which produces antibodies in response to microbes.[2] The alveoli in the lungs also contain

- cells which produce further antibodies to attack any microbes present; and
- further cells (*macrophages* and *polymorphonuclear lymphocytes*) which engulf small particles, such as any food substances accidentally inhaled, or also invading microbes.[3]

Other functions of the upper airway

The upper airway has several important functions, such as acting as a heat and moisture exchange system. When we breathe out, heat and moisture are retained from the exhaled air, and then transferred to the relatively cool and dry air we breathe in, which prevents the lungs from becoming too dry.[4] Overall, the lungs and upper airway require a high degree of moisture to function normally, which is why the air we breathe out is saturated with water vapour—even though the upper airway extracts and retains as much of this as possible.[5]

The Chinese medicine functions and effects

In Chinese medicine, the upper airway and nose are considered to be an extension of the lungs; i.e. that all are part of the same organ—the lungs. And through practical observation of signs and symptoms and the responses to treatment, the *Nei Jing* authors (or their ancestors) worked out the functions and effects[*] of the lung, which are that it

1. takes in air, with assistance from the "kidneys";
2. contributes to immunity;
3. has a close association with the nose and sense of smell;
4. influences the quality of the skin and hair;
5. supports the voice; and
6. has mental and emotional functions.

1. Takes in air, with assistance from the "kidneys"

This is a combination of a function and an effect. The fact that the lungs take in air is clearly a function, but the fact that they require the assistance of the "kidneys" to do this is an indirect effect (of the "kidneys"), as explained below (p.128).

The *Nei Jing* authors theorized that the lungs inhale air and obtain clear influence (*qing chi*) from it. This corresponds with the main lung function in contemporary physiology—the clear influence corresponding to oxygen.

There was no notion that the lungs exhale "waste air"

It was also stated that the lungs were responsible for inhaling and exhaling, but there was no notion that the exhaled air contained waste matter of any sort—such as anything that could be considered analogous to CO_2. Breathing was only considered in the context of taking in clear influence. The *out* breaths were merely considered to be part of the same process, to be a necessary part of the breathing cycle. After all, you cannot repeatedly breathe in unless you breathe out as well. Apart from this, breathing out was not seen as serving any function. The only other context that breathing was mentioned in, was when irregular breathing was symptomatic of ill health.

> **Extract from *Su Wen*, Chapter 17**
> As for the five [*yin* organs (*zang*)], they are the guardians of the centre. When the centre has abundance and when the [*yin* organs] are full and when the [influence] dominates and one is harmed by fear, when the voice sounds as if words came out of a room, this is *dampness* of the central [influences].[6]

This extract may seem incomprehensible because of its reliance on such phrases as "guardian of the centre" and notions such as "the centre having abundance", which do not mean anything to today's readers. However the following commentary is helpful:

[*] See page 64 for an explanation of the term "effects" in this context.

Wang Bing (in 762 AD) commented on the above extract

The [influences] overpower exhalation and inhalation, causing them to change to panting breath. That is, when the [influences] abound in the abdomen, when the lung ... is filled and when the [influences] overpower the patient's breathing so that it changes to panting, in this condition the patient tends to be harmed by fear and his voice cannot be emitted; it is as if it were in a room.* All this results from *dampness* [influence] in his abdomen.[7]

Extract from *Su Wen*, Chapter 32

The patient cannot take deep breaths. The head aches unbearably. Sweat leaves the body and the patient feels cold.[8]

Wang Bing (in 762 AD) Commented on the above extract

The lung is situated above the diaphragm. The [influence] rules the chest. If it changes the direction of its movement repeatedly, this results in coughing. Also, [the lung] stores the [influence] and rules ex- and inhalation. The back, in turn, is the palace of the chest centre. Hence the patient pants and coughs, pain moves into [their] chest and back and the patient cannot take deep breaths.[9]

It was understandable that the *Nei Jing* authors did not consider what function exhaling might serve, since there was no practical observation that could have alerted them to the need for any such function. It is notable that in all the various *Nei Jing* theories of metabolism, not one of the authors ever theorized about the *production* of anything like "waste influence" or "turbid influence"—at least, not as a part of metabolism. It was theorized that the lungs obtained clear influence (*qing chi*) from the inhaled air. The notion that this clear influence (or "oxygen") was needed everywhere in the body to enable the energy to be released from food influence (analogous to glucose), is notably absent. There was no notion that anything like this essential chemical process even existed, and certainly no notion that it produced a waste substance (CO_2) which needed to be expelled from the body (pp.33-48). And again, there was no reason why they *should* imagine any of this—at that time.

However, today's Chinese medicine has added a new lung function, that of expelling waste along with the exhaled air.[10] It appears it was added as one of the many attempts to reconcile the *Nei Jing* with contemporary physiology. Yet the curious fact is that this recently added function has no clinical application in Chinese medicine, so it is difficult to see the merit of adding it. Why modify the *Nei Jing* theories when the "corrected" theory adds nothing? Surely it would be better to accept that *Nei Jing* theories are often untrue and embrace all the positive aspects, such as the many practical observations that still enable clinical results in many areas that contemporary medicine cannot yet equal (in the treatment of IBS, hay fever, asthma, the many stress-related conditions, mental and emotional conditions, and others).

There is no definitive Nei Jing theory of metabolism

As stated throughout Chapter 2, the *Nei Jing* authors theorized about how the food taken

* I.e. the voice is in a room but we are outside the room, listening through the walls.

in by the stomach, and the air taken in by the lungs were used to produce the resources the body needs, which theories also included notions about the defence against pathogens. But different *Nei Jing* authors produced different, contradictory theories about the fine detail, so that there is no single, definitive *Nei Jing* theory of metabolism.

All agreed that the lungs inhaled clear influence (*qing chi*) from the air, which was then stored in the lungs and heart, where it was then known as chest influence (*zong chi*), whose sole role was to assist the lungs and heart to function (p.41). And it was considered that several other types of influence were extracted from our food; i.e. food influence (*gu chi*), constructive influence (*ying chi*), and defensive influence (*wei chi*); and that liquids (*jin* and *ye*) were also extracted and converted into blood. But some said the conversion into blood took place in the stomach, some said in the "meridians" and collaterals*. And there was even wider disagreement over the circulation route of the influences; some said this was from the stomach to the pancreas, which then circulated them to the meridians; some said the stomach produced a "steam" which rose to the lungs, and that the lungs then passed all the influences (which were akin to vapours) to the "meridians", thus beginning their circulation from the lung "meridian"; and others said the stomach passed the food influence to the pancreas, which then circulated it to the other organs, meanwhile somehow converting it into constructive and defensive influences, and that these influences were finally passed to the "meridian" network (pp.24-48).

Chinese medicine textbooks of the past few decades only tend to mention one of these conflicting theories—that it is the lungs that circulate the influences through the meridians.[11]

The Nei Jing theory that the lungs circulate influences

One of the competing *Nei Jing* theories was that the lungs circulate the constructive influence (*ying chi*) and defensive influence (*wei chi*) via the network of "meridians" and collaterals, which then enables these influences to nourish the skin, muscles and organs.

> **Extract from *Nan Jing*, Section 24**
> The great-yin conduit is associated with the lung. It transports influences and warmth to the skin and its hair.[12]

> **Extract from *Ling Shu*, Chapter 81**
> The stomach and the intestines receive grain; the upper [section of the *san jiao* (i.e. the heart and lungs)] releases [the influences]. It is to them to supply the partings of the flesh with warmth, and to nourish the bones and the joints, as well as to penetrate the skin structures.[13]

It was noticed that when a person had poor lung function (p.143), they tended to suffer from general weakness, felt the cold, had cold extremities and were more vulnerable to attack from airborne pathogens (*cold, wind, dampness*, and so on).[14]

At that time, the only circulatory system known was the "meridians", and there was no separate knowledge of the blood circulatory

---

* The "meridians" being artery-like tubes, which were thought to lie deep beneath the *pathways on the skin* (what we today call the meridians); and the "collaterals" being the superficial veins and arterioles that were used for bloodletting; see page 31.

system as it is known today (it was assumed the blood also circulated in the "meridians"—p.42), and certainly no knowledge of the chemistry of the body, nor knowledge of the immune system. Therefore, when theorizing about the above lung-related signs and symptoms, it seems reasonable that the *Nei Jing* authors deduced that when the lung function was normal, the constructive influences (*ying chi*) and defensive influences (*wei chi*) were circulated (via the "meridians") to the skin and muscles, which then nourished them to enable their normal function; hence the skin was warmed, strength was provided to the muscles and the person was protected from environmental factors—due to the warmth of the skin and muscles (p.44).

This all seems to make perfect sense—based on the limited knowledge available at that time. And even to sensitive people today, the notion of the lungs spreading "nourishment" around the body via the meridians can still seem convincing. People who practise one of the martial arts, or any activity that involves an awareness of breathing or the energy in the body (such as yoga or tai chi), tend to be aware of the apparent direct connection between breathing and the nourishment circulating the body. Each time we breathe in, air enters the lungs, and on each out breath, nourishment seems to spread around the body. It is as though the process of the lungs spreading this nourishment can be consciously felt. It even seems to be possible to deliberately direct this nourishment to any part of the body, such as the hands or any other part, by focusing the mind on that part while breathing out—which seems to cause the hands to start tingling, so nourished are they. These experiences certainly seem to confirm this lung function of spreading the influences (*chi*) around the body, and would have no doubt convinced the *Nei Jing* authors that this was, indeed, what was happening.

So, again, it is perfectly understandable that *some* of the *Nei Jing* authors believed the lungs circulated the influences (*chi*) in the "meridians". But today, we know that no detail of this theory is true. The constructive and defensive influences do not even exist (pp.42-47), and every detail of metabolism is different from how they imagined it.* In contemporary metabolism, glucose is the body's main fuel; this is extracted from food by the combination of the stomach, pancreas and small intestine, the last of which absorbs the glucose into the blood. Oxygen is extracted from the air by the lungs and also circulated in the blood; and glucose and oxygen are combined in every cell of the body to produce the energy each cell needs.

Accepting that this account in contemporary physiology is true, how is it that it can appear to energetically-sensitive people (as well as to some *Nei Jing* authors) that the lungs *do* circulate nourishment through the meridians on each out breath?

Even though this mixing of glucose with oxygen takes place in every cell of the body, the process requires oxygen, which is supplied by the lungs. Admittedly, the oxygen is circulated via the blood, but the process still requires the active involvement of the lungs.

* It is true that in the *Nan Jing*, "constructive influence" is equated with blood (p.44), which certainly does exist; however, the blood was considered to flow in the "meridians", which do not equate to the arteries of today's circulatory system, so that, again, what was imagined to be happening was untrue.

With each breath, the blood is oxygenated by the lungs, and this oxygen then becomes available to every part of the body soon after, when fresh energy may be released in the cells of the local tissue. To sensitive people who are aware of the energy in their body, this process could give the impression that the lungs spread nourishment to every part of the body each time we breathe out—simply because the two experiences are linked; we breathe out, then feel the muscles tingling with energy.

In fact, the lungs *do* obtain the oxygen, which enables the release of energy in the body's cells; and if we stop breathing, no part of the body can survive for long. And when this part of the lung function is merely weak, this has a noticeable impact on every system and part of the body.

The lungs dominate the influences

In today's Chinese medicine, this first lung function is often described as "dominating the influences (*chi*) of the whole body".[15]

The simple way to understand this idea in the context of contemporary physiology is that the lungs supply the oxygen, which is essential to enable the release of energy in the body. The energy is released within every cell, but this process can only work when oxygen is present, along with the glucose extracted from our food (p.336). The lungs are the only source of oxygen in the body, and oxygen is not stored, which is why we need to continuously breathe to stay alive. Hence, the lungs enable the release of energy in every cell of the body.

I have said that the influences (*chi*), as imagined by the *Nei Jing* authors (i.e. vapours that circulate in the "meridians" to provide nourishment), do not really exist (pp.41-47), so how could the lungs be thought to "dominate the influences", if the influences are imaginary?

To be able to accept this statement as valid (in contemporary physiology), it would be necessary to think of the constructive influence (*ying chi*) as being analogous to the glucose circulating in the blood; and the oxygen supplied by the lungs (which also circulates in the blood) then enables the glucose to be used—so that the lungs therefore enable the "constructive influence" to nourish the body, and thus "dominate the influences". And the same also applies to the defensive influence (*wei chi*), which could be thought of as analogous to the active components of the immune system (p.46), which, like any other cells in the body, require the presence of oxygen to be able to function, so that, again, the lungs "dominate the influences".

The kidneys assist the lungs to breathe in

The *Nei Jing* authors noticed that when a patient suffered from asthma or shortness of breath, of the type where it was hard to breathe in (rather than being hard to breathe out), they also had poor kidney function (p.174), and once the "kidneys" were successfully treated, the patient's breathing problems cleared.[16] From this it was deduced that the kidneys assist the lungs to breathe in.

This observation is reinforced by the fact that asthma attacks of this type most often occur at around five a.m., which is the time of day when the kidney function is at its weakest (p.379); and also by the fact that when treating a patient, their relief usually begins during the acupuncture session, as soon as the kidney function is normalized. Various key kidney acupoints can be used to do this, such as Kidney-6 (*Zhaohai*), and when any of these are needled, the relief from shortness of breath often occurs within a few seconds. Or in patients who had not complained of shortness of breath, when such acupoints are needled on them, I have often found that during the treatment they will comment that they can breathe more easily since that particular acupoint was needled.

Contemporary anatomy and physiology has not yet explored this functional relationship between the "kidneys" and lungs, and since there is no known mechanism to account for the relationship, it must be regarded as an indirect effect (of the "kidneys") rather than a direct function.

2. Contributes to immunity

This is a direct function rather than an effect.

The *Nei Jing* authors noticed that patients with poor lung function tended to be more vulnerable to airborne pathogens (such as *wind*, *cold*, and any pathogens carried on the wind),[17] and also tended to feel the cold more than other people[18]; and that once their lungs were successfully treated, these patients tended to no longer feel the cold as much and suffered less from colds or flu.

From these observations it was deduced that our "immunity" from attack by airborne pathogens was provided by the lungs. It was theorized that defensive influence (*wei chi*) performed the protection. This, like all forms of influence, was thought to be a vapour-like substance, but in this case it circulated on the *outside* of the "meridians", perhaps akin to an enshrouding mist. It spread to the spaces between the muscles and skin, providing warmth to the muscles and skin; and it was this warmth that was thought to protect us from the harmful effects of wind and cold (pp.44-47). And it was thought that the lungs were responsible for circulating this defensive influence.*

As with many *Nei Jing* passages, it is generally only the aspects based on practical observations that are true. The theoretical aspects tend to be untrue. And in the case of defensive influence (*wei chi*), every aspect of the theory is untrue. No substance akin to defensive influence flows in the "meridians", or indeed in the *pathways on the skin*, which is what we today call the meridians (p.44), and our protection from attack by external pathogens does not take place in the space between the muscles and skin.

However, the original observation (that people with normal lung function suffered less colds) was fact based, so it ought to be possible to account for it using contemporary physiology.

In such terms, our protection from external pathogens takes place in two locations. Since the lungs breathe in air from outside, any pathogens carried by the air tend to affect the lungs first, so the body's first line of defence takes place in the nose, upper airway, and within the lungs themselves. Amongst other measures, these structures contain lymphatic tissue which produces antibodies in response to microbes; and in the alveoli of the lungs, there are also other cells which engulf small particles, such as inhaled pathogens (p.123).

The second location of our defence is the immune system generally. But in Chinese

* See the extract from *Ling Shu*, Chapter 81, on page 126.

medicine terms, the equivalent of this is the constitution, which is considered to be provided by the "kidneys", so this aspect is described in the chapter on the kidneys (p.156).

Hence, the *Nei Jing* authors correctly deduced the involvement of the lungs in the protection from external pathogens, but got the location of the physiology wrong—which is understandable when considering the absence of any significant knowledge of the body's internal anatomy.

3. Has a close association with the nose and sense of smell

This is an indirect effect rather than a function, since the lungs have no functional link with the sense of smell. Instead, as an indirect consequence of the lung function, the sense of smell and ability to breathe through the nose are affected.

The *Nei Jing* authors noticed that when a person had normal lung function, they had a good sense of smell and were able to breathe easily through their nose; while when they had poor lung function, they usually had a poor sense of smell (or sometimes none at all) and were unable to breathe easily through their nose.[19] It was also noticed that when a person suffered a cold (which is an attack on the lungs), their signs and symptoms would usually be focussed on their nose, with either congestion or a streaming nose, the inability to breathe through their nose, and sneezing.[20] From these observations it was deduced that the lungs have a close association with the nose and sense of smell.

In clinic, this association is often evident. When treating a patient's lungs using the lung acupoints (which are nowhere near the nose), patients will often report they can suddenly breathe more easily through their nose; and will also often return for a follow up treatment and comment on the marked improvement in their sense of smell, raving about all the things they can now smell which they were unaware of before, and even complaining that the world now seems *too* smelly to them. The fact that these effects are achieved without treating the nose but instead only treating the lungs, indicates a clear association between the lungs and sense of smell. However, it is not possible to explain this using contemporary physiology, since it has not yet been explored in such terms.

The lung meridian flows into the large intestine meridian which then ascends to end on either side of the nose[21] (the relationship between the lungs and large intestine is discussed on page 137 below). And this meridian connection between the lungs and nose provides a possible mechanism to enable the lungs' health to be reflected in the sense of smell and ability to breath properly through the nose. When an organ is stressed, its related acupoints become tender, which could only be due to some aspect of the local tissue ceasing to function properly (p.369); and in the same way, the local tissue at the nose (including the olfactory nerves[22]) may also cease to function properly when the lungs are stressed. In other words, for the sense of smell to work properly, it is necessary for the lung function to be healthy.

4. Influences the quality of the skin and hair

This is an indirect effect rather than a function, since there is no direct functional link between the lungs and the skin and hair. Instead, these effects are an indirect consequence of the lung function.

When a patient has poor lung function, they are often prone to skin problems, such as rough, dry or flaky skin, psoriasis or dermatitis; and are also prone to having poor quality body hair. But when a person's lung function is normal they tend to have good quality skin and hair. From these observations, it was deduced that the lungs influence the quality of the skin and hair.

Chapter 10 of the *Su Wen* states "The correlate of the lung is the skin; its splendour appears in the body hair."[23]

> **Extract from *Nan Jing*, Section 24**
> When the [lung meridian] is cut off from the movement of the influences, the skin and its hair will be scorched. The [lung meridian] it transports influences and warmth to the skin and its hair. When the skin and its hair are not supplied with influences, they will be scorched. When the skin and its hair are scorched, the liquids leave. When the liquids leave, the skin and the joints will be harmed.[24]

The theoretical aspect to the above extract (in the explanation of *how* the lungs influence the skin and body hair; i.e. by sending a supposed vapour-like substance through the "meridians", etc) is untrue (p.47). However, the significant fact is that the *Nan Jing* author (or their ancestors) associated the signs of poor skin and body hair with poor lung function, which must have been noticed through practical observation, then the theory came later (p.261). Hence, the associations are valid, even if the theory is not.

The Nei Jing notion that the lungs manage the circulation of body fluids to the skin

It was noticed that when a patient had poor lung function, their perspiration may become disrupted (either be excessive or absent) and their skin become too dry.[25] It may have been these observations that inspired the theory that the lungs play an active part in the circulation of body fluids to the skin and muscles, and in the body generally. And this notion may have also been reinforced by the observation that when a patient suffered a cold (an attack on their lungs), this would usually result in a major disruption in the circulation of body fluids, with excess moisture accumulating in their nose, and their body skin becoming dry.

> **Extract from *Su Wen*, Chapter 21**
> Beverages enter the stomach. Overflowing essence [influence] is transported upward to the [pancreas]. The [pancreas influence] spreads the essence, which turns upward to the lung. The [lung] frees and regulates the paths of the water, it transports the water downward to the urinary bladder.[26]

It should be noted that there was considerable disagreement between different *Nei Jing* authors on matters related to metabolism, so that theories such as the above should not be understood to be stating universally held views. Contradictory theories were often stated by different *Nei Jing* authors (pp.33-48).

However, in contemporary physiology, body fluids are circulated in the blood and lymph (p.165), and the lungs' involvement in this process is more passive. The normal function of the lungs, upper airways and nose has a high demand for fluid; and when the lung function is disrupted (such as in a cold, flu, or when the patient has poor lung function), the handling of this large through-flow of fluid would also be disrupted, which is enough to account for the accumulation of fluids in the nose, airways, and sometimes the lungs. In other words, the body's normal management of body fluids is disrupted due to this log-jam in the lung system and also the consequent loss of fluids from the nose—all of which greatly reduces the fluids normally available to the rest of the body, producing such signs as dry skin. Hence, the lungs do play a roll in the circulation of body fluids, but this is more passive—is due to the fact that the normal lung function has a high demand for fluids.

5. Supports the voice

This is an indirect effect rather than a function, since there is no anatomical link between the lungs and vocal cords. Instead, when the lung function is poor, one indirect consequence is that the function of the vocal cords is impeded.

The *Nei Jing* authors noticed that when patients suffered a cold, they would sometimes lose their voice. At other times, with patients who had poor lung function it was noticed that they tended to have a weak voice, were often disinclined to talk, and when they *did* talk for some time, this tended to drain their energy and cause them to lose their voice. From these observations, it was deduced that good lung function was necessary to enable the voice to function.

Extract from *Ling Shu*, Chapter 33

When the sea of [influence] has an insufficiency, then the breath [influence] will be diminished and [is] not enough to allow one to speak.[27]

Extract from *Su Wen*, Chapter 17

When the speech is feeble and when it takes an entire day before he speaks again, this is [influence] deprivation.[28]

The "sea of influence" is also known as the "chest centre" which is also the name of an acupoint, Ren-17 (*shanzhong*).[29] This acupoint tends to become tender when the patient experiences shortness of breath. The "sea of influences" can be understood as referring to the resources obtained by the lungs; or, in other words, the state of having good lung function. Or, it could also be understood as meaning the availability of chest influence (*zong chi*), which, in other words, also means the state of having good lung function (along with good heart function).

Patient example

Male, aged 56. This patient initially sought treatment to help him give up smoking and to improve his energy and sleep. His lung function was low, and when he needed to talk a lot during his work this made him tired. See the full case history on page 246.

In contemporary physiology, the sound is produced by the vocal cords; but these, along with any part of the airways right up into the nose, are considered in Chinese medicine to be an extension of the lungs, which does *appear* to suggest a correlation between this *Nei Jing* lung effect and contemporary physiology. However, the fact that the function of the vocal cords may rely on the good function of the lungs has not been explored in contemporary physiology, therefore it could not currently be regarded as a function, and must be regarded as merely an effect, unexplainable in contemporary physiology.

6. Has mental and emotional functions

In contemporary physiology, the main function of the lungs is to take in oxygen from outside, so that this can be transported to every cell in the body where it is combined with glucose to produce the energy the cells need to both survive and perform their functions; and then to expel carbon dioxide, which is a waste product of this process. In other words, the lungs' main function is to obtain air from outside, separate the precious oxygen, utilize this within the body and then expel the waste. This could be summarized as: *to take in something intangible from outside, sort the good from the bad, incorporate the precious and let go of the waste.*

This wording also summarizes the lungs' intention (since its physical function and its intention are one and the same—p.93).

The early primitive creature did not possess a lung

The creature I have so far considered at the early stages of evolution would not have possessed a lung at all. Since life began in the sea, the creature would have first developed gills; and at a later stage the first embryonic lungs would have evolved, which were also concerned with taking in oxygen from the outside (just as the gills were). Initially, this was perhaps a measure to obtain extra oxygen by gulping in air from the surface when the water was not oxygenated enough—hence both gills and the primitive lungs may have existed in the creature at the same time. Once the creature became land based, the gills were no longer needed and the lungs became the primary organ for taking in oxygen.[30] It is the intention of the lungs at this stage and onwards that my descriptions here refer to. Though it should be noted that both gills and lungs perform the same role (extracting oxygen and performing *gas exchange**) so that it seems possible that the first lungs may have evolved as an extension of the already existing gills, and thus shared much of the same biology of the gills. In other words, that both organs had the same intention.

The lung function is used to process our thoughts

Over millions of years, each organ evolved logic to enable it to carry out its functions and coordinate these with the other organs (p.91). And once our conscious mind started having complex thoughts about the world around us, it is possible that this pre-existing organ logic may have been used to process such thoughts. Today, this notion is supported by the clear two-way associations between the lung function and certain of our mental processes, as described in the remainder of this chapter.

The thoughts produced by the lung function

The lung function could be summarized as: *to take in something intangible from outside, sort the good from the bad, incorporate the precious and let go of the waste.* And when the lung logic associated with this function is used to process our thoughts, what thought patterns might result?

* Gas exchange is defined on page 183.

Appreciating quality in things

The lungs take in air (something intangible) from around us and extract the precious oxygen from it. In our mental world, there are countless opportunities for this same processing to be applied. For example, this happens when the brain processes our *visual* "thoughts". When we look at a landscape in nature, most of us would experience a pleasurable sensation within our chest (in the region of the lungs); a feeling as though we were breathing unusually clean air, or a feeling akin to a sigh of relief. This is the finding of something precious in an intangible thing (the sight) and incorporating it within us.

The same happens when we look at a fine painting or photograph, or when we see certain clothes, the design of a fine building, or furniture and objects that *we* consider "fine". This, of course, is different for different people. For example, some people may appreciate the design of a particular car, whereas others might say one car looks the same as another to them.

In all these situations the eyes take in rays of light. From a pure physics point of view, one image is the same as another; it is simply a large mass of "dots" of one colour or another. But the brain assembles these dots into an image and in the contents of *some* of those images, we are able to find great pleasure.

To us, that pleasure seems to enrich us; it is as though we were taking in visual food, which makes us feel good and thus even seems to have a nutritional value for the body. When our conscious mind becomes aware of these images, it is the lung function that "takes in" the image (just as it breathes in air), finds something precious (in the same way that it manages to separate out the valuable oxygen) and incorporates this precious substance within us—to nourish us (just as it does with oxygen). And the same is true of sounds, tastes, and even smells. These mental "images" are processed in the same way by the lung logic and when it manages to find something precious within them, this is incorporated within us to nourish us. In other words, it is perceived by us as "quality", which makes us feel good.

The other significant aspect of our mental experiences which the lungs process in this way is our perceptions of other people—their behaviour towards us and to others; the things they say or the way they say them in. All these thoughts are processed by the lung logic which searches for quality, and when found, this produces our sense of pleasure in the company of that person. Some people we find great pleasure in (the people who are "quality" in our eyes) while if we can find no such qualities in a person, then, by definition, our mind regards them as being the *opposite* of "quality" and we reject them.

If a photo or picture does not please us, we reject it; if a cityscape does not please us, we reject it. While many of us can readily find beauty in a natural landscape, many of us would recognise urban landscapes as "poor quality" and the lung function would reject these. For this reason most of us feel we can breathe better in a natural landscape; the air seems cleaner. We feel this because the lungs are literally working better. When the lung logic processes what we see, and detects quality, this reinforces that logic—simply because our mind has focused on it and used it successfully. And there is a two-way connection between the lungs' logic and their physical function, so that what happens in the one is immediately duplicated in the other (p.94). What was reinforced in our mind was the lungs' ability to *sort the good from the bad and incorporate the precious.* Therefore this same function would be reinforced in the lungs—their ability to extract the precious oxygen from the air and circulate it. Hence we could literally breathe better, and the air seemed cleaner, more oxygenated. The fact that this effect was not produced by the air simply being cleaner could be confirmed by looking at a picture of that landscape while at home, when the same feeling of being able to breathe more easily would usually be induced—even though the air you were breathing had not changed.

The health implications of this process

As said on page 111, in most people, one of the five main organs tends to be dominant; and in people whose lungs are dominant, this tendency to seek quality becomes exaggerated. This would produce in them a keen awareness of the flaws in such things as common cultural experiences (TV programmes, film, music and song) and also in everyday experiences such as in the meaning of other people's comments, or their sentence construction or logic, or the way other people dress, behave, talk, and in the décor of the home, workplace, and every similar experience they encounter from day to day. They would detect and take exception to flaws that would go unnoticed by most other people. They would certainly be regarded as perfectionists and would usually also extend their high standards to themselves, which might cause them to carefully control what they allowed themselves to do or say, which may cause other people to simply find their conduct puzzling.

It should be noted that we all posses these same tendencies to seek quality, to cherish the good and reject the bad, but in people who are lung-dominant the tendencies become excessive. It is as though they no longer have the sense of proportion that other people do.

> **Patient example**
> Male, aged 57. This patient was a perfectionist and drove himself hard in his business. Over many years this caused him to develop a wide range of health issues, eventually affecting all his main organs. See the full case history on page 250.

Disappointment regarding quality, depresses lung function

When a person is lung-dominant, their mind is constantly occupied with this lung function of identifying quality. But the more they look for quality, the more this quest is doomed to fail—and instead they notice the bad qualities in the other person, or in the activity, landscape, cultural or other experience. This has the following consequence. Every aspect of the lung function is represented in its logic (p.91), and any state in this logic is immediately duplicated in the lungs' physical function (p.94). Therefore, when this aspect of the lung function fails in our mind, this causes the same aspect of the lungs' physical function to act as though *it* had failed—as though the lungs had failed to extract oxygen from the air around us. And when this mental disappointment becomes an almost constant companion of our waking hours, this has a depressive and weakening effect on the lung function.

Apart from depressing their lung function, this constant feeling of disappointment gives lung-dominant people an air of sadness, an apparent tendency towards introversion and an appearance of always being serious.[31]

This same depressive effect in the lung function routinely happens in all of us though. Whenever we are in the company of a person, situation, or in an environment we find lacking in quality, this would induce in us the feeling that we "cannot breathe". You may feel you "cannot breathe" when around a certain person, and so on—which is literally what is happening.

Separating the good from the bad and letting go of the waste

Another aspect of the lung function is to *sort the good from the bad, incorporate the precious and let go of the waste.* When this function is working properly, we are able to see the good and the bad in proportion; we are able to separate them and let go of the bad (the waste). But in people who are lung-dominant and focus too much on seeking quality, this eventually weakens their lung function, so that the mental aspect *also* does not function correctly, and they often lose this sense of proportion.

In relationships, they might spot one bad quality in an acquaintance and reject the friend, overlooking all their friend's good qualities or the benefits to themselves of having that friendship—which is why lung-dominant people are often loners. And being unable to *sort the good from the bad*, they might also have difficulty identifying when something had become detrimental to them and would persist with it. They would hold on to unfulfilled ambitions, or resentment, or bear grudges for past wrongs, and would continue doing these things long after other people would have given up and moved on. They are unable to let go of the "waste" and instead hold on to it.

The lungs feel loss and grief

Because the lungs provide us with the ability to discern quality, to *sort the good from the bad and let go of the waste*, they play a central role in the process of grieving or feeling loss. When a person close to us dies, or a relationship ends, or a cherished job is lost, our conscious mind is faced with the problem of letting go of something we greatly cherish. We must somehow now come to see this as waste and let go of it. Of course this is a painful process. It creates a great conflict within us; we are naturally reluctant to regard as "waste" such a cherished thing, so our conscious mind (and other organs such as the heart) resist the process. This then tends to block the normal lung function (prevents the lungs from letting go of the waste—in other words, from breathing out properly), which gradually weakens the lungs, since breathing out is an important part of the breathing cycle. Hence, in grief, it is primarily the lungs that suffer—that "feel the loss". I said above that the feeling of disappointment tends to depress lung function. And grief is disappointment to an extreme degree, so this weakens the lungs much more than mere disappointment does. Our conscious mind is overwhelmed by the absence of such a cherished person or thing, which we simply cannot let go of, so the lung function is continuously and heavily impeded and the lungs are unable to find quality in anything.[32]

Another clinical observation that helps to clarify the lungs' role in all the above is this. In today's Chinese medicine, it is recognised that the inability to breathe normally (in other words, asthma) has two possible causes.

When the person finds it hard to breathe in, the cause is usually a weakness in their kidney function (p.176), but when they find it hard to breathe out, this is due to a weakness in their lung function. [33] This indicates that when a person's lungs are weak, the most noticeable sign would often be their inability to breathe out, which indicates that the action of breathing out is no mere passive activity (such as the relaxing of muscles) but one that requires the active, purposeful effort of the lungs. The *letting go of the waste* is an active role that the lungs perform, and when the lungs are weak, their inability to let go may become life threatening (people can die of this type of asthma).

In the same way, on the mental level, when a person's lung function is weak, they are less able to mentally let go of things that are, in effect, waste; and this would also affect their ability to grieve normally. Even though grief and sadness weaken a person's lung function, if they had normal lung function *before* their loss occurred, they would be able to go through the normal process of grieving and eventually let go of their loss and move on. However, in people whose lung function is usually weak, they may find it impossible to go through the normal grieving process and be left with constant feelings of denial, anger, resentment, or other such self-destructive feelings.

The role played by the large intestine

The organs are paired in various patterns. One pattern is that each *yin* organ (*zang*) is functionally paired with another *yin* organ, and the same with the *yang* organs. These are known as the "six channel" pairings (p.397).

For example, as shown on page 398, the lungs and pancreas are paired (both are part of the *taiyin* channel), and there appears to be close cooperation between them, so that any impairment in the function of one tends to affect the other. This is often seen in clinic. When a person suffers a cold, for instance, their digestion is often affected. Whatever the explanation, this could be visualized as follows. It is as though the two organs share a single pool of resources, and when the lungs are weakened, the pool is drawn on by the lungs—to fight off the illness—and the pancreas is left with insufficient resources, so symptoms of poor pancreas function start to appear, such as having a weak sense of taste, loose stools, a bloated and tender abdomen. On the other hand, when this "shared pool of resources" is already low, and the person eats a meal, the resources are drawn on by the pancreas—to help digest the meal—and the person then suffers symptoms of poor lung function, such as a runny nose.

With all these "six channel" pairings, there appears to be no physiological reason for the close cooperation between the organs; however, there is a close relationship between their meridian paths (as described on page 398), so that the explanation for their interaction may involve this meridian relationship.

The other pattern of pairing is where each of the *yin* organs (*zang*) is paired with a *yang* organ (*fu*) (p.348). Some of these pairings appear to be due to the obvious functional relationship between the two organs, such as the liver being paired with the gallbladder, the kidneys with the bladder, and the pancreas with the stomach. But with the other pairings the functional relationship is less clear. For example, the lungs are paired with the large intestine, but there does not seem to be an anatomical connection between them, and, on first appearance, there is also no apparent functional relationship between the two. And they are even situated in different locations in the torso, the lungs in the upper and the large intestine in the lower part. However, when this book's approach to defining the organ intentions is used, the functions of these two organs then appear to be remarkably similar. They both sort the good from the bad and expel the waste from the body. The lungs separate the oxygen from the air we breathe, absorb the oxygen and expel the CO_2 (the waste) on every out breath; and the large intestine (in contemporary physiology) separates out any remaining liquid and nutrients from digested food, absorbs those and expels the waste during a bowel movement.

Physically, then, there are similarities between the functions of these two organs, and therefore both organs *could* play some of the same roles in our mental activity. There is an observable connection between this aspect of our mental activity (sorting the good from the bad and letting go of the waste) and the physical function of both these organs. I have described the mental role played by the lungs, but the large intestine could also be involved in this same role. When a person tends to hold on to grudges, cannot seem to forgive and move on, or to let go of any failed ambitions or desires, these people often also suffer from chronic constipation—their large intestine is also unable to let go of the waste.

I have also noticed an example of this mental function in myself. I usually do my writing in the mornings and when I am still working on a problem, almost without fail this is marked by the absence of a bowel movement; but as soon as I solve the problem and hence let go of it, within a few seconds a bowel movement usually follows. On letting go of the problem, I feel a "tingling" sensation in my abdomen, as though the energy to my large intestine had been suddenly switched on, and a few seconds later the waste is let go of. It is as though the mental process of holding on to the "waste" prevents this physical function in the large intestine from taking place.

It might be argued that another factor in this example is the liver. The creative thinking involved in problem solving causes the liver function to stagnate, which can be another cause of constipation (p.113). But in the example I have given I am convinced the effect is produced by my mind's holding on to the problem and then suddenly letting go of it, rather than as a by-product of the creative process. It is my mind's *awareness* of the problem, and my determination to solve it, that translates to a physical inability to *let go of the waste*. My conscious mind has overruled this function, *by* my determination to hold on to the problem (which is seen as something undesirable; i.e. as waste), which overruling continues *until* I have solved the problem.

The explanation for this close relationship

There are close functional ties between three of the *yin-yang* paired organs (the pancreas and stomach; the liver and gallbladder; and the kidneys and bladder), where the *yang* organ (*fu*) services the *yin* organ (*zang*) in some way, and the *yang* organ also communicates more directly with the outside of the creature (p.391). These close ties are enough to explain these *yin-yang* pairings. But what is the explanation for the pairing of the lungs with the large intestine?

The end section of the lung meridian is joined to the first section of the large intestine meridian, which suggests that there ought to be a functional relationship between the two organs—as there is with all other such paired organs*. The intentions of the two organs are very similar (almost identical), and since an organ's intention and its function are one and the same (p.93), this appears to confirm that their *functions* are similar. Admittedly, the substances they process are quite different (air and respiratory waste; and food and digestive waste), but it is in the *nature* of that processing where the similarity lies. And this functional similarity is enough to explain the pairing of these two organs.

To support this notion, there is also historical evidence of this similarity. Since life began in the sea, the earliest creatures would not have possessed a lung. In terms of the organ intentions, a fish's gills could be considered the forerunner of the lungs. And gills not only excrete respiratory waste into water, but also diffuse some other types of excretory products—such as salt, electrolytes, ammonia, urea.[34]

This demonstrates that the *letting go of the waste* aspect of the lung function was not always restricted to respiratory waste only, which reinforces the similarity between the intentions of the lungs and large intestine.

Interestingly, fish do not possess a true large intestine, as exists in mammals. Their small intestine connects directly to their rectum, through which digestive waste is excreted.[35] This implies that both the lung and large intestine evolved much later than the other organs—when the creature finally ventured onto dry land. At this stage, the evolution of a large intestine was necessary to enable us to preserve as much of the body fluids as possible, which is one role the large intestine performs: to extract water from the digestive matter before excreting it (p.149). When still living in water, there was no such need. The fact that these two organs were the last to evolve, and they evolved for the same, joint purpose—to enable us to live on land—suggests a further (though circumstantial) explanation for their association.

Improper function

The lungs take in air directly from outside and are therefore particularly vulnerable to attack by harmful factors from outside the body. For this reason Chinese medicine refers to the lungs as the "tender organ". This situation produces the commonest lung condition.

Invasion by airborne pathogens

The *Nei Jing* authors (or their ancestors) noticed that when a person was exposed to airborne pathogens such as *wind* and *cold*, and their body was unable to resist the pathogens, their lung function became impaired and the person could suffer any of the following symptoms:

A. sneezing, cough, build up of mucous, nasal obstruction, watery nasal discharge, possible fever and chills, aching body, an aversion to wind and drafts, and headache.

* Page 208 explains the association of the heart with the small intestine.

And in some instances, the following signs and symptoms could also occur:

B. thirst, yellow mucous, sore throat, sweating, rapid pulse, and a red tongue with a thin yellow coat.

The normal function of the lungs requires a large amount of body fluids and when the lung function is impaired (due to its reaction to the invading pathogen), the lungs' management of these body fluids is disrupted which produces the typical congestion, nasal obstruction and streaming nose.

Extract from *Su Wen*, Chapter 60

Huang Di asked: I have heard, the wind is the origin of the one hundred diseases. To treat it with needles, how to proceed?

Qi Bo responded: When wind enters the body from the outside, it lets a person shake from cold. Sweat leaves the body and the head aches. The body feels heavy and has an aversion to cold. Treat this at [Du-16 (*Fengfu*)].[36]

In contemporary physiology this condition is known as a cold or influenza, which is considered to be a viral infection. In today's Chinese medicine the condition is known as a "wind invasion", together with a description of the signs and symptoms as "cold" or "hot". If the symptoms are largely those from list "A" above, this is known as a "Wind cold invasion", but if they include some signs or symptoms from list "B", the overall condition is termed a "Wind heat invasion".

Extract from *Su Wen*, Chapter 32

When the lung has a heat disease, at first the patient shivers, there is receding [influence] and the finest body hair rises. The patient has an aversion to wind and cold. The upper surface of the tongue is yellow. The body is hot. When the heat is fought [by the lungs[37]], then the patient pants and coughs. Pain moves into the chest, the breast, and the back. The patient cannot take deep breaths. The head aches unbearably. Sweat leaves the body and the patient feels cold.[38]

The above extract describes the signs and symptoms of a "Wind heat invasion" in detail; and every aspect of it would be recognizable to most people today. This suggests that the information was gained from practical observation, rather than through theorizing, and was therefore fact based, which explains why, over two thousand years later, it still seems factual.

In contrast, it is the theoretical content of the *Nei Jing* that is often untrue. In this case, the theory was that when a strong or cold wind strikes us, if the skin and muscles have not been sufficiently "warmed" by the circulating defensive influence (*wei chi*), then the wind is able to penetrate the skin and lodge within us. Inside us, it exists in the form of a vapour, known as "evil influence" (*xie chi*), which is then able to travel the body through the "meridians". It can be expelled or released from us by acupuncture treatment, but if it is not expelled, it could eventually reach the organs, where serious illness could result.

Extract from *Su Wen*, Chapter 38

Skin and body hair are the correlates of the lung. Skin and body hair are the first to receive evil [influence]. This way, the evil [influence] enters the lung from its correlates.[39]

The theoretical aspects of the above are simply untrue (p.44). However, the condition being described, and the account of the signs and symptoms (in the extract from *Su Wen*, Chapter 32, above), are all factual.

Since the condition is factual, does this mean that the Chinese medicine terms of *wind* and *heat* refer to viruses? And what exactly is meant by *wind* or *heat* in this context—how are these terms being used?

These questions are dealt with fully in Chapter 16 (p.307), which also tackles such questions as "Can acupuncture treat a viral or bacterial infection?" But for now I have simply translated the Chinese medicine concept of a "wind invasion" into: "invasion by airborne pathogens", which covers all possibilities—including viruses.

Treatment

When the lung function is impaired in this way the key lung-related acupoints tend to become tender, such as Lung-1 (*Zhongfu*) or Bladder-13 (*Feishu*). When one of these acupoints is stimulated, this encourages the organ to cancel out the malfunction in itself that caused the tenderness (p.372), and the organ returns to normal function.

If the patient has a sore throat, the acupoints Lung-5 (*Chize*) or Lung-10 (*Yuji*) would also tend to be tender and would be needled—for the same reason. And other features of the body's reaction to the condition would cause other acupoints to become tender, such as Bladder-12 (*Fengmen*) and Large-intestine-4 (*Hegu*), which are acupoints commonly used to treat a cold*, as is the one recommended in the extract from Chapter 60 of the *Su Wen*, on page 140 above, which could be added or used as an alternative. In acupuncture, there are often several different acupoints that could each successfully treat the same problem, and their use is often a matter of the practitioner's personal preference.

If the treatment is performed in the early stages of the cold, this can often prevent the cold developing any further and the patient returns to feeling well immediately after the treatment.

Extract from *Su Wen*, Chapter 19

The wind is the chief cause of the one hundred diseases. Now, when wind and cold settle in a person, they let this person's entire finest body hair stand up straight. The skin closes and develops heat. At this time, the wind and the cold can be effused through induced sweating. In some cases block, numbness, swelling, and pain result. At this time, it can be removed through hot water and poultices, as well as through fire cauterization and piercing. If no cure is achieved, the disease enters the lung and lodges there. It is now called "lung block". It develops cough and rising [influences (*chi*)].[40]

I have often found (as they clearly knew, well over two thousand years ago) that in the early stages of a cold, a hot bath, which is hot enough to induce sweating, can prevent the cold developing. At other times, I have found that simply needling the left Large-intestine-4 (*Hegu*) on myself, can have the same effect.

* In Chinese medicine terms, these acupoints are said to expel such pathogens from the body, but this is an oversimplification; see page 308 for a discussion of this topic.

In contemporary physiology, how could such a result be explained? It may be that the acupuncture treatment returns the main organs to their normal function, including the lungs and "kidneys" which are responsible for providing immunity (p.156), and the body is then able to fight off the cold to prevent it developing any further. If this is the explanation, then it seems that relaxing in a hot bath may also sometimes have a similar effect on the organs (but this may depend on how stressed a person's organs are in general).

However, if the cold is not treated until about two or three days after the initial sneezing began, and the main symptoms are now fully developed, the treatment can only usually make the person feel more comfortable and speed up their recovery.

Retention of phlegm in the lungs

This condition tends to occur after suffering repeated attacks of colds or flu without properly recovering from each attack.

A simple cold can affect the body heavily. In a healthy person with a strong constitution, they are able to recover quickly, but many people will ignore a cold and simply continue with their normal stressful lives, not allowing themselves the opportunity to properly recover. When this pattern is repeated for years, all the main organs are likely to be affected. Such a person may develop poor functioning of the pancreas, lungs, kidneys (from constantly drawing on adrenaline to support their stressful lifestyle—p.174), and also stagnated liver function (due to the prolonged stress—p.113). With all the main organs affected, phlegm builds up in the lungs, which are unable to shift it.

In contemporary medicine, this condition would tend to be called either chronic bronchitis or bronchial asthma.[41]

The signs and symptoms could include any combination of the following:

- recurring or persistent cough with lots of white or frothy sputum, or a cough that is loud, barking and painful, with yellow mucus which may be blood stained and strong smelling;
- shortness of breath, rattle in the throat; and
- fullness or stuffiness in the chest, sometimes with loss of appetite, nausea and vomiting, and finding it uncomfortable to lie down.

Treatment

The treatment would focus on returning the affected organs to their normal function, including the lungs, pancreas, kidneys and liver. The key acupoints to do this would have become tender, and needling them encourages the respective organs to resume their normal function.* This then enables the lungs to clear the phlegm, and the digestive organs to function properly, which aids the patient's recovery. However, with any condition that is the result of chronic deficiencies (weaknesses in

---

* These acupoints might include: Lung-9 (*Taiyuan*), Lung-1 (*Zhongfu*), Bladder-13 (*Feishu*), which strengthen lung function; Stomach-40 (*Fenglong*), which clears phlegm; Lung-7 (*Lieque*), Ren-22 (*Tiantu*), Ren-17 (*Shanzhong*), which clear cough; Bladder-20 (*Pishu*), Ren-12 (*Zhongwan*), Stomach-36 (*Zusanli*), which strengthen the digestion; Bladder-23 (*Shenshu*), which improves kidney function; Large-intestine-11 (*Quchi*), Lung-5 (*Chize*), Lung-10 (*Yuji*), which clear the *heat* signs and symptoms.

the function of the main organs), the condition may be slow to respond to treatment, which means that "strengthening" treatments could be required for several weeks, along with advice to the patient on changes in their lifestyle (including avoiding "damp-inducing" foods, as listed on page 81) which would enable them to recover more quickly.

Poor lung function

The *Nei Jing* authors noticed that when a person had poor lung function (also called "Lung chi deficiency"), they could suffer any of the following signs and symptoms:

- shortness of breath which is worse on exertion[14,20,42];
- weak cough with clear, thin sputum[18];
- poor energy and pale complexion,[43] with an even greater energy lag between three and five p.m.;
- lack of desire to talk, having a quiet voice, and tiring quickly when having to talk a lot[44];
- spontaneous daytime sweating[45];
- frequently suffering colds and flu, and generally being easily affected by external pathogens[17];
- tending to feel the cold and having a dislike of being in the wind or cold[18];
- a poor sense of smell[19], blocked nose[20,46] and sinuses; and
- pain or discomfort anywhere along the lung or large intestine meridian.[47]

Face colour and tone of voice

Chapter 10 of the *Su Wen* states "If the complexion is generated by the lung, it resembles red wrapped up in white silk,"[48] meaning that if a person has a pronounced or chronic lung condition, their complexion would tend to be whitish.

Chapter 5 of the *Su Wen* associates the lungs with a "weeping" tone of voice.[49] When a person is prone to poor lung function, their voice can have a "weeping" quality, as though they were constantly sad, or about to cry.

The causes of poor lung function

This condition would tend to be present whenever the lungs are affected by an illness; or it could develop when the constitution is weakened through years of working excessively while failing to maintain an appropriate balance in life.

> **Patient example**
> Male, aged 56. This patient had poor energy due to the poor function of both his pancreas and lungs, which developed after years of driving himself too hard, which also produced poor kidney function. See the full case history on page 246.

The condition may also be present due to constitutional factors. In people who are lung-dominant, the lung function tends to become poor due to mental factors (p.135).

> **Patient example**
> Male, aged 57. This patient was a perfectionist and drove himself hard in the running of his business. Over many years this caused him to develop a wide range of health issues, eventually affecting all his main organs. See the full case history on page 250.

The lungs are also weakened due to grief or prolonged sadness (p.136), in which case poor lung function would be present. Grief is not only felt due to the loss of a loved one, but can also be felt due to the loss of anything the person cherishes, such as their job, career, social status, material possessions or wealth, and so on. When such a loss occurs, it is important that the lungs are treated to enable the person to recover from the loss; that is, to let go of the thing they cherished and move on. When a person has poor lung function, they would find it particularly difficult to go through this normal grieving process and would tend to hold on to the memory of whatever it is they had lost.

> **Patient example**
> Female, aged 65. This patient's lung function was already weak when she suffered a series of losses; first a close friend died, then her career ended, then her son died, which all affected her lung function. See the full case history on page 254.

Another factor that can lead to poor lung function is overuse of your voice. As said on page 132, the lungs support the voice. When the lung function is weakened by illness, this can often result in the voice failing. Conversely, overuse of the voice tends to weaken the lung function.

In my practice I have treated many teachers and almost all of them had health issues related to poor lung function. Teachers not only must use their voice excessively, and often project it over a resistant and vocal class of children, but also the defensive aspect of their lungs is continuously taxed due to the prevalence of colds amongst children, and also the fact that teachers can sometimes feel "under attack" by their students—which has the same effect on us that physical pathogens do and would certainly also tax our immunity. Their lungs would also be taxed due to them having to constantly assess the quality of their students' work (teachers, by definition, are perfectionists), which also tends to weaken the lungs (p.135).

Another symptom that reflects the prevalence of lung issues amongst teachers is the fact that many teachers tend to suffer an energy lag around three p.m. This is the time of day when the lung function is at its weakest (p.379), hence the energy lag felt by people with poor lung function. This energy lag, along with any other signs and symptoms related to poor lung function, tends to clear after a few treatments (which I mention to demonstrate that this energy lag is not merely due to the fact that three p.m. is near the end of most teachers' working day).

> **Patient example**
> Male, aged 24. This patient sought treatment for migraines. He was a newly qualified teacher. He had a poor constitution due to inheriting poor kidney function, and he also had poor lung function, which caused him to experience an afternoon energy lag while at school. See the full case history on page 249.

Helpful lifestyle changes

With people whose poor lung function is not due to them overusing their voice, and are constitutionally quiet and reluctant to speak, one very effective way to improve their lung function is by using their voice more. Singing or playing a wind instrument are particularly effective.

Treating the mental factors

When there is a mental factor to the patient's condition, these usually also respond well. When a person's lung function is poor, the lung's mental functions would also be impeded and the person may find it harder to *take in something intangible from outside, sort the good from the bad and incorporate the precious* (p.133). This may cause them to become obsessed with seeking quality, since their ability to identify it is impeded, which would only drive them to seek it more. And any further failure to find it would weaken their lung function further, which would only fuel their obsession and lock them into a self-destructive cycle.

When a person is trapped in such a pattern of mental activity, it can be extremely difficult to break the pattern. But one of the strengths of acupuncture is that it prompts the physical organs to return to normal function and does this without involving our conscious mind. In effect, acupuncture seems to "get under the radar" of our conscious mind. And once the organ functions are normalized, this tends to also normalize each organ's mental functions; and after a few treatments patients often describe the changes they have spontaneously adopted in their mental behaviour.

Treatment

The following acupoints tend to become tender when the lung function is poor. When one of these acupoints is stimulated, this encourages the organ to cancel out the malfunction in itself that caused the tenderness at the acupoint (p.372), and the organ returns to normal function:

- Lung-1 (*Zhongfu*), Bladder-13 (*Feishu*). These tend to become tender when the lungs are affected by any condition, hence they can be used to treat most lung conditions.
- Bladder-42 (*Pohu*). When the lungs are weakened by mental or emotional factors, such as grief or loss, this acupoint is often tender.

In this way, as with all acupuncture treatments, the problem is corrected by the organ itself (p.78).

Asthma

Asthma is the contemporary term usually used to refer to all instances of breathing difficulties, but in today's Chinese medicine it is recognised that the underlying cause may lie in the function of either the lungs or kidneys. When the patient finds it hard to breathe out, this is usually due to poor lung function and would be treated as above. But when the patient finds it hard to breathe in, this is usually due to poor kidney function.[50] In this case the kidneys would be treated (p.176), and treating the lungs would have no effect on the underlying cause of the condition.

The *Nei Jing* notion that the lungs control the liver

In my own practice, I have frequently noticed that when a patient has stagnated liver function and also poor lung function (Lung chi deficiency),[*] and I needle a lung acupoint, such as Lung-1 (*Zhongfu*), this often frees up the liver function immediately, which is evident in the pulses.

[*] Which is indicated by a deep and weak lung pulse, even though it may not be producing any significant symptoms in the lungs.

This is reminiscent of a relationship predicted by five phase theory. The five phases are each associated with one of the *yin* organs (*zang*), and the phases progress in a cycle. There is said to be a "domination" (or "control") relationship between each phase and the phase two places ahead of it in the cycle (p.263). This means that the phase of Metal (which is associated with lungs) is thought to dominate the phase of Wood (which is liver). But the relationship is also said to work in reverse, so that if the lungs failed to dominate the liver, then the liver would "take revenge" and "insult" the lungs—meaning that an "excess" liver would be capable of suppressing lung function, particularly if the lungs were "deficient". But does this theory apply in practice? In other words, is it true?

In the following extract and commentary, it should be noted that Wood is said to normally dominate Earth (or soil), while Metal normally dominates Wood.

Extract from *Su Wen*, Chapter 67

When the [influence] has a surplus, then it restrains that which it normally dominates and insults that which it normally does not dominate. When it is inadequate, then that which it normally cannot dominate insults and harasses it and it is treated lightly and insulted by that which it normally dominates. That which has insulted is affected by [harmful influences] in turn.[51]

Wang Bing (in 762 AD) commented on the above

When the wood [influence] has surplus, it restrains the soil [influence] and thinks lightly of the metal [influence]. Since the metal does not take up a fight, the wood relies on its surplus and insults the metal. Also, when the wood [influence] is diminished and when the metal [influence] dominates, the soil [influence] contrary to its normal relationship insults the wood because the wood [influence] is insufficient to dominate the soil. Hence the soil turns reckless and insults the wood.[52]

Does the clinical situation mentioned above (where treating the lungs appears to benefit the liver), fit this scenario? There was stagnated liver function (an excess, or "surplus of influence") and poor lung function (a deficiency of influence), and correcting the lung function, immediately corrected the liver function.

The theory is that the stagnated liver function (being an "excess condition") was not being controlled by the lungs (the Metal did not "take up a fight", as Wang Bing put it), therefore the liver reversed its normal relationship of being "dominated" by the lungs, and instead insulted the lungs, producing (or worsening) the poor lung function.

This theory could be taken to imply that the poor lung function was partly (or even primarily) responsible for establishing the stagnated liver function, or perhaps for worsening it. However, many patients who have stagnated liver function, do not also have poor lung function. In fact, a person whose liver is habitually stagnated (due to their personality makeup), would usually have a loud voice (p.111), which implies strong lung function. It could be argued that in such people, their lung function is strong *because* it is attempting to control their stagnated liver function, which would then fit five phase theory.

However, the fact that treating the lungs often immediately corrects stagnated liver function, does seem, on first sight, to support the theory. But there is a reasonable explanation for this relationship, which is described below.

In developed countries today, it is common for people to have stagnated liver function, poor pancreas function,[*] and also, though less commonly, poor lung function.

This is the natural order of things—when living under today's stresses (stress stagnates the liver function; overthinking weakens the pancreas function, which in turn would tend to weaken the lung function—due to the "six channel" association). And there is no reason to imagine that Chinese society of two thousand years ago was any different. In fact, the *Nei Jing* depicts it as being remarkably similar in this respect (p.227).

Therefore, this common pattern of organ malfunction lends itself to five phase theory—and may even have been instrumental in forming the notion of these control relationships in the theory. But when these same control relationships do not then exist between all the other organs around the five phase cycle, the theory cannot be said to be true. If this is the case, then it is simply a coincidence that the theory fits the pattern of liver "excess" and pancreas and lung "deficiency".

The control relationship between the liver and pancreas is analysed on page 103, where there is an equally common scenario that occurs in clinic, which is usually described as "Liver invading pancreas"[†]. As with the clinical observation of the relationship between the lungs and liver, there is no doubt that a similar relationship exists between the liver and pancreas. But this five phase domination cycle theory only appears to exist in the liver (and then only in certain circumstances), and seems not to exist between the other organs, therefore it cannot be regarded as a valid rule.

For example, the theory caters for the situation of the liver having insufficient influences, so that the pancreas could then insult the liver and somehow further diminish its function. But the notion of the liver being dominated by the pancreas is difficult to imagine, and certainly not one I have seen in clinic, along with the supposed control relationships between the other organs.

Pages 263-277 analyse the overall five phase theory and demonstrates that many of its correspondences and relationships are arbitrary, and simply do not apply in reality.

If the above clinical situation (where treating the lungs immediately corrects stagnated liver function), is not the result of the five phase control theory, what is the explanation?

Since the relationship clearly exists, it ought to be possible to account for it using contemporary physiology, and the following provides a simple, possible explanation.

When the lung function is weak, this would tend to limit the lungs' ability to extract oxygen from the air we breathe. The liver is energy hungry. It is said that *each* liver cell contains between 1,000 to 2,000 mitochondria, which are the energy factories of the body's cells (p.336 and 386). A mitochondrion produces energy via a chemical reaction, which is fuelled by the burning (or *oxidizing*) of glucose in the presence of oxygen. The glucose and oxygen are transported via the blood into each mitochondrion, to fuel the production of energy. Clearly, when

[*] Also called "Spleen chi deficiency".

[†] Also called "Liver invading spleen".

there is a reduction in the availability of oxygen (due to poor lung function), the mitochondria would be less able to produce energy, which means the liver may not have sufficient energy to drive its functions; hence the liver functions would tend to stagnate. But once the lung function is normalized, this would immediately increase the supply of oxygen, which would then restore the energy production in the liver cells and thus enable the liver to perform its functions more smoothly.

Clearly there is a "control" relationship of some sort between the lungs and liver, as there is between the lungs and every other organ. But this does not prove the five phase control theory. Far from it. In the theory, the lungs are said to control the liver, but, by definition, to not have the same control relationship with the other organs. Yet in reality, if they can be said to control the liver by ensuring a supply of oxygen, they must also be said to control every other organ in this same way. And this would then contradict the five phase control theory.

However (interesting though the above explanation may be), it is not able to account for the control relationship noticed in clinic. Oxygenated blood from the lungs passes back to the heart and is then pumped outwards via the *aorta artery*; this descends, and at the abdominal part of the aorta, the *coeliac artery* branches off, then divides into the *hepatic artery* which supplies the liver (amongst other organs).[53] On average, blood circulates at around twelve centimetres per second (p.404). This means that freshly oxygenated blood from the lungs would take about five or six seconds to reach the liver. But in clinic, when I have monitored the effect of Lung-1 (*Zhongfu*) on remedying stagnated liver function, the effect seems to happen more quickly than this. But also, the blood-oxygen level does not vary much anyway; and in the patients where I noted this lung-controlling-liver effect, I do not believe there would have been any significant change in their blood-oxygen level during the treatment—since they experienced no energy or breathing problems beforehand. So, something else must explain the effect.

Other possible explanations

Similar relationships exist between organs that share a "six channel" meridian (p.397). For example, in clinic it is common to experience a "pericardium controls liver" effect, where a pericardium acupoint may clear stagnated liver function, due to both organs sharing the *jueyin* meridian (p.398). I have also routinely experienced a "heart controls kidneys" effect, where Heart-7 (*Shenmen*) can greatly increase kidney *yin*, since both organs share the *shaoyin* meridian. And the same relationship can often be seen symptomatically between the lungs and pancreas (p.137), which share the *taiyin* meridian.

Note that in these "six channel" examples, "control" simply means that when the function of one of the organs is corrected, this tends to also correct the function of the other organ, rather than there being any *active* "control" between the organs. And this may also be the case in any other context, such that the concept of "control" may be a misnomer.

These "control" effects are reliable and are clearly fact-based, yet they contradict five phase theory. According to that theory (p.263), heart should control lungs, *not* kidneys. It is the pancreas that should control the kidneys, though I have never seen evidence of this relationship in clinic. As for the pericardium controlling the liver, five phase theory does not even cater for the pericardium, since it only has room for five organs, so one needed to be left out—which is another problem with five phase theory overall (p.272). And as for any "control" relationship between the lungs and pancreas, five phase theory rules this out, yet the relationship clearly exists in reality.

The above relationships can be accounted for due to the "six channel" association (and all appear to contradict, and therefore disprove, the five phase control theory). And due to the speed of the "control" effect of the lungs on the liver, it is assumed that this may also be explained by a meridian relationship. It is said that an internal branch of the liver meridian connects with the lungs,[54] which may provide a possible explanation, but this is less clear cut than with the "six channel" organ relationships.

It is clear that there are such "control" relationships between the organs, but they are most easily accounted for by meridian paths, and most of the relationships contradict five phase theory.

As said above, it is possible that the *Nei Jing* authors noticed this apparent control relationship between the lungs and liver, and between the liver and pancreas, and that this inspired the creation of the five phase control theory, which was then arbitrarily applied to every other organ around the five phase cycle, even though in practice there are no such relationships between the other organs. In other words, that the theory is simply untrue and there are other explanations for the apparent relationships that *do* exist.

See also page 267, which describes critical comments made by ancient Chinese physicians on the misapplication of five phase "control" theory. They describe the practice as "empty talk" and compare it to demonology or astrology, rather than to real medicine.

Large intestine conditions

Functions of the large intestine

In contemporary physiology, the large intestine receives the processed food and liquid from the small intestine, moves this downward while absorbing water from it, then expels the remainder (the waste) from the body.[55]

In Chinese medicine terms, the *Nei Jing* notions of the large intestine functions are suggested by the following extracts.

Extract from *Su Wen*, Chapter 8, with commentary by Wang Bing (writing in 762 AD)

The small intestine is the official functioning as recipient of what has been perfected. The transformation of things originates in it. [WB: i.e. "The small intestine takes orders from the stomach to receive and hold the waste. Once it has received the waste, it transforms them anew and transmits them into the large intestine."] ... The large intestine is the official functioning as transmitter along the Way [WB: i.e. transmitting the "unclean" along its path]. Changes and transformations originate in it [WB: i.e. "change and transformation of the physical appearance of things"].[56]

This passage suggests the notion that the "unclean" part of the processed food is passed on from the small intestine, and the large intestine transforms it further. And the following extracts describe observed symptoms related to large intestine function, and theories as to their cause.

> **Extract from *Ling Shu*, Chapter 35**
> In the case of a large intestine swelling, the intestines have noises and they ache. There is a gurgling sound. When the patient was struck by severe cold in winter, he discharges undigested food.[57]

> **Extract from *Su Wen*, Chapter 23**
> When the [influence] in the five [*yin* organs (*zang*)] have a disease: .... In the large intestine and in the small intestine it causes outflow.[58]

> **Commenting on the above passage, Wang Bing (in 762 AD) theorized**
> The large intestine is the [*yang* organ (*fu*)] representing a transmission route; the small intestine is the [*yang* organ] of accepting riches. When the abundant [influence] received by the small intestine is depleted and when the marshal of the transmission routes is not restrained, then this results in outflow.[59]

Hence, the *Nei Jing* authors considered the normal function of the large intestine to involve "transmitting the unclean along its path". In other words, excreting the unusable part from digested food. There was no notion of the large intestine absorbing liquid from the stool and recycling this, as in contemporary physiology. However, in some of today's Chinese medicine textbooks, this new function is added, perhaps in an attempt to "update" or "correct" the *Nei Jing* to try to reconcile it with contemporary physiology. But this added function is incompatible with the other *Nei Jing* notions of metabolism, so that such corruptions (even though well meant) would only seem to make it even harder for students to appreciate the *Nei Jing*.[60]

Improper function

Just as in ancient times, the most common problems related to the large intestine are either constipation or diarrhoea. These may occur for a number of reasons, most of which are due to problems in the function of other organs. For example, poor pancreas function often causes loose stools and sometimes diarrhoea (see pages 65-67, which discuss the treatment of IBS); stagnated liver function can cause constipation (p.113); and general signs of *heat* in the body (p.307) would also tend to dry the body fluids and lead to constipation. In all these situations, the organs involved would be treated (the pancreas, or any other organ affected), which then tends to solve the problem. But at the same time, acupoints related directly to the large intestine are also often needled, such as any of the following:

- Bladder-25 (*Dachangshu*) and Stomach-25 (*Tianshu*). Both these acupoints treat the large intestine directly by normalizing the function of the organ and they can thus be used for any condition affecting the large intestine.
- Pancreas-15* (*Daheng*). This acupoint also regulates the large intestine and

* Also called Spleen-15.

can treat either constipation or diarrhoea.

Problems due to mental factors

As with all the abdominal organs, the large intestine has mental functions. There is a close link between the large intestine and lungs (p.137). In contemporary physiology, the two share the same function, which is to *sort the good from the bad, incorporate the good and let go of the waste,* so the large intestine is often *also* affected, as well as the lungs, when this mental function is impeded (p.136). Hence, when a person cannot mentally *sort the good from the bad* and *let go of the waste,* this failure of function is duplicated in the large intestine and the person becomes constipated.

As ever with acupuncture, by treating the organ, this would often enable the person to unconsciously make the necessary changes in their mental patterns, and once they were able to mentally *sort the good from the bad and let go of the waste,* their large intestine function would also tend to return to normal.

Damage due to improper food intake

It was noticed that when a person ate excessive amounts of raw and cold foods, or "unclean" foods (dirty water or rotten foods), this could produce any combination of the following signs and symptoms:

- abdominal pain;
- stools that have a foul smell with blood or mucus, *or* diarrhoea with yellow, watery stools (the diarrhoea starts suddenly and urgently, and the desire may continue afterwards, even though the bowels are empty);
- burning sensation in the anus; and
- there may also be thirst, fever, dark urine, and a rapid pulse and red tongue with a yellow coating.

In Chinese medicine terms, the condition is known as "Damp heat invading the large intestine" (see pages 76 and 181 for an explanation of the terms *dampness, heat,* and *damp heat).* In today's Chinese medicine, it is theorized that the "unclean" food injures the stomach, pancreas and intestines, and these effects produce the signs and symptoms listed above. In particular, when *damp heat* is present, this is theorized to injure the blood vessels of the intestines, which produces the blood and mucus in the stools, and that it is the retained *dampness* in the large intestine that impairs its function, producing the diarrhoea with yellow, watery stools and the burning sensation in the anus (all of which are indicators of the *heat* produced by the *dampness*).[61]

In contemporary medicine, this same condition would probably be called bacillary dysentery.[62]

Treatment

The acupoints mentioned above—Bladder-25 (*Dachangshu*), Stomach-25 (*Tianshu*) and Pancreas-15 (*Daheng*)—may be used to treat any condition affecting the large intestine, including this one, but in particular, the following acupoint would usually also be added:

- Stomach-37 (*Shangjuxu*). This acupoint has been found to treat a wide range of conditions affecting the large intestine, and in particular to alleviate diarrhoea and dysenteric disorder.[63]

Chapter 8. Kidneys and bladder

Attribution of Chinese medicine organs

To work out the functions and effects of an organ, the *Nei Jing* authors used practical observation of the signs and symptoms present when that organ was diseased. This indicated that the "kidneys" had the functions and effects listed on page 156 below. But when considering the functions of the adrenal glands and gonads (in contemporary physiology), it is clear they are amongst the functions attributed to the "kidneys" by the *Nei Jing* authors. What might explain this?

Each organ has its own separate meridian, and there are only twelve main meridians, one for each of the organs listed in Table 6 on page 348. There are no meridians for the adrenal glands or gonads. But when considering the function of the "kidneys", this equates to the primordial "intention" of the "kidneys" (p.93), therefore it seems that all three of these structures serve this same primordial intention. This suggests that at an early stage of evolution, there may have been just a *single* organ responsible for all the kidney-related functions and effects mentioned above, but that later on, perhaps as the separate functions became more specialized, the organ may have split into these three separate structures—the kidneys, adrenal glands and gonads. Of course, such an explanation could only be speculation. However, the scenario also makes sense anatomically, since these other two structures are located very close to the kidneys. The adrenal glands are attached to the top of each kidney, and the gonads are nearby (in a male embryo, the testes are initially in the same location as the ovaries, and only later descend into the scrotum).[1]

For all these reasons, when we treat the kidneys in Chinese medicine, we are normalizing the function of the kidneys, adrenal glands and gonads collectively (including the hormonal activity of each), and when we diagnose a problem with the "kidneys", it may involve signs and symptoms produced by any (or all) of these three structures.

Functions of the three kidney-related structures

The kidneys

In contemporary physiology, the kidneys

- Filter out various toxins from the blood, and also some of the waste products of the normal chemical activity in the body (such as urea).[2]

- Regulate the amount of water that circulates in the blood plasma by either recycling water back into the plasma to increase the level, or excreting any excess in the urine.[3,4]
- Recycle other vital nutrients in the body, such as glucose and amino acids (the kidneys reabsorb these so they can be reused).[5,6]
- Martial the body's resources in times of stress. The kidneys secrete the hormone *angiotensin*, which constricts the blood vessels, resulting in an increase in blood pressure, which is one of the body's measures to enable us to deal more effectively with the stressful situation[7] (and other measures are produced by the adrenal glands, as described below).
- Regulate the amount of red blood cells. When this falls too low, the kidneys secrete the hormone *erythropoietin* which instructs the bone marrow to produce more red blood cells.[8]
- Regulate the acid level (pH) in the body. Many chemical processes take place in the body and for these to function normally, pH must be maintained at a certain level. The kidneys work closely with the lungs to maintain this—the kidneys by regulating the bicarbonate and hydrogen levels, and the lungs by regulating the carbon dioxide concentration in the blood.[9]

The adrenal glands

The adrenal glands are also known as the *suprarenal glands*, since they are located at the top of each kidney, which also means that each person has two adrenal glands. Each gland is divided into two parts, the outer portion, known as the *adrenal cortex* (from where the name "adrenal gland" comes), and the inner portion, known as the *inner medulla*.

The adrenal cortex secretes various hormones which have a wide range of functions, largely concerned with regulating the bodily resources. One such hormone is *aldosterone*, which helps to keep salt and water balanced in the body. And another is *cortisol* (also known as *hydrocortisone*). This is one of the key hormones in the body, and it has the following functions.

In the non-stressed state

Under normal conditions (that is, when we are not stressed), cortisol is secreted throughout the day, but the amount varies according to the time of day. The level peaks at around eight a.m. and is at its lowest at around midnight (which roughly coincides with the peak activity of the digestive organs—p.379). Under these "normal" conditions, cortisol

- Regulates the body's energy usage and mobilizes its energy stores. It does this by selecting, at any one instant, whether carbohydrate, fat, or protein should be used as the energy source to meet the particular demands on the body.[10]
- Regulates the blood glucose level, by counteracting insulin.[11,12]
- Plays a significant role in enabling the conversion of glycogen to glucose in

the liver, kidneys,[13] and muscle tissue, which releases stored glucose to be used as energy; and also mobilizes the energy stored in the body's fat reserves for use elsewhere, such as in the active muscles.[10]

- Is necessary for the development and maintenance of normal immunity.[14]
- Enables the brain to create short term memories; cortisol works with adrenaline to do this.[15]

In the stressed state

The inner medulla secretes hormones in response to stress; one of these is *epinephrine*, which is also known as adrenaline, and one of the actions of adrenaline is to increase the secretion of cortisol. Therefore, when we experience stress (that is, when the body has recognised an important situation that must be urgently dealt with), cortisol secretion increases, which then marshals the bodily resources to deal with the situation. This includes

- Suppressing the bodily functions that deal with our long-term survival, such as the immune system (the production of B-cell antibodies is reduced) and bone formation. It also slows down the healing of wounds, and shuts down the reproductive system, so that more of our energy resources can be focused on solving the urgent situation.
- Actively increasing the immediate supply of energy. It does this by increasing the conversion of proteins into energy via the process of *gluconeogenesis* in the liver.
- Raising blood pressure levels by increasing the sensitivity of the blood vessels to adrenaline, causing them to contract[16].

The gonads

The gonads are the testes (in men) and the ovaries (in women). Between them they secrete hormones that control the body's development at each stage of life—as we pass from childhood into puberty and on into adulthood and old age:

- *Testosterone* stimulates the male reproductive system to grow to full size and become functional; stimulates the formation of sperm; determines the male sexual behaviour[17]; stimulates the development of characteristics such as the growth of a beard, deepening of the voice, enlargement of the genitalia, broadening of shoulders, enlarged and stronger bones and muscles[18]; and even changes the development of the brain to produce some of the recognised differences in the mental characteristics of males and females.[19,20]
- *Oestrogen* stimulates the female reproductive tract to grow to full size and become functional; stimulates the production of ova; and stimulates the characteristics such as enlargement of the breasts, broadening of the pelvis, depositing of fat in the thighs, and the onset of the menstrual cycle.[18]
- *Progesterone* suspends ovulation during pregnancy; causes the foetus to fix to the uterine wall; forms the placenta and controls the development of the foetus in the uterus.[21]

- *Relaxin* relaxes the cervix of the uterus and ligaments of the pelvic girdle to prepare for birth.[22]

The Chinese medicine functions and effects

As said above, when the term "kidneys" is used in Chinese medicine, this refers to three structures collectively—the kidneys, adrenal glands and gonads.

In Chinese medicine the "kidneys" are seen as an extremely important organ which has a wide range of vital functions and a profound influence on our long-term health.

The functions and effects* are as follows; the "kidney"

1. plays a key role in providing the constitution;
2. regulates and enables the functioning of the other organs;
3. guides the growth and sexual development of the body;
4. enables the development of bones, bone marrow, the formation of blood, and supports the brain's health;
5. coordinates the circulation of body fluids;
6. assists the lungs to breathe in;
7. has a close association with the ears, sense of hearing and balance; and
8. has mental and emotional functions.

* See page 64 for an explanation of the term "effects" in this context.

1. Plays a key role in providing the constitution

This is a direct function rather than an effect, though caveats need to be applied, as described throughout this section. The function is produced by the combination of the kidneys and adrenal glands.

The *Nei Jing* authors (or their ancestors) noticed that we were each born with a particular constitution.

Chapter 47 of the *Ling Shu* states that we all have the same organs and substances, which we were "supplied with by heaven" (i.e. were born with), but some people may live a long life while being exposed to many pathogens and never becoming seriously ill, while "there are those who never leave the protection of their home, and who never are depressed by fear, and yet they cannot escape disease."[23]

The author went on to theorize that a person's constitution was accounted for by the physical qualities of the organs they were born with. He suggested that the *yin* organs (*zang*) may vary in their location, size, whether hard or brittle, whether they "stand upright" or are "inclined". And the *yang* organs (*fu*) may vary in size, length, thickness, whether "curved" or "straight", relaxed or tense. He stated that it is these qualities that determine the good or bad function of each organ; and that by examining a person's complexion, external body shape and the quality of their skin, it is possible to determine the particular shape of their organs.

The theory (which was formulated at a time when knowledge of the anatomy of the organs was scarce—p.16), is clearly untrue. The organs do not exhibit the variety of shape, position and texture described here, and their good or bad function is determined by other factors. However, the author's fact-based observations were that each person was born with a particular constitution, and the author also listed variations in each organ's function, including the mental and emotional aspects, which appeared to be due to that person's particular constitution.[23]

Chapter 50 of the *Ling Shu* stated that people may look the same from the outside, but when exposed to a violent wind and to heavy rain, some fall ill while others do not; and that these different responses depend on the above mentioned constitutional differences in the physical characteristics of the organs they were born with; and which could be detected in a person by examining their complexion and the thickness of their skin and flesh. Also, it was believed that a person's courage depended on these same constitutional aspects. It was said that in those who were courageous, their skin structures were horizontal, their heart stood upright, their liver was big and firm, and their gallbladder was full.[24]

Chapter 54 of the *Ling Shu* describes the beginning of a human person. It states "Longevity and early death are unequally distributed among humans. Some die early, others have a long life," and that this depended, in effect, on well-functioning organs being passed on from our parents. It stated that "The [influences] of one's mother constitute the basis. Those of the father serve as shield." This was in the context of a new human life forming in the womb, and the chapter stated "...when the five [*yin* organs (*zang*)] have assumed their complete form and function ... then a person is completed too."

But there appeared to be no notion of an inherited "substance" of any sort that determined the makeup of the organs (as there is understood to be today). It was only stated that this happened in the mother's womb. There was also no suggestion that the organ makeup was a copy of any similar state in our parents' organs. There was simply no mention of a specific mechanism of inheritance (which notion, it must be assumed, had not occurred to the authors).[25]

At the time of the *Nei Jing*, the term *ming men* 命門("gate of life") was used to refer to the eyes,[26] but in the later *Nan Jing*, a new meaning was ascribed to the term.

Extract from *Nan Jing*, Section 36

The two kidneys are not both kidneys. The one on the left is the kidney; the one on the right is the gate of life. The gate of life is the place where the spirit-essence [*shen jing*] lodges; it is the place to which the original influences [*yuan chi*] are tied. Hence, in males it stores the essence [*jing*]; in females it holds the womb.[27]

Hence, by now the notion was introduced that the kidneys stored the constitutional factors passed on to us from our parents. In the context of the phrase "in males it stores the essence", the term "essence" was being used to mean "seminal essence".

These ideas were argued over by commentators for more than a millennium, with various theories being offered.[28]

Then, in 1269, Li Chiung theorized: "The essential influences flow from the five [*yin* organs (*zang*)] and six [*yang* organs (*fu*)] and leak into the kidneys. The [*yin* organ] of the kidneys receives and stores them. Each of the five [*yin* organs] contains essence [*jing*].

Whenever necessary, the [*yin* organs] pour it into the kidneys. The kidneys are the location from which the city gates are controlled. The essence [*jing*] of the body is stored here."[29]

Some four centuries later, Li Chung-tse (died 1655) produced a new theory which combined ideas from previous commentators. He theorized that the kidneys, pancreas* and stomach were the most important organs in the body. The kidneys were seen as the "root of early days". He theorized that the kidneys existed before a foetus assumed any form, so that the kidneys were the root of all the organs. But if the foetus, or later, the body, received no nourishment, it would die. And as soon as the body assumed its physical form, it required the influences contained in food. Food entered the stomach and was then freshly stored in the six *yang* organs (*fu*). The foods then released their influences, which were blended in the five *yin* organs (*zang*), to form blood. And for the entire course of our life, we depend on these influences; hence the pancreas and stomach were considered the "root of later days."[30]

In today's Chinese medicine, these notions are summarized as follows.

> Essence (*jing*) is the material base of the human body and of many of its functional activities. Kidney essence (kidney *jing*) consists of two parts: congenital and acquired. Congenital essence is inherited from the parents, and acquired essence is transformed from the essential substances of food by the [pancreas] and stomach.[31]

As with many theories in Chinese medicine, from the *Nei Jing* onwards, none of the above theories are literally true. For example, the substance *jing* was considered to be akin to influence (*chi*). Therefore it would have been imagined to be something akin to a vapour containing some "flavour" of the person or organ that it originated from; and this vapour (like all influence) was imagined to circulate in the "meridians", along with the blood. Today, it is known that no such substances circulate in the "meridians" (since the *Nei Jing* considered these to be imaginary artery-like tubes, which do not exist; nor even circulate in the *pathways on the skin*, which is what we today call the meridians; see page 29), nor even exist in the body—if the Chinese medicine texts are to be interpreted literally.

But again, as with most Chinese medicine theories, there were usually fact-based observations that came first—then the theories were developed to attempt to explain them. From the content of *Ling Shu* Chapters 47 and 50 (summarized on page 156 above), it is clear that the authors observed the concept of a person's constitution—that different people were born with a different degree of stamina and resistance to illness. This was true, but their theory to explain this was untrue (i.e. that it was determined by differences in the size, shape, position and texture of the person's organs).

From the content of Section 36 of the *Nan Jing* (p.157), it is clear that its author had observed that the kidneys play a key part in determining a person's constitution. In other words, when a person was born with poor kidney function, they had a weak constitution. This observation was true (as is repeatedly confirmed in clinic today); however their theory to explain it could only be considered

* Also called the spleen in Chinese medicine.

untrue, since it relies on the existence of *jing* and its transport through the "meridians".

Likewise, the theories of Li Chiung, Li Chung-tse, and today's Chinese medicine rendition of these, are also not literally true, though the observations they attempt to explain are fact based.

It is true that the constitution is passed on to us from our parents, and that our general health, stamina and resistance to illness rely on this, but also on the food we eat and our ability to digest it. And it is true that the strength of the "kidney" function is central to our constitution, in that when this is weak, or if we were born with poor kidney function, we tend to suffer colds or flu more frequently than other people and may also suffer from allergies to pollen, animal fur, dust, and so on.

Though the Chinese medicine explanations are not literally true, they are a close analogy to the underlying mechanisms in contemporary physiology.

Chinese medicine had, and has, no concept of "immunity", as we think of it today (pp.44-47). However, their notion of a person's "constitution" includes some concepts that, in contemporary physiology, would be attributed to the immune system—such as our resistance to illness.[32] And it is recognised today that the adrenal glands (one of the kidney-related structures) play an essential role in the development and maintenance of normal immunity.

It is also recognised that very many states in the body, including the functioning of the main organs, may be inherited from our parents, and that the information that determines this is passed on via the gonads, which are another of the kidney-related structures.

Patient example
Male, aged 45. I treated this patient for hay fever which was present from childhood, since he inherited poor kidney function. And after a course of treatments he was completely clear of symptoms, despite it being mid hay-fever season. See the full case history on page 255.

2. Regulates and enables the functioning of the other organs

This is a direct function rather than an effect—the function being produced by the kidneys and adrenal glands in combination.

In today's Chinese medicine, it is said that the kidneys

1. are the foundation and source of the *yin* and *yang* of the entire body, and that
2. "kidney *yang*" warms the organs and tissues and thus promotes their functioning.[33]

What is meant by these statements? Though some parts of these theories may not be literally true (particularly item "2"), the practical observations that inspired them were fact based, therefore any such statement in Chinese medicine ought to be explainable using contemporary physiology, or at least be analogous to such an explanation.

The *yin-yang* rule is simply a universal balancing law that applies to all things in nature (p.345). The statement that the kidneys are the foundation of the *yin* and *yang* of the body could thus be interpreted to mean that the kidneys play a key role in balancing (or regulating) every aspect of the body.

In contemporary physiology it is recognised that the kidneys regulate the amount of body fluids and blood in circulation, and the pH level; and the adrenal glands regulate the body's energy supply, both in normal and stressed states. Hence the "kidneys" are seen as playing a key role in regulating and balancing both the blood and body fluids (the *yin*) and the energy (the *yang*) aspects of the body, which corresponds with the Chinese medicine description—only the terminology is different.

It is also stated that the kidneys are the *source* of the *yin* and *yang* in the body. This could be interpreted to mean the kidneys play a key role in the supply and circulation of the body fluids and the production of the blood (the *yin*), which is covered in function "4" below; and also the generation of our energy (the *yang*), which is covered by the interpretation of the second statement:

> "Kidney *yang*" warms the organs and tissues and thus promotes their functioning.

"Kidney *yang*", as used in the above quote, is understood to be derived from kidney essence. In other words, kidney essence, like all phenomena, has a *yin* and *yang* part; and when its *yang* part is considered separately, this would equate to the theoretical substance known as "kidney *yang*". As described on page 177, the term kidney essence could be considered analogous to the hormonal activity of the three kidney-related structures—the kidneys, adrenal glands and gonads. Hence "kidney *yang*", or any other substance derived from kidney essence, could also be considered analogous to this same hormonal activity, but to represent, perhaps, a particular effect achieved by the hormones. For example, some hormones may help produce the blood, while others may "energize" the organs, or enable the immune system to function. Therefore the above statement could be interpreted as stating that it is, in fact, this *hormonal activity* that "warms" the organs and tissues and enables the functioning of the organs.

But what is meant by "warmed"? This statement is generally interpreted by today's acupuncturists to mean that this element of the kidneys acts as a "spark" that "ignites the fire" under the organs—much like a pilot light in a gas boiler. But to interpret the statement using concepts from contemporary physiology, it could be understood as meaning the "kidneys" are the initial source (the starting point) of all the energy in the body, since the adrenal hormones (and cortisol in particular) regulate and enable the activity of the digestive organs in converting the food we eat into fuel (mainly glucose) which all the cells in the body can then use to release energy, and it is this energy that enables the organs and bodily tissue to function—and in the process, to become warm (p.154). Looked at another way, this description using contemporary physiology is also confirming that the kidneys are responsible for *warming* the organs and bodily tissue (in enabling the energy supply) and in doing this, also *promoting* the activity of every structure in the body.

Hence, again, though the Chinese medicine description is not literally true, it is possible to regard it as being metaphorical, in which case it corresponds with the fact-based descriptions in contemporary physiology. However, it should be noted that the original authors would not have intended their statement to be metaphor and instead would have believed it to be literally true. But today, the generosity of regarding it to be metaphor is necessary to be able to accept it as valid.

3. Guides the growth and sexual development of the body

This is a function rather than an effect, the function being produced by the gonads and adrenal glands in combination.

The stages of growth and sexual development were described in Chapter 1 of the *Su Wen*.

> **Extract from *Su Wen*, Chapter 1**
>
> In a female, at the age of seven, the [influence] of the kidneys abounds. The first teeth are substituted and the hair grows long. With two times seven, the heaven *gui* arrives, the controlling vessel is passable and the great thoroughfare vessel abounds with [influence]. The monthly affair moves down in due time and, hence, a woman may have children. With three times seven, the [influence] of the kidneys has reached its normal level. Hence, the wisdom teeth emerge and females grow to their full size. ... With seven times seven, the controlling vessel is depleted and the great thoroughfare vessel is weak and its contents are diminished. The heaven *gui* is exhausted. The way of the earth is impassable. Hence, the physical appearance is spoilt and a woman can no longer have children.[34]

The same progression is then described for males. The theory depicted is that the influence of the kidneys plays a key role in this process—since it is described as increasing in level until the age of twenty-one (in women). But the "heaven *gui*" is also described as guiding the sexual development through its entire cycle, which terminates at the age of forty-nine (in women). But what does "heaven *gui*" refer to? In the commentaries to Chapter 1 of the *Su Wen*, this was debated for two millennia. It was variously interpreted as menstrual blood (or, in males, semen), as "*yin* essence", or "essence influence".[35] However, the significant detail, from this book's point of view, is that sexual development was thought to be guided by the kidneys.[36]

In clinic today, patients with poor kidney function will often display such symptoms as infertility, lack of sex drive, or premature ejaculation in men (along with other kidney-related signs and symptoms), all of which symptoms usually improve when the kidneys are treated.

The above *Su Wen* extract also features another observation made by the *Nei Jing* authors, which was that the stages of development occur in seven and eight year phases (seven for women and eight for men), so that key stages of development tend to occur at the end of each phase. For example, puberty would normally occur in women at the age of fourteen, and in men at the age of sixteen. And in clinic when I take a case history of a new patient, if they describe decisive moments in their life (such as when they completely changed career, or when other such life-changing events happened to them) these often occurred at the end of one of these phases. In men, this would typically be at the ages of twenty-four, thirty-two, forty, forty-eight or fifty-six, or very close to these ages; and in women, the corresponding ages would be twenty-one, twenty-eight, thirty-five, forty-two or forty-nine. Another function of the kidneys (described below, on page 168) is to provide our drive and ambition, and identify and pursue our goals for the future; and it may be that we are most likely to heed this inner voice of the kidneys (or that this inner voice is most strong) around the anniversaries of these seven and eight year phases, which would account for us tending to make big changes in our lives at these points.

In contemporary physiology, the stages of sexual development and the growth of the body are under the control of the sex hormones secreted by the gonads and adrenal glands, which coincides with these *Nei Jing* descriptions, since these structures are part of the "kidneys".

4. Enables the development of bones, bone marrow, the formation of blood, and supports the brain's health

This is a combination of functions and effects, as described below.

It was noticed that patients with poor kidney function sometimes had

- aching in the lumbar region[37];
- weak knees and joints[37];
- poorly developed bones, such as in spinal defects[37];
- poorly developed teeth, or teeth that were too loose[38]; and
- poor short term memory, poor concentration, dizziness,[39] a feeling of emptiness in the head,[40] and dull headache which affects the whole head.[41]

Poor kidney function is common in old age, when people often suffer a selection of the above signs and symptoms; but it can also occur earlier in life. This tends to happen in people who drive themselves too hard for many years, allowing themselves no opportunity for daily or weekly rest—people who run on adrenaline, which then exhausts that aspect of the kidneys (the emergency reserves), so that the kidneys *overall* become exhausted.[42] This can also happen in people who have sex too often, particularly when their kidney function is already poor (as a person ages, if they are sensitive to their body's needs, their desire for sex would decline).

Extract from *Ling Shu*, Chapter 4

When one uses all his strength to lift something heavy, or when he enters the women's chamber excessively [i.e. has sex too often], or when he sweats and takes a bath in water, this will harm the kidneys.[43]

And some people are born with poor kidney function which they inherited from their parents. In all these cases, such people would tend to suffer a selection of the above signs and symptoms (the typical signs of old age) throughout their life.

When considering the connection between poor kidney function and the above signs and symptoms, the *Nei Jing* authors theorized that

A. the kidneys were responsible for generating the bones and marrow[44]—so that poor kidney function would be unable to generate strong bones; and that
B. the marrow filled the spinal cord, which then flowed up to create the brain[45]—so that poor kidney function would be unable to properly produce the marrow and hence the brain, which would cause the symptoms of poor memory and concentration, dizziness and empty headedness.

In contemporary physiology, the kidneys secrete the hormone *erythropoietin* which instructs the bone marrow to produce red blood cells (p.153); and the bone marrow is necessary to nourish the bones (as well as playing a crucial part in providing immunity). This recognises a direct link between the kidneys and the quality of the bones, marrow, and the production of the blood, which correlates with part "A" of the *Nei Jing* theory. To have worked out this association over two thousand years ago, using pure logic, was impressive.

As to part "B" of the theory, like many other *Nei Jing* theories, the observation (the association of those symptoms with the kidneys) was fact based and therefore true, but the theory that strived to explain the symptoms was untrue. The spinal cord is in no way connected with bone marrow, and there is no connection or resemblance between the brain and bone marrow. At the time though, the explanation clearly seemed convincing, and this is understandable; there was no knowledge of the nervous system, nor anything like it; on crude dissection, the brain may have *appeared* like bone marrow; and their theory would have *seemed* to account for the symptomatic associations. However, the association of these brain-related symptoms with poor kidney function is seen repeatedly in clinic today, so there is no doubt that the *Nei Jing* symptomatic observations were true.

In contemporary physiology, the hormones *cortisol* and *adrenaline* enable the brain to create short term memories (p.154). These hormones are produced by the adrenal glands, which are one of the kidney-related structures, so this recognizes the link between poor kidney function and poor short term memory.

But with the other brain-related signs and symptoms (such as the development and health of the brain, and such symptoms as poor concentration; the feeling of empty headedness; whole-head headaches; and the brain-related signs of old age, such as dementia) the link between these signs and symptoms and "kidney" function has not yet been explored in contemporary physiology. For this reason, the fact that the "kidneys" *support the brain's health* must currently be regarded as an indirect effect rather than a function. Whereas the fact that the "kidneys" *enable the development of bones, bone marrow, and the formation of blood* are functions—of the literal kidneys.

5. Manages the circulation of body fluids

This is a direct function rather than an effect—the function being produced by the literal kidneys.

The *Nei Jing* authors noticed that when a patient had poor kidney function, they could develop swelling of the body (oedema); this could be in the body generally or focussed on the lower legs and ankles. These latter swellings are a common symptom of old age, when poor kidney function is common, which helps to reinforce the association between these signs and the kidneys.

The following *Nei Jing* extract suggests a theory to explain these signs.

Extract from *Su Wen*, Chapter 61

The kidneys constitute a female depot. When the [influence] of the earth rises, it associates with the kidneys and generates water fluid. Hence, it is called "extreme *yin*".

> When one does something with resolve and taxes oneself to the extreme, then sweat leaves from the kidneys. When sweat leaves the kidneys and encounters wind, internally it cannot enter the [organs] and externally it cannot transgress beyond the skin. It settles in the dark palaces [i.e. the pores] and moves inside the skin. Its transmission leads to *fu*-swelling. This is based in the kidneys. The name is wind water....
>
> As a fact, water diseases, below they cause *fu*-swelling in the upper abdomen, above they cause panting exhalation.[46]

> **Wang Bing (in 762 AD) commented on the above**
>
> When water resides in the kidneys below, then there is a *fu*-swelling in the region from the abdomen to the feet. When above it enters the lung, then pant-breathing, hasty and tense, as well as strong exhalations result.[47]

This theory could not have been based on knowledge of the body's internal anatomy, since at that time any such knowledge was too limited for this purpose, so instead it had to be constructed from logic alone. The original observation was fact based; that is, that when the kidney function is poor this often leads to swellings in the body, particularly in the lower part. But the *Nei Jing* theory that attempts to explain *why* this happens, is untrue in every detail.

In the first paragraph of the above extract, the statement "When the [influence] of the earth rises, it associates with the kidneys and generates water fluid" could be interpreted to be referring to *Nei Jing* metabolism. The "earth" may refer to the stomach and pancreas (which are the Earth phase in five phase theory), meaning that the stomach takes in liquid and grain; and then a variety of things are theorized to happen next—depending on which of the contradictory theories of metabolism are applied. The influences (including liquid) are either then passed to the lungs, which then circulates them in the "meridians"; or passed directly to all the other organs, which then circulate them in the "meridians"; or passed to the pancreas, which then circulates them (pp.41-47).

The kidneys are associated with water

However, the statement in this first paragraph is simply suggesting that the liquids from ingested food, once they have been separated ("When the [influence] of the earth rises"), the part that "associates with the kidneys" then becomes "water fluid". This theory does not trouble itself with the detail of *how* the water gets from the stomach to the kidneys, but merely relies on the fact that the kidneys are associated with water (which is a fundamental *Nei Jing* deduction[48]) and does not feel the need to get involved in the metabolism argument. Instead, those details are left vague.

Is this fundamental deduction true? When taking the broad view, Yes it is. In contemporary physiology, the kidneys do process the part of the body fluid that is contained in the blood (see below), so they could be said to be "associated with water". The *Nei Jing* authors were not aware of the fluid element in the blood, and certainly did not imagine that the kidneys filter blood (pp.42-44 and p.47), but as an overall concept, keeping the details vague, their deduction was true.

The second paragraph of the above extract, though, is untrue in every detail. The theory assumes that when a person "does something with resolve and taxes oneself to the extreme, then sweat leaves from the kidneys." This is untrue. With such *Nei Jing* statements, it is tempting to try to find some metaphorical or analogous interpretation, so that the statement could be interpreted sympathetically. But when comparing this with similar passages, I believe it was meant literally; and that this author believed that sweat could be produced by *any* organ, whenever that organ was working hard.[49]

This is simply untrue; in contemporary physiology, sweat is not produced in this way but is produced in the sweat glands beneath the skin, which are stimulated by sympathetic nerves in response to raised body temperature or fear.[50]

The theory then goes on to conjecture that when the "sweat leaves the kidneys and encounters wind" (i.e. a pathogenic obstruction), "internally it cannot enter the [organs]" (which is probably expressing the idea that "sweat" circulates inside us, passing to the organs, to perhaps moisten them) "and externally it cannot transgress beyond the skin" (i.e. leave the skin as sweat normally does). Note that the author would have assumed that this internal transport of the "sweat", and also the obstruction by pathogenic *wind*, took place within the "meridian" network, which was thought to consist of artery-like tubes that lay deep beneath the *pathways on the skin* (which is what we today call the meridians), and which the blood and vapours (influence, or *chi*) were also thought to flow within (p.29). Every detail of this description is untrue.

The theory then conjectures that the sweat "settles in the [pores] and moves inside the skin," thus producing the observed swelling. This is also untrue. In contemporary physiology, the swelling that occurs due to the accumulation of body fluid is certainly not the result of liquid accumulating in the pores of the skin; but rather, oedema is the accumulation of excess fluid in the body tissue generally.[51]

Every detail of this theory is therefore untrue. It is only the original symptomatic observation that is fact based (that poor kidney function can result in swelling), and also the notion that the kidneys are associated with water.

Nonetheless, studying such *Nei Jing* passages provides a fascinating insight into the thinking of the ancient Chinese physicians. And it is possible for today's practitioners to still apply this same type of reasoning in their approach to diagnosis and the choice of acupoints if they choose to, and this will in no way reduce the effectiveness of their treatments. But it is important to be aware of which parts of the *Nei Jing* are fact based and which are not, so that the practitioner at least stands a chance of being able to communicate with patients—and also with anyone else not familiar with Chinese medicine.

In contemporary physiology, the kidneys regulate the amount of water that circulates in the blood plasma by either recycling water back into the plasma to increase the level, or excreting any excess water in the urine; and they also regulate blood pressure (p.153). Normally, fluid from the blood plasma enters the body tissue through the capillaries, and the process is regulated by the hydrostatic pressure in the capillaries (the blood pressure). The fluid accumulates in the interstitial space—the space between individual cells in the tissues. In humans, 20 litres of plasma is released into the interstitial space of the tissues each day due to this capillary filtration. Of this, 17 litres is reabsorbed directly by the blood vessels, and the excess is returned to the bloodstream via the lymphatic system. And it is recognised that poor kidney function is a common cause of oedema.[52] This correlates with the *Nei Jing* symptomatic observations, and confirms that "managing the circulation of body fluids" is a direct kidney function rather than an effect.

Frequent and urgent urination

It was also noticed that when the kidney function was poor, patients could also suffer from frequent and urgent urination, or incontinence,[53] which could be considered another aspect of this function.

6. Assists the lungs to breathe in

This is an effect rather than a direct function.

The *Nei Jing* authors noticed that when patients suffered shortness of breath or asthma of the type where it was hard to breath in, the patient would usually also have poor kidney function, and that once the kidneys were successfully treated, these signs cleared.[54]

Around a millennium later it was discovered that the kidney function is at its weakest between the hours of five and seven in the morning (p.379),[55] and in my own clinical experiences, patients are most likely to suffer a kidney-related asthma attack between these hours, which confirms the involvement of the kidneys. And I have also noticed that when I needle a kidney acupoint on patients with poor kidney function, they often comment that they can suddenly breathe more easily. Some patients even link this to that particular needle being inserted—which is often Kidney-6 (*Zhaohai*).

In today's Chinese medicine, it is theorized that the "kidneys" assist the lungs to breath in,[56] but no detail has ever been suggested of the mechanism that might be involved—in physiological terms. The symptomatic observation of the *Nei Jing* authors is borne out by the evidence routinely seen in clinic today, which confirms that it was fact based. But there is no knowledge in contemporary physiology to explain this observation; that is, no evidence of cooperation between the "kidneys" (i.e. any or all of the three kidney-related structures) and lungs where the cooperation assists the lungs to breathe in. Therefore the observation must be regarded as an indirect effect rather than a function.

7. Has a close association with the ears, sense of hearing, and balance

This is an effect rather than a direct function.

The *Nei Jing* authors noticed that patients with poor kidney function tended to have poor hearing and low pitch tinnitus (hearing rumbling or swishing sounds),[57] both of which cleared once their kidneys were successfully treated—which suggests that the sense of hearing is dependent on good kidney function.[58]

> **Extract from *Ling Shu*, Chapter 29**
> The kidneys rule the outer regions. They are engaged to listen to far-away places. One inspects the ears to find out whether their hearing ability is good or bad, and from this one may recognise [the health of the kidneys].[59]

Extract from *Ling Shu*, Chapter 33

When the sea of bone marrow has a surplus, then one feels light and vigorous, and overexerts himself. When the sea of bone marrow has an insufficiency, then the brain revolves, and there are noises in the ears.[60]

Poor kidney function can be experienced at any stage of life; however it is extremely common in old age. Normally, the kidney function gradually weakens later in life, and the resultant poor kidney function that exists in most old people was observed to be responsible for all the classic signs of old age, one of which is poor hearing or total deafness.[61]

Another common symptom suffered in old age is loss of balance,[57] and the association of this symptom with the kidney function can also sometimes be illustrated earlier in life. In developed countries today, when a patient's kidney function is affected by pharmaceuticals (either purposefully or inadvertently) many can experience loss of balance.[62]

Inherited poor kidney function

In my clinical practice I have noticed that when younger patients experience poor hearing, they usually have poor kidney function which they inherited from their parents. They usually also have other kidney-related symptoms which were present from childhood, such as asthma or hay fever. And it often transpires that the patient was the last child of several to be born, often with a gap after the previous child—so that their parents were middle-aged, which is when their own kidney function and fertility would be waning; or that both their parents tended to drive themselves hard and were particularly exhausted around the time of conception—which again meant that their own kidney function was poor.

Patient example

Female, aged 29. This patient inherited poor kidney function from her parents, due to them both being in their late forties when she was conceived, and also being in the habit of driving themselves very hard. When born, she was deaf in her right ear, had only partial hearing in her left; and now also had a wide range of serious symptoms, affecting all five of her main organs. See the full case history on page 246.

Patient example

Male, aged 45. This patient's father was 48 when the patient was conceived, and the patient was born with poor kidney function, which caused him to suffer pronounced hay fever in childhood. See the full case history on page 255.

While writing this chapter, I had an experience that graphically demonstrated the association between the kidneys and ears. When out walking, a dog suddenly barked aggressively at me and I felt a surge of energy around my ears; it started below my ears, around the acupoint Lymphatic-system-17* (*Yifeng*), and surged up into my ears on both sides and I then immediately felt the hairs on the back of my neck rising—at the location where the bladder meridian descends.

In contemporary physiology, this type of reaction is known as an adrenaline release. The adrenal glands are one of the kidney-related structures, which confirms the association between the "kidneys" and this type of experience.

* Also known as San-jiao-17, or Triple-burner-17, etc. (p.211).

It seems that the emotion of fear (which is produced by the kidneys—p.169 below) and the "flight response" are most readily invoked by sounds. If you recall the last time you felt fear due to a sound, you might recall yourself physically jumping, being aware of the effect of the adrenaline (your increased pulse rate, etc.) and the sense of alarm. And this type of experience seems a further reflection of the association between the ears and kidneys—and the kidney-related phenomena of fear and adrenaline.

The kidneys are also connected to the ears via the bladder meridian. The kidney and bladder meridians are consecutive, and from the main bladder meridian on the head, a branch descends to encircle the ear.[63] This meridian relationship provides a possible mechanism that could enable the kidneys' health to be reflected in the hearing. When an organ is stressed, its related acupoints become tender, which appears to be due to some aspect of the local tissue ceasing to function properly in response to the organ stress (p.369). And in the same way, the local tissue at the ears may also cease to function properly in response to poor kidney function. In other words, for the hearing to work properly, it is necessary for the kidney function to be healthy.

These practical observations aside—contemporary physiology is unable to explain this association between the "kidneys" and the sense of hearing and balance. Therefore this association must be regarded as an indirect effect rather than a direct function. In other words, it could not be said that the hearing is a function of the "kidneys", but rather that the "kidneys" have clear functions, and as an indirect consequence of one or more of those functions, the sense of hearing is affected.

8. Has mental and emotional functions

Over millions of years, each organ evolved logic to enable it to carry out its functions and coordinate these with the other organs (p.91). And once our conscious mind started having complex thoughts about the world around us, it is possible that this pre-existing organ logic may have been used to process such thoughts. Today, this notion is supported by the clear two-way associations between the kidney function and certain of our mental processes, as described in the remainder of this chapter.

The thoughts produced by the kidney function

In contemporary physiology the "kidneys" (considering all three kidney-related structures as a whole) are mainly concerned with our self-preservation, both in the present and the future. Amongst other functions, the kidneys coordinate our growth and development, from conception through to adulthood; are the key reproductive organ, being responsible for fertility and our sexual behaviour, which thus provides us with our engagement in life, the desire to go on living and the tendency to form goals and have the determination to see them through. They regulate the body's energy usage, so as to ensure the proper function of all the organs, thus enabling us to function at our best in the present and also enabling us to deal with stressful situations; and they manage and support immunity.

Considering all these factors, the kidneys' physical function could be summarized as: *to* (produce the desire to) *want to be alive and continue living; to reproduce, set goals for the future and pursue those goals; and to recognise threats and find a solution to them* (which is the role played by immunity).

When the kidneys' logic associated with this function is used to process our thoughts, what thought patterns might result?

Our motivation in many areas of life

The kidney function to *reproduce, set goals for the future and pursue those goals* produces every aspect of our sexual behaviour, all our actions and thoughts concerning our attraction to others and making ourselves attractive to *them*. This could cause us to modify our appearance or seek such things as status or certain achievements, all of which we may consider—even if only subconsciously—could enhance our attractiveness. And when the kidney function drives us *to set goals for the future and to pursue them*, we may often feel the desire to be doing or producing something that we feel is "worthwhile", or wanting to achieve something that makes us feel good about ourselves. Both these are very similar motivations to that of wanting to improve our status or attractiveness. But at other times, our only motivation may be seeking to enjoy the simple pleasure of being alive, which is produced in us by the kidney function *to want to be alive and continue living*. And another common motivation is the desire to leave something behind, which is produced by this same function: the kidneys' desire for us to go on living.

The kidney function *to recognise threats and find a solution to them* was originally evolved to protect us from predators. This still applies today, on the occasions when we might be faced with an actual predator (such as an aggressive animal or person), but this also applies to other threats, such as illnesses (causing us to avoid an ill person) or dangerous situations. And this also applies whenever any aspect of our status, or the safety of anything or anyone we care about is threatened. In any of these situations, this kidney function produces our feeling of fear and also focuses our resources (by releasing adrenaline) to enable us to tackle the threat.

The kidneys produce fear

Through practical observation, the *Nei Jing* authors noticed that the emotion of fear was produced by the kidneys.[64]

Just as whenever the *liver* function is obstructed and the liver produces the emotion of anger to attempt to remove the obstruction; so, when the kidney function is undermined (perhaps some element of our safety or status, or a cherished person or thing, is threatened), the kidneys produce the emotion of fear to cause us to take urgent action to remedy the situation. This might be to flee from the danger or take evasive action to remove the threat. Fear is produced in two main situations.

1. When the kidney function becomes weak

When the kidney function is poor, this makes us less resilient, reduces our stamina, weakens the function of *all* the organs, as well as reducing the availability of energy generally. All these things are regulated by the "kidneys"; hence any weakness in the kidney function could produce these effects. This places us in a vulnerable state. One of the kidney functions is *to want to be alive and continue living*, and when we feel vulnerable, this undermines this function, so the kidneys produce the emotion of fear to prompt us to address the situation.

This would start as a state of general fearfulness, rather than a sudden fright, but it would also be accompanied by a release of adrenaline. This state can be frequently seen in people. When they become drained (often through driving themselves too hard), they tend to become jumpy, and their sensitivity to sounds may also become more acute—hearing is the sense the kidneys are most closely associated with (p.166).

This is a defensive state; we are made more alert, so we can watch out for danger and are able to respond quickly to it, should we spot it. Ordinarily, this is intended only as a short-term measure, but when this state becomes almost constant, it only weakens the kidneys further—through overuse of these emergency reserves. This then only increases our fearfulness, increases our general depletion and inhibits the good function of all the organs, all of which diminishes our long-term health.

The stage of life when poor kidney function is common is old age, which is why old people are often fearful—which constant state of fearfulness only tends to weaken their kidney function even further. If longevity is a concern of yours, then avoiding fearful situations at *all* stages in life would be beneficial.

2. When we notice a threat

Another of the kidney functions is *to reproduce, set goals for the future and pursue those goals*. This also goes hand in hand with its function *to want to be alive and continue living*.

When we notice anything that threatens our own physical safety, or that of our loved ones, or threatens our social position or our achievements, this undermines these kidney functions. In response, the kidneys produce the emotion of fear to prompt us to address the threat—and the degree of fear would reflect the urgency of the threat.

In contemporary physiology, the adrenal glands are heavily associated with the "flight" response, and since the adrenal glands are one of the three kidney-related structures, this also supports the associations between fear, flight, self preservation and the kidneys.

The kidney function is also used to *process* the threatening situation. One part of its function is to *recognise threats and find a solution to them*. It is possible that this kidney logic (in other words, the "logic" of the immune system) is then used to quickly process the situation and present a solution to our conscious mind.

The "immune system" can also process our thoughts

Supposing the threat were to our physical safety, the solution might be the idea that we should flee the danger, should move aside and dodge it. Or, if the threat was from another person or an animal that we could combat, the solution may be to fight it. Or the threat may be a comment a person made which appeared to put us in jeopardy in some way. This may be by threatening our position, our notions of our own status or worth, or the security of our job or our relationships or something else we cared deeply about. In this situation, the kidneys' solution may be to work out a lie for us to tell to fend off the danger, and this lie would then pop into our mind. It is common to see people reacting in this way, when they will clearly enter an adrenaline-fuelled state and spontaneously lie to protect themselves from any perceived threat.

In other situations, people may respond to a threat by working out a course of action to discredit the person who appears to be attacking them. If this course of action occurs to them spontaneously, within a second or so of them perceiving the threat, it would have most likely been worked out by the immune-system aspect of their kidney function. But sometimes, people can dwell on such threats for hours or days, until the solution eventually pops into their mind. In this situation, the solution would have probably been worked out by their liver function, using the liver's creative ability—to remove this "obstruction to the flow of their thoughts" (p.108).

Another way the kidney function may be utilized mentally is in spotting opportunities to further its goals. These might be in the workplace or socially. Suppose you were in a work situation and your superior said something, and in response an idea popped into your head about something you could say or do that would advance your position, either in the eyes of your boss or your company generally. This idea, which appeared to spontaneously occur to you, was produced by your kidney function. The same situation may occur to us socially. Your partner, or an admired friend, may say or do something, and in response an idea may spontaneously pop into your head about something you could say or do to curry favour with them. Again, this idea would have been produced by the logic of your kidneys.

This type of spontaneous idea is often accompanied by a release of adrenaline, which reinforces the notion that the idea originates in the "kidneys".

We have all experienced this phenomenon, but as to whether or not we act on the idea is another matter—some people do and some do not. Another common example is when we see an object unattended, which we regard as having value. It might be money, or a phone or laptop computer or item of jewellery or simply an object that only we cherish and which is of little value to anyone else, such as an object of no intrinsic value but which we consider collectable. In this situation, the idea may pop into our mind to commit an opportunistic theft—and may be accompanied by a surge of adrenaline, which may be proportionate to the value the object has in *our* eyes. Such ideas are produced by the kidney function. We have all experienced this, but, again, whether or not we act on the idea would be determined by other "voices" within us. These may be produced by the logic of the lungs, liver, or heart—which consider such matters as quality, including the quality of our own behaviour in *our* eyes; our sense of obeying the rules, of what is wrong or right; and our feelings towards other people. And it is also these same "voices" that determine whether or not we act on this type of spontaneous idea in social or work situations.

If a situation is urgent, the kidneys tend to respond—since they are mostly concerned with our self-preservation and dealing with immediate threats. Whereas if the situation is not urgent, but a niggling preoccupation, then it would be the liver that tends to respond—since it is primarily concerned with keeping substances moving in the body and removing any obstructions to that flow; and here the "substances" are our ideas and thoughts—p.108.

How this affects our health

On the mental and emotional level, the role of the kidneys is to, in effect, manage the balance between fear and drive. Sometimes our drive is in response to fear. For example, we may fear losing our job if we do not work excessively hard and long hours, or we may fear losing a friendship or romantic relationship if we do not constantly work hard at it. This type of drive is unhealthy; it would be accompanied by an adrenaline release, which would assist us to perform but over time would tend to weaken the kidneys (through overuse of this emergency resource) which in turn would produce poor kidney function with a *selection* of the physical signs and symptoms listed on page 174 below.[65]

> **Patient example**
> Male, aged 57. This patient drove himself hard. He ran his own business, and due to the responsibilities he took on single-handedly, he felt unsupported. This produced a sense of fear for his long-term survival which impeded his kidney function and also caused serious low-back problems. See the full case history on page 250.

Once a person has poor kidney function, the mental and emotional functions of the kidneys would also function poorly, causing the person to see threats in situations which other people would not consider threatening. This would only cause them to work that much harder (whether in a social or work context), which would tend to weaken their kidney function even further, causing extra or stronger physical symptoms, and possibly causing the work or social relationships to become strained. This would then only increase the perception of danger and the tendency to drive themselves too hard.

On the other hand, drive can often be healthy, provided it is not excessive. When we are driven to do a certain thing through pure excitement alone, or interest in that activity, this can be invigorating. It evokes the kidney function of *regulating and enabling the functioning of the other organs*—in other words, providing our "spark". It can make us feel energized and alive. This type of drive has no element of fear and is usually only beneficial, provided an appropriate balance is practised in every area of your life—including allowing yourself enough relaxation and an appropriate amount of physical exercise and an adequate diet. But when the drive becomes excessive (even though driven by excitement alone) this would also weaken the person's kidneys and could produce any of the signs and symptoms of poor kidney function.

When our spirit is defeated

Another common health problem related to the mental aspect of the kidneys is when our spirit is defeated. The kidney logic identifies our goals in life, our ambitions, and fosters our ideas about our worth, status, or position in life; and the kidneys then drive us to achieve these ambitions. But when any of our ambitions are defeated, or our status or position in life is taken away, this undermines these kidney functions in our thoughts, which undermining is duplicated in the kidneys, impeding their physical function.

Extract from *Su Wen*, Chapter 77

[When] the patient was formerly of noble rank and later fell to low rank, even though he was not hit by [harmful influence from the outside]; his disease emerged from within. It is called lost [constructive influence]. [When] the patient was formerly wealthy and later became poor, this is called lost essence [i.e. this weakens the "kidneys"].... When a man of noble rank is stripped of his power, even though he was not struck by a pathogen from outside, his essence and spirit have been harmed inside [i.e. his "kidneys" have been harmed by the loss of status].[66]

In this situation, the person's "spark" would be clearly diminished; they would become gloomy, dispirited. The kidney function of regulating the production of energy would become poor and consequently the other main organs would function poorly. The person would become sluggish, would certainly be melancholic or in a depressive state (as though their body had been shut down) and they may feel like giving up on life, having no drive or spirit.

In such patients, the kidney acupoints on their chest would tend to be tender when pressed, and needling these can often visibly restore the patient's spirit during that session. The key acupoints are Kidney-24 (*Lingxu*) and Kidney-25 (*Shencang*). Historically, in China acupoints were known by names, rather than using the numbering system we use today, and the names often indicate the use of the acupoint. Interestingly, in the case of these two acupoints, these were called "spirit ruin" and "spirit storehouse" respectively, indicating that they tended to become tender when a person's spirit was damaged, and could therefore be used to rectify the situation. That is, to normalize the aspect of the kidney function that was undermined by the mental or emotional shock.

Patient example

Male, aged 51. This patient took a break from treatment for three years. When he next came, he was like a broken man and seemed noticeably aged. He had been through a divorce and felt the financial loss greatly. The acupoint Kidney-24 (*Lingxu*) was very tender when pressed. I needled this, and other acupoints, and at the end of the session he looked about five years younger and the sparkle had returned to his eyes; he said he felt like a new person.

Dietary factors

The *Nei Jing* authors noticed that salt "resonates" with the kidneys.[67] In other words, salt nourishes the kidneys and a certain amount of salt intake is essential for the kidneys to remain healthy. Because of this, people with poor kidney function often crave salty foods. But as with all aspects of Chinese medicine, balance is the key. If too much salt were eaten this would have a depleting effect on the kidneys. However, many people in developed countries have been mislead into thinking that *all* salt is bad and should be avoided at all cost. This is equally wrong. Apart from the fact that correct seasoning enhances the taste of food and so increases the pleasure we gain from it, salt is an essential mineral for our health.

Drinking too much water can also damage the kidneys, and many people have also been mislead into thinking they must drink a large amount of water each day. In general this is also wrong and would tend to weaken the kidneys. Extra water should be drunk only when you feel thirsty.

In contemporary physiology, salt deficiency is called *hyponatremia*, and is recognised as being associated with such conditions as poor mental development in children and poor mental function and brain damage in adults (all of which the *Nei Jing* authors associated with poor kidney function), and it is also recognised that this condition can be caused in adults by drinking too much water, which again correlates with this ancient (but forgotten) knowledge.[68]

Improper function

In Chinese medicine, the main condition that affects the kidneys is poor kidney function (also called "Kidney chi deficiency", or other terms—listed on page 176 below), which would tend to produce a *selection* of the following signs and symptoms:

A. Soreness and weakness of the lower back (lumbar region), and weak knees or stiff joints[37]; frequent and urgent urination (it cannot be put off), and dribbling of urine after urination, or incontinence (enuresis)[53]; premature ejaculation in men; hay fever and other allergies, frequent colds and flu[32]; dizziness[39] or lightheaded feeling (particularly after sex in men); oedema, particularly in the lower half of the body[69]; low-pitch tinnitus (or rumbling or swishing sounds)[57]; deafness or being hard of hearing[58]; loss of balance[57,70]; tendency to feel fearful[64]; craving salty food.[67]
B. Shortness of breath, asthma (where it is difficult to breathe in*).[54]
C. Insomnia; poor short term memory; thirst, afternoon fever (hot flushes) and night sweating,[71] dry mouth, hot hands and feet.[72]
D. Cold limbs, aversion to cold; low energy and apathy.[73]
E. Slow physical development, poor skeletal development, brittle bones, poorly formed or loose teeth[38]; slow mental development; mental dullness, premature senility, dementia[40]; premature greying and hair loss; impotence, infertility.[74]

Face colour, tone of voice, and food craving

Chapter 10 of the *Su Wen* states "If the complexion is generated by the kidneys, it resembles violet wrapped up in white silk,"[75] meaning that if a person has a pronounced kidney condition, this particular hue would tend to be visible in their face, particularly beneath the eyes.

Chapter 5 of the *Su Wen* associates the kidneys with a "groaning" tone of voice.[76] Again, when a person is prone to poor kidney function, this "groaning" tone can often be clearly heard in their voice as a constant background tone. Such factors are so distinctive that with practice it is often possible to make a fairly reliable diagnosis from simply hearing a person speak, with no other information about them at all—such as when hearing a stranger talk in a nearby room, or on the radio.

* Difficulty in breathing *out* is due to poor lung function (p.145).

Such a patient would also tend to crave salty food, since salt was recognised to benefit the kidneys.[77] Some patients, though, may tend to feed their craving to excess, which would then only tend to overwhelm the kidneys and have a negative effect.[78]

Causes of poor kidney function

In most people this condition develops as a normal part of the aging process. Indeed all the classic signs of old age are due to poor kidney function (deafness, loss of teeth and hair, infertility, low back ache, weak knees, brittle bones, incontinence, frequent urination, low energy or "slow movements", lack of drive, poor short term memory, senility, dementia). But the kidney function can also be weakened for the other reasons mentioned above (p.172 onwards): through driving ourselves too hard; by our spirit being defeated; or the condition can be inherited from our parents.

> **Patient example**
> Male, aged 24. This patient had a ten-year history of migraines. He inherited poor kidney function from his parents, which caused childhood hay fever and poor hearing, and also left him with a weak constitution, which made him prone to migraine attacks later in life. See the full case history on page 249.

Treatment

When the "kidney" function is poor, this causes various acupoints to become tender. When one of these acupoints is stimulated, this encourages the "kidneys" to cancel out the malfunction in themselves that caused the tenderness (p.372), and the "kidneys" return to normal function. In this way, the problem is corrected by the organ itself (p.78). The key acupoints are:

- Kidney-3 (*Taixi*),
- Kidney-6 (*Zhaohai*),
- Kidney-1 (*Yongquan*),
- Ren-4 (*Guanyuan*),
- Bladder-23 (*Shenshu*),
- Du-4 (*Mingmen*), and
- Heart-7 (*Shenmen*).[79]

The Ren and Du meridians are extra meridians which are not directly associated with any of the twelve organs but which contain many key acupoints associated with those organs. Page 359 describes how the nearby presence of an organ may be able to create an acupoint on any meridian that passes over that location, and this may explain how these key organ acupoints are created on the Ren and Du meridians as they pass over the locations of those organs.

Moxibustion

Moxibustion is a technique that is very effective when treating the kidneys. This is the application of heat to the acupoints using a stick containing powered *mugwort*, which is often used in addition to needling those acupoints. The energy contained in the heat seems to be communicated to the associated organ, greatly increasing the strength of its function. With "deficient" conditions, moxibustion tends to be a very effective addition to the treatment.

General prognosis

Due to the nature of poor kidney function (it being a condition where the patient's core resources have become depleted, or where they were born with inadequate core resources) recovery tends to be slower than with conditions related to the other main organs. Still, with many patients great success can be achieved after a course of about six treatments. This is even the case when the condition has developed as a part of the aging process; I have treated many elderly patients who have gained relief from many of their kidney-related symptoms. But with patients who inherited poor kidney function from their parents, it is sometimes not possible to *permanently* normalize their kidney function. In these cases, after the initial course of treatments, the patients may need to return for a maintenance treatment once a month or so if they wish to maintain good health (p.79). This would depend on each patient; the more they were able to adjust their lifestyle to match their limited physical resources, the less they would require further treatments. This often happens spontaneously anyway, since the treatments seem to make patients more aware of things in their life that are wrong for them—and they start to make appropriate changes. With *all* patients, the more they were able to do this, the less they would require follow-up treatments—though maintaining the perfect balance in life is not an easy task in developed countries, where many aspects of life can often be stressful.

Asthma

The underlying cause of asthma is often poor kidney function.[54] This would be the case when the patient finds it hard to breathe in. When patients find it hard to breathe out, this would usually be due to poor lung function. It is important to establish which of these two types the patient has, so the condition can be effectively and quickly treated. If the kidney function is the problem, the patient would be likely to also suffer a selection of signs and symptoms from those listed on page 174 above, and the shortness of breath would often be worse between five and seven a.m., which is when the kidney function is at its weakest (p.379).

Other Chinese medicine terms used for kidney conditions

In today's Chinese medicine, poor kidney function is usually called "Kidney chi deficiency". And when certain signs and symptoms predominate, several other terms are also used. For example, most patients would tend to suffer *some* of the signs and symptoms from list "A" on page 174 above, but if they *also* suffered some from one of the other lists, then a different Chinese medicine term may be used to describe the condition instead. If symptoms from list "B" were also suffered, the term "Kidney failing to receive chi" could be used; or if symptoms from list "C", the term "Kidney yin deficiency" could be used; or if symptoms from list "D", the term "Deficient kidney yang" could be used; or if signs and symptoms from list "E", the term "Deficient kidney essence" or "Deficient kidney jing" could be used.

It should be noted that the above terms were not used in the *Nei Jing* or *Nan Jing* and have been adopted more recently (p.449).

However, each of the terms is simply indicating that the patient has poor kidney function with signs and symptoms in a certain area tending to predominate. And in all cases the treatment is almost identical anyway, so (in line with the general *Nei Jing* practice—

p.449) this book simply lists a single kidney condition: poor kidney function.

Analogies in contemporary physiology for the kidney-related concepts

In Chinese medicine, the notions of kidney essence (kidney *jing*), original influence (*yuan chi*), essence (*jing*), essence influence (*jing chi*), kidney *yang*, and "*ming men* fire" were all used at different times and by different authors to describe kidney-related concepts (p.25). Some of these terms were used interchangeably by different authors, and they are all related to theories that attempt to explain some aspect of kidney function. But the *Nei Jing* and *Nan Jing* theories that utilize these terms were (like many other *Nei Jing* theories) not literally true. The meaning they intended was that these substances consisted of vapours circulating in the "meridians" * which produced all the various effects they attributed to them. But like most other forms of influence (*chi*), nothing akin to these imagined vapours circulated in the "meridian" network (pp.40-47), and the network itself was also imaginary (p.29). Therefore any theory that relies on this notion can also only be untrue. However, these theories would have been derived to attempt to account for symptomatic observations that *were* usually true, so that the concepts themselves (of the effects these imaginary substances were thought to have) may be considered valid, in which case it ought to be possible to find an analogy for them in contemporary physiology. This section demonstrates how the term "kidney essence", as used in the following quotations, is analogous to the hormonal activity of the three kidney-related structures.

The nature of kidney essence is usually described in the following ways:

> Kidney essence is responsible for managing growth and sexual development, producing in us all the changes in the body that occur as we pass from childhood into adulthood and old age.[80]

In contemporary physiology, this is clearly referring to the sex hormones secreted by the gonads and adrenal glands, which perform these same functions (p.155).

> Kidney essence is made up of two parts; one part is inherited from our parents at conception (the congenital part) and the other is manufactured in us from the food we eat (the acquired part), which replenishes the essence.[81]

In this description, the *congenital* part of kidney essence relates to the "blueprint" passed on to us from our parents. In contemporary physiology, this could only mean the genetic blueprint passed on to us via our *parents'* gonads, which determines the strength of the overall kidney function, so that the quote is simply stating that one aspect of the kidney function is the constitution inherited from our parents. However, the notion of the genetic blueprint may be an over-simplification, since contemporary physiology does not yet allow for the "energetic blueprint", which is another mechanism for inheritance. This relates to the energetic influence that our parents' (largely our mother's) organ functions

---

* That is, in the deep, artery-like tubes that were thought to follow the same paths as the *pathways on the skin* (which are what we today call meridians); see page 29.

have on our own organs while in the womb and afterwards. Genetics clearly determine *some* of our qualities, but I believe the energetic influence plays a much larger part than genetics in determining our personality and general health. Page 364 describes the influence one person's organ functions can have on another person's organ functions; and this influence would clearly be far greater between a mother and her unborn baby, even possibly affecting the physical development of the baby's organs. However, whatever the mechanisms of inheritance, the above Chinese medicine quote is still simply stating that the strength of the kidney function is dependent on our inherited constitution.

The reference to the *acquired* part of kidney essence could be interpreted to be referring to the hormonal activity of all three kidney-related structures. This "essence" is replenished when those structures are nourished by the food we eat—as is every other part of the body. In other words, glucose is extracted from the food we eat, which is used to release energy in the body's cells, which enables the kidneys, adrenal glands and gonads to function; and in functioning, they secrete hormones. Therefore these hormones are the "kidney essence" which is "replenished" by the food we eat.

> The congenital and acquired essence rely on and promote each other. Before birth, congenital essence has prepared the material base for acquired essence. After birth, acquired essence constantly replenishes congenital essence.[81]

Again, this is merely stating that the constitution we were born with (which was inherited from our parents) determines the strength of the "kidney" function—as it does the strength of all the organs. And after birth, the "kidneys" (i.e. the three kidney-related structures) release hormones to regulate most key systems in the body, including the digestion, which enables every structure in the body to be properly nourished, including the "kidneys" themselves, which, in turn, strengthens their function. But this regenerative ability is dependent on the constitution we inherited.

> Kidney essence is the material base of the human body and of many of its functional activities.[82]

This could be interpreted to mean that the hormonal activity of the three kidney-related structures regulates the digestion, production and use of energy, and many of the important functions of the main organs (pp.153-155), and in doing so enables the body to flourish, both physically and functionally. Therefore, again, "kidney essence" could be understood as being analogous to these hormones.

> Kidney essence determines the basic constitutional strength and resistance to exterior pathogenic factors.[83]

The relation between the "kidneys" and the constitution is discussed on pages 156-159. But the above notion of the "resistance to exterior pathogenic factors", in relation to the "kidneys", is largely an invention of some of today's Chinese medicine textbooks.[84] In the *Nei Jing*, this "resistance" was provided by the lungs circulating defensive influence (*wei chi*) which then warmed the skin and muscles, and this warmth was thought to provide the resistance to external pathogens, such as *wind*. Chinese medicine had, and has, no concept of "immunity", as we think of it today (pp.44-47). However, their notion of a person's "constitution" includes some concepts that, in contemporary physiology, would be attributed to the immune system—such as the resistance to illness. Therefore, it is in this context that "kidney essence" *could* be interpreted to provide the "resistance to exterior pathogenic factors". Therefore, again, the reference to kidney essence in the above quote is consistent with the function of adrenal and kidney hormones. The adrenal hormones play a key role in producing immunity (p.154), as do kidney hormones, in signalling the production of red blood cells in the bone marrow, which are a key component of the immune system (p.153).

> Kidney essence is not tangible, as blood is; it is derived from the more solid substances but is a more refined manifestation.

This is also consistent with a description of hormones, which are certainly less tangible than blood. They are "derived from the more solid substances" in that glucose (extracted from ingested food) enables all the organs to obtain the energy they need to function, and the functioning of the "kidneys" produces the "kidney"-related hormones.

Hence, in all the above quotes, kidney essence could be considered analogous to the hormonal activity of the three kidney-related structures. And the same applies to all other kidney-related terms, such as original influence (*yuan chi*), kidney *yang*, and "*ming men* fire", since these were considered to originate from kidney essence.

Bladder conditions

In contemporary physiology, the function of the bladder is to temporarily store and then excrete urine, which is produced by the kidneys. The kidneys filter out various toxins from the blood, and also some of the waste products of the normal chemical activity in the body, such as urea (p.153). These are excreted in the urine, which passes down the *ureter* (a thirty centimetre tube) to collect in the bladder.[85] Normally, the urine consists of about 96% water, 2% urea, and the remaining 2% is made up of other substances.[86]

In *Nei Jing* terms, the bladder was considered a storage place for body liquids. Chapter 8 of the *Su Wen* states "The urinary bladder is the official functioning as regional rectifier.[87] The body liquids are stored in it."[88]

Extract from *Nan Jing*, Section 31

The [*san jiao*] encompasses the passageways of water and grain in the body. It represents the conclusion and the start of the course of the influences.... The lower section of the [*san jiao* (i.e. the kidneys, intestines, and bladder)] begins exactly at the upper opening of the bladder[89] and extends downward. It is responsible for separating the clear from the turbid portions. It masters discharge but not intake, and it serves as a transmitter.[90]

Commenting on the above, Li Chiung (in 1269) wrote

The lower section of the [*san jiao* (i.e. the kidneys, intestines, and bladder)] separates the water and the grains which were taken

> in through the upper* section of the [*san jiao*]. The clear portions become urine; the turbid portions become faeces. They are then transmitted to the outside.[91]

The *san jiao* has always been a controversial organ, with different authors disagreeing on its definition. However one interpretation is that its three sections simply serve as a summary of the functions of the organs in each section of the torso, where the lower section summarized the functions of the kidneys, intestines and bladder—as indicated in brackets in the above quotes.[92] Hence, the *Nei Jing* (and *Nan Jing*) notion of the bladder was that it served to store and excrete the clear part of the "dregs" from the digestion. And the following extract adds further detail.

> **Extract from *Ling Shu*, Chapter 18**
> The lower [section of the *san jiao* (i.e. the kidneys, intestines, and bladder)] discharges into the curved intestine and pours out into the urinary bladder where its liquids seep in. The fact is: Water and grain are regularly present together in the stomach. There they are transformed to dregs and together they descend into the large intestine, where they constitute the lower [section of the *san jiao*], where its liquids seep in. A separate juice is secreted along the lower [section of the *san jiao*] and seeps into the urinary bladder.[93]

This passage conveys the clear notion that the urine originates in the large intestine. It was theorized that the "dregs" from the stomach (the result of the stomach's processing) were passed on to the large intestine, and the large intestine separated out the "clear" portion (which was the "urine"), then passed this to the bladder.

This theory, like many aspects of *Nei Jing* metabolism, is untrue. Urine does not originate from the digestion at all, and it certainly is not produced by the large intestine; instead, it is produced by the kidneys, which filter it from the blood (p.153). But further, not only were the *Nei Jing* authors unaware that urine is produced by the kidneys, but nowhere in the *Nei Jing* or *Nan Jing* is there the notion that the blood needed to be filtered at all.

The *Nei Jing* notions of metabolism were contradictory and largely untrue (pp.33-47), so any further theories built on those foundations could not be expected to be factual. For example, the blood was not thought to serve the transport purpose that is known today—transporting all substances extracted from food, plus the substances related to the body's cellular communication (such as hormones), and also its chemistry (such as urea). Therefore, it would not have occurred to the *Nei Jing* authors that the blood might contain "debris" that needed to be filtered out—so that their mistake regarding this aspect of metabolism was understandable.

Treating the bladder

In practical terms (which are the *Nei Jing's* greatest assets), it was recognised that the strength of the bladder function was dependent on the strength of the kidney function. When the kidney function was poor, the patient would suffer such symptoms as frequent and urgent urination and incontinence; and after the kidney function was treated, these symptoms would clear.[53] This symptomatic association between the two organs is so

* The "upper section" was said to relate to the functions of the heart and lungs, so this was probably meant to say the "middle section".

strong that, in Chinese medicine terms, such symptoms are seen as symptoms of poor kidney function, rather than of poor bladder function. And due to this symptomatic link between the two organs, the bladder is usually regarded as merely an extension of the kidneys, with no need for it to be treated, or considered, separately. However, one fairly common bladder condition requires separate mention.

Burning sensation on urination

The usual symptoms are: burning sensation on urination, with cloudy, deep yellow, strong smelling urine; and there is usually also poor kidney function, which may cause various other signs and symptoms from the list on page 174 above. The condition is usually treated with a selection of the following acupoints:

- Bladder-23 (*Shenshu*),
- Bladder-28 (*Pangguangshu*),
- Ren-3 (*Zhongji*),
- Pancreas-6[*] (*Daheng*), and
- Pancreas-9[†] (*Yinlingquan*).

In my experience, the treatment is extremely effective and the main symptom (the burning sensation on urination) is often cleared with a single treatment.

In today's Chinese medicine, this condition is called "Damp heat in the bladder", which can understood as follows.

The terms "heat" and "damp heat"

The Chinese medicine term of *dampness* was explained on page 76, and is summarized as follows. In contemporary physiology, this may be visualized as the improper regulation of the glucose, fats and proteins circulating in the blood, which then denies the organs and systems of the body proper nutrition, which, in time, may impede certain aspects of the kidney function, resulting in oedema.

In Chinese medicine, this state is regarded as pathogenic; that is, the *dampness* itself is regarded as a pathogen. Simplistically, this could be visualized as the "soup" of nutrients in the blood being too thick.

The Chinese medicine term *heat* simply means any unusual warmth in the body—which could be generated by the body's reaction to a pathogen, or by the malfunction of the organs or bodily tissue (p.307). The warmth is generated by our own body and is often accompanied by redness and swelling.

When such *heat* is produced in response to *dampness*, the condition is known as *damp heat*. Regarding the symptom of "burning on urination", the *heat* would be the symptom produced in the "kidneys" and/or bladder due to their function being impeded by the *dampness* (i.e. the improper regulation of the organs' nutrition).

The acupoints I mentioned above are used to remedy the condition as follows. Pancreas-6 (*Daheng*) and Pancreas-9 (*Yinlingquan*) strengthen the digestion, so that less *dampness* is produced, and the accumulated *dampness* clears more quickly; Bladder-23 (*Shenshu*) and Bladder-28 (*Pangguangshu*) are used to strengthen the "kidney" and bladder functions respectively; and Ren-3 (*Zhongji*), which is directly over the bladder, *appears* to directly

[*] Also called Spleen-6.
[†] Also called Spleen-9.

vent the *heat* from the bladder (but see the topic on page 308, which considers whether acupoints can vent pathogens).

> **Patient example**
> Female, aged 32. This patient sought treatment for issues related to her menstrual cycle, primarily acne but also PMS and painful periods; and she also had recurring thrush, with a burning sensation on urination. In this case the thrush was due to *damp heat*. See the full case history on page 252.

One of the assets of Chinese medicine is that it can treat such conditions by referring to general concepts such as *heat* and *damp heat*, without having to define the condition in microscopic terms. Instead, it simply prompts the organs to return to normal function, and the organs themselves make any chemical, hormonal, or other adjustments necessary.

In contemporary physiology, such a condition is said to be caused by a bacterial or viral "infection", which appears to suggest that such a condition ought not to respond to having an acupuncture needle inserted in the skin. However, the treatment is extremely effective and has been used for thousands of years, which highlights one of the common problems encountered when attempting to understand this ancient healing system using concepts from contemporary physiology.

In Chapter 16 (p.307), I describe in more detail the interpretation of Chinese medicine concepts such as *heat* in the context of contemporary physiology, and also explain (in this same context) how acupuncture successfully treats bacterial and viral infections.

Chapter 9. Heart and small intestine

The heart functions

In contemporary physiology, the heart provides the force to move the blood, while the blood vessels are the physical structures that contain and circulate the blood. The largest blood vessels are the arteries, which carry the blood away from the heart. This begins with the *aorta* artery, which leaves the heart; it then branches off into the other arteries which supply the head, organs and limbs. The veins are similar to arteries, only they have a thinner wall, and their function is to return the deoxygenated blood back to the heart—at a lower pressure. As the arteries branch, they become smaller, and the smallest ones are termed *arterioles*. The smallest of these break up into minute vessels called *capillaries*. The wall of a capillary consists of a single layer of endothelial cells through which water and other small-molecule substances can pass. These form a bed which is the site of the exchange of substances between the blood and the tissue fluid which baths the body's cells. In this way, nutrients (such as oxygen) are transferred from the blood into the cells, and any waste products (such as CO_2) are transferred from the cells back into the blood, which process is known as *gas exchange*.[1]

In Chinese medicine, the functions and effects of the heart are that it

1. works closely with the lungs,
2. has a close association with the tongue and faculty of speech, and
3. has mental and emotional functions.

1. Works closely with the lungs

This is a direct function rather than an effect.

The *Nei Jing* authors (or their ancestors) noticed that when the heart function was poor, the following symptoms (amongst others) could occur:

- shortness of breath,
- profuse sweating,
- chills, and
- listlessness or lassitude (p.196).

They also noticed that when the lung function was poor, the following, similar symptoms could occur:

- shortness of breath,
- sweating,
- feeling cold, and
- lack of energy (p.143).

When stressed, either of the organs could produce these very similar symptoms. The main factor that differentiates between the two organs is that if the lungs produce the symptoms, the patient also has a cough; but if the heart produces the symptoms, the patient has palpitations.

Since both organs could produce very similar symptoms, it must have seemed to the *Nei Jing* authors that the function of the two organs was inextricably linked. And this idea was expressed in their metabolic theories.

Extract from *Ling Shu*, Chapter 71

The five grains enter the stomach. The dregs, the *jin* and *ye* liquids and the [chest influence (*zong chi*)] are separated to enter three channels. The [chest influence] collects in the chest, it leaves the chest through the windpipe. It penetrates the heart vessels, and it is responsible for ex- and inhalation.[2]

It should be noted that the *Nei Jing* authors had no notion of the blood circulatory system known today. The "meridians" (*jing mai*) were thought to be deep, artery-like tubes, which both the blood and influences (*chi*) flowed through, but rather than following the paths of the literal arteries (as known today), they were thought to lie deep to the *pathways on the skin*, which is what we today call the meridians (p.29). The term "collaterals" referred to the superficial veins or arterioles (as known today) which were used for bleeding a patient. And they were thought to branch off from the "meridians". Both the blood and influences (*chi*) were thought to flow throughout this whole network, but the blood was considered to be a purely nutritive substance (p.42); hence this system could not be said to equate to the blood circulatory system known today. These differences in the meanings of these common terms (meridian, collateral, artery, vein) cause much confusion when interpreting *Nei Jing* passages today.

The term *mai* 脈 ("vessel") was used to refer to the "meridians" (*jing mai*) or the collaterals (*luo mai*), but when the term was used alone, its meaning could be referring to either (p.16). Therefore the term "heart vessels" in the above extract may refer to the "meridians" related to the heart (though such terms in *Nei Jing* passages are often open to interpretation). But the important point is that the passage seems to encapsulate the notion of the heart and lungs both sharing the chest influence (*zong chi*), which was thought to enable the function of both organs.

Extract from *Su Wen*, Chapter 10

When the five [influences] enter the nose, they are stored by heart and lung. When heart and lung have a disease, the nose is not free as a result.[3]

Ma Shi (in 1586) commented on the above

Of the five [*yin* organs (*zang*)], only heart and lung are located above the diaphragm and receive these five [influences]. Hence when heart and lung have a disease, the nose is impassable as a result.[4]

And Zhang Zhenyu (in 1984) commented

The character 肚 should be interpreted as 深 "deep". This is to say, the clear [influence] that is inhaled enters deep into the heart and the lung.[5]

Extract from *Nan Jing*, Section 32

The heart is associated with the blood; the lung is associated with the influences. The blood is occupied with constructive functions; the influences are occupied with [defensive] functions. They follow each other, moving up and down in [the body]. They are called constructive and [defensive] influences. They proceed through the [meridians and collaterals] and circulate through the body's external regions.[6]

This *Nan Jing* passage introduces extra confusion to the *Nei Jing* theories on metabolism. The term "constructive influence" is now being used to refer to the blood,[7] whereas in the *Nei Jing*, the term usually referred to something extracted from ingested food—the *yin* part of "food influence" was separated to become "constructive influence", while the *yang* part became "defensive influence" (p.24); whereas the blood was formed separately from the liquids extracted from ingested food (p.42). However, the passage encapsulates the notion of the heart and lungs working closely together. And this is reinforced in the following commentary on the above passage.

Yü Shu (in 1067) commented on the above extract

The heart masters the blood; the blood is occupied with constructive functions. The lung masters the influences; the influences are occupied with [defensive] functions. The flow of the blood relies on the movement of the [defensive] influences; the movement of these influences depends on the flow of the blood. Blood and influences proceed through [the body] in mutual dependency.[8]

The notion of the blood and influences being interdependent, reinforces the notion that the function of the heart and lungs were considered to be interdependent. Or perhaps it was the other way around, and it was the realization that the heart and lungs work closely together that inspired the theory that the flow of the blood and influences are interdependent.

In contemporary physiology, there is also close cooperation between the heart and lungs, in the *pulmonary circulation*. The deoxygenated blood from the body returns to the heart via the *venae cavae* (the two largest veins in the body) and enters the right *atrium* of the heart. It then passes to the heart's right *ventricle* and is pumped into the *pulmonary artery*. This carries the deoxygenated blood to the lungs (the pulmonary artery divides into two, to supply each lung). Within the lungs the pulmonary arteries divide into smaller arteries, *arterioles* and *capillaries*. Gas exchange takes place between the air in the *alveoli* of the lungs and the blood in the capillaries (oxygen passing from the air into the blood, and CO_2 passing from the blood into the air). The capillaries which contain the oxygenated blood, join up to form two veins in each lung, the *pulmonary veins*, which then leave each lung and return the oxygenated blood to the left atrium of the heart. This passes into the left ventricle and is pumped out into the *aorta*, which is the first artery of the general blood circulation in the body.[9]

This validates the *Nei Jing* authors' observations. Having no knowledge of this close "plumbing" between the heart and lungs, they managed, over two thousand years ago, to deduce that this close cooperation existed by merely observing symptoms. It is true that in

Nei Jing metabolism there was no notion of the blood being oxygenated, but instead it was imagined that the close cooperation consisted of the blood and influences flowing together and interdependently in the "meridians". Every aspect of these details was untrue; the "meridians" were imaginary vessels, which were not related to today's blood circulatory system, and a vapour-like substance known as "influence" (*chi*) does not flow in these imaginary "meridians", and, strictly speaking, *chi* cannot even be said to exist (p.49). But nonetheless they deduced that close cooperation existed between the two organs.

The function of "circulating the blood"

In today's Chinese medicine, it is often stated that the heart is responsible for circulating the blood "just the same as in Western medicine", and that this circulation takes place in the same arteries and veins known today.[10] No such notions existed in the minds of the *Nei Jing* or the *Nan Jing* authors, nor in the minds of Chinese commentators for most of the two thousand years that followed. Neither the lungs or the heart were thought to provide any pump-like action (p.42). And the blood was considered to flow in the network of "meridians" and collaterals, along with the influences. It is true that the collaterals were the same veins and arterioles known today, and that these were thought to flow into deeper artery-like tubes, which were know as the "meridians". However, these "meridians" could not be considered to be the literal arteries known today (since they were imagined to follow the same routes as the *pathways on the skin*, which is what we today call the meridians; therefore the actual "meridians" imagined in the *Nei Jing*, did not really exist), and since the heart was not considered to serve any pump-like action, the two systems could not be considered equivalent.

This is perhaps a little confusing, but the confusion only arises when *Nei Jing* terms are considered to have the same meaning that those terms have today. To properly understand the *Nei Jing*, I feel it is better to not fall into this trap.

The *Nei Jing* notions of metabolism were often contradictory (being based on theory alone), so that it is difficult to make any single, definitive statement on any aspect of it. It was theorized by some *Nei Jing* authors that the influences found their way into the "meridians" via the lungs, but others theorized that the influences took other routes; and in most passages, it seems likely that the intended meaning was that influences were self-propelling. In which case, the same notion must have applied to the blood. It seems that the notion of these substances being propelled along the "meridians" by some outside force did not occur to the *Nei Jing* authors—and why should it? Influences were thought to consist of a vapour-like substance, and when such substances were seen in nature, why would the observer imagine some separate force was required to propel them? It seems more likely that they considered such phenomena to be inherently self-propelling, just as a river or stream might have seemed to be.

In the above extract from Section 32 of the *Nan Jing* (p.185), there is no notion portrayed of either the blood or influences requiring any propulsive force outside of themselves. It is merely stated that "They follow each other, moving up and down in [the body]…. They proceed through the [meridians and collaterals] and circulate through the body's external regions." And in the commentary that follows the quote, the notion portrayed is that the flow of the blood and of the defensive influences (*wei chi*) each depended on the flow of the other.

The notion that the heart propels the blood, and that this causes the blood to travel through the network of the literal arteries and veins, this notion is invented by today's Chinese medicine (the ideas clearly adopted from contemporary physiology) and are alien to the Chinese medicine of the *Nei Jing*, and of most of the two thousand years that followed.

Of course, when interpreting the *Nei Jing*, it is tempting to see meanings in the text that are informed by today's knowledge of anatomy and physiology. But it seems to me that this tendency only makes Chinese medicine even harder to understand. The theories of the *Nei Jing* are muddled enough already; they are not improved by modifying parts of them to attempt to reconcile them with contemporary anatomy and physiology. This only reduces clarity, rather than improving it.

The heart's relationship with the "vessels"

In Chapter 9 of the *Su Wen*, it is said "The heart... Its effulgence is in the face. Its fullness manifests itself in the blood vessels."[11]

The task of interpreting such an apparently simple statement provides a good insight into the "muddle" of the *Nei Jing*. The first part "Its effulgence is in the face," is straightforward. When a person's heart is healthy, you can clearly see this in their complexion; or more notably, when a person's heart is stressed, their complexion becomes distinctly lacklustre. Since this is so obvious in clinic today, it is safe to assume that the *Nei Jing* authors also made this same clinical observation—so that the statement is therefore fact based and straightforward. However, the second part of the quote "Its fullness manifests itself in the blood vessels," is problematic.

Today, it might be tempting to interpret "blood vessels" as referring to the literal arteries and veins. But since the *Nei Jing* authors considered the blood to flow in the "meridians" (imaginary, artery-like tubes) together with the influences (p.42), this cannot be the case.

Wang Bing (in 762 AD), commented on this *Su Wen* passage: "The heart nourishes the blood; it rules the movement in the vessels. Hence the text states: *Its fullness manifests itself in the blood vessels.*"[12]

This interpretation now seems to make the passage consistent with the extract from Section 32 of the *Nan Jing* (quoted on page 185 above), which states that the "heart is associated with the blood" and that the blood and influences move together through the "meridians". Hence, Wang Bing's comment "The heart nourishes the blood; it rules the movement in the vessels," *could* be understood as saying that good quality blood is required for there to be good "movement in the vessels".

But now another problem arises. What did Wang Bing mean by "The heart nourishes the blood"? The *Nei Jing* authors theorized that the blood was formed from liquids extracted from ingested food, and that the manufacture took place either in the stomach or in the "meridians", depending on which author you choose to follow (p.42), so how could the heart "nourish the blood"? If taken literally, this notion seems incompatible with the other

Nei Jing notions of how blood is manufactured.

And what did the *Nan Jing* passage (quoted on page 185) mean by "The heart is associated with the blood"? What is the connection between the heart and the blood? In *Nei Jing* metabolism and physiology, the blood is manufactured by the digestive organs (either the stomach or the stomach and pancreas combined); the blood then flows in the "meridians"; the heart has no pump-like function (as we think of it today) and the blood is therefore assumed to be self-propelling; so how, exactly, is the heart associated with the blood? It has nothing to do with its manufacture or propulsion.

The task of finding a concrete meaning in an apparently simple *Nei Jing* statement can sometimes be daunting. If the statement is considered in isolation, a suitable interpretation may present itself, but when the statement is then compared with the various (often contradictory) notions of *Nei Jing* metabolism and physiology, your interpretation may no longer stand up to scrutiny.

For example, the *Nei Jing* term "blood vessel" usually refers to the collaterals—that is, the superficial veins (p.29). Bearing this in mind, if we then consider the statement that "the heart is associated with the blood," this now seems to make sense, since, in contemporary physiology, the heart pumps the blood which circulates in the veins, therefore by looking at the blood in the veins (as visible through the skin), we might consider that we can detect the effects of the heart's pumping action. But if we then consider this statement in relation to *Nei Jing* metabolism and physiology, those same veins (collaterals) would now be considered to branch off from the "meridians", to carry both blood and influences (just as the "meridians" were thought to), and for these substances to be self-propelling—so that there would now be no association between the heart and the blood that flows in these veins.

This type of problem may stem from the fact that the *Nei Jing* notions of metabolism were mainly theoretical and not based on any *useful* knowledge of internal anatomy or physiology—and sometimes based on no knowledge of this at all. This probably explains why different authors made contradictory statements, and also perhaps why the language is often vague and open to interpretation.

When interpreting *Nei Jing* passages, it is helpful to be aware of which statements appear to be based on practical observation and which seem to be theoretical—and therefore possibly untrue.

Wang Bing's statement "The heart nourishes the blood; it rules the movement in the vessels" may be theoretical, though its vagueness makes it difficult to be certain. If the statement *does* refer to a practical observation, the following is the only observation I can think of that *might* fit the words.

What the *Nei Jing* authors called a "movement in the vessels" (related to a particular "meridian"), in today's Chinese medicine, is called an organ's "pulse". And when the heart has an "excess-type" condition (p.454), its "pulse" would usually be "full" and strong. Hence, when the heart is in an "excess" condition, this produces an "excess" movement in the vessels. It is possible that this simple observation is what the statement was referring to. Wang Bing could not have meant that the heart literally "nourishes the blood", since this contradicts all *Nei Jing* notions of metabolism, so he may have meant that the heart's state is merely *reflected* in the blood as it flows through the "meridians".

It could be argued that the state of *all* the organs are reflected in the organ "pulses". But at the time of the *Nei Jing*, bloodletting was a common therapy, and there was a connection between heart stress and the heart "pulse" being "full" and therefore the "meridian" needing to be incised to let out the excess blood. It is true that other organs can also adopt an "excess" state in this same way, but perhaps Wang Bing was most familiar with this concept in relation to the heart. If so, this may have been the practical observation he had in mind, and what he meant by "the heart nourishes the blood" was simply that the heart produces an excess which is apparently present in the blood, and hence in the "movement in the vessels". And note that this interpretation would also fit the *Su Wen* statement that Wang Bing was striving to explain: "The heart... Its fullness manifests itself in the blood vessels" (p.187).

An author, who is perhaps primarily a healer, could be forgiven for not being a good writer and hence producing a vague or sloppy description which lends itself to misinterpretation. This is a common scenario today, so it would not be surprising to find examples of such writing in ancient China.

Lastly, if Wang Bing's statement *were* interpreted literally today, it could have little *practical* application anyway, since, in reality, the blood cannot be "nourished" by the heart, and the "movement in the vessels" (i.e. the organ pulses) are determined by the health of the particular organ associated with each meridian. Therefore the statement could only be seen as being either theoretical and unrelated to reality,[*] or being badly expressed and having some meaning other than the obvious literal interpretation that might occur to us today.

2. Has a close association with the tongue and faculty of speech

This is an indirect effect rather than a function.

The *Nei Jing* authors noticed that when a person had poor heart function, they would often also have speech defects (such as stammering or stuttering) which cleared once the heart was successfully treated,[13] and this association is still routinely encountered in clinic today. This suggests that the good function of the heart is essential for the speech to work smoothly.

The heart is said to be connected to the tongue via a meridian that ascends from the heart and travels to the root of the tongue.[14] This meridian connection provides a possible mechanism to enable the heart's health to be reflected in the speech. There is also an explanation in the heart's mental function (p.194), but this supposed[15] meridian link could contribute to any effects by impeding the tongue's mobility, as follows. When an organ is stressed, its related acupoints become tender, which could only be due to some aspect of the local tissue ceasing to function properly (p.369); and in the same way, the local tissue at the tongue may also cease to function properly when the heart is stressed.

[*] See also pages 276-277 for an analysis of passages where Wang Bing used five phase theory to construct explanations that are clearly untrue.

However, the above explanations are currently only hypothetical. And beyond the practical observations (mentioned in the second paragraph above), there is no knowledge in contemporary anatomy and physiology to explain the association between the heart and speech. Therefore the association can only currently be regarded as an indirect effect of some aspect of the heart function.

3. Has mental and emotional functions

In contemporary physiology, the main physical function of the heart is to circulate blood to every other organ and part of the body, through the system of arteries and veins.

This book's approach to explaining the mental functions of the organs is to start by considering the intention of the organ. The heart's physical function appears to be simple, but to properly understand the intention behind it, it is necessary to consider how this system of blood vessels may have evolved.

If we again imagine a hypothetical creature at the stage when the embryonic organs began to evolve—there must have already been primitive blood vessels connecting the heart to the other embryonic organs (by an "embryonic" organ, I mean the earliest *functional* mass of tissue that would later evolve into the organ we recognise today). And since the other embryonic organs could not have existed in a substantial form *without* there being a blood supply to nourish their tissue, it seems likely that this embryonic network of blood vessels must have gradually formed at the same time that the embryonic organs were forming.

One possible scenario is that all the embryonic organs, together with the embryonic network of blood vessels, may have initially existed in a single "mass of activity", concerned with digesting food particles and converting them into usable energy and other nourishment. And over (perhaps) millions of years, this "mass of activity" gradually developed specialist areas within it, as the processes demanded. And as these separate, specialist areas first formed, there may have been the rudimentary beginnings of the blood vessels which connected *one* of these specialist areas (the one which would later become the heart) to all the other specialist areas (the other embryonic organs) within the mass of tissue.

By the time this hypothetical stage was reached, the embryonic heart's intention must have already come into existence; and the connection of itself to the other embryonic organs—so that it could supply nourishment to them—was a "design" that must have been created by this intention. Or possibly the other way around; that is, the fact of this connective network being required, dictated the heart's intention.

This intention could be summarized in words as: *to reach out to those around it and spread nourishment to them.* As regards the evolution of the organ system, the term "those around it" refers to the other organs. This wording also summarizes the heart's function (since its physical function and its intention are one and the same—p.93).

The heart function is used to process our thoughts

Over millions of years, each organ evolved logic to enable it to carry out its functions and coordinate these with the other organs (p.91). And once our conscious mind started having complex thoughts about the world around us, it is possible that this pre-existing organ logic may have been used to process such thoughts. Today, this notion is supported by the clear two-way associations between the heart function and certain of our mental processes, as described in the remainder of this chapter.

The thoughts produced by the heart function

The heart function could be summarized as: *to reach out to those around it and spread nourishment to them.* In our mental and emotional lives, there are two main situations in which this function is applied. The first is when we feel concern for other people or feel affection for our friends or loved ones; and the second is when we feel the desire to share our knowledge or good fortune with others.

When we feel concern for another person, we can often sense that this emotion originates from the heart; and when sensing this, some people even physically clutch their chest over the heart region. This knowledge has clearly existed in society for a long time, since it is fossilized in our language, in phrases such as "my heart goes out to them". And whenever we care for someone in this way, we may also experience a "warm glow" in the heart. Why do we feel this sensation?

The heart function is *to reach out to other people and spread nourishment to them*, and when this function is used to process our thoughts, this produces our concern for other people. This concern is probably the strongest mental expression of the heart function we could make; and this emphasizes the heart function in our thoughts. This emphasis is then duplicated in the heart, causing us to feel that warm glow. That is, the heart feels unusually energized. This is similar to the way the heart may feel after a bout of physical exercise; that is, a bout of vigorously spreading nourishment to those around it (the other organs).

This effect happens even if we only *think* fondly of another person, so that just the idea itself is able to enhance the heart function and produce that warm glow within it.

When we simply talk to other people, a similar effect happens. Again, we are *reaching out to other people and spreading nourishment to them.* In the human context, this nourishment simply involves information about the world. In creatures who do not have the faculty of speech, the sounds they produce would constitute "nourishment" in some other way. Much of the animal sounds that have been understood by us (including bird song and the sounds produced by many mammals) are clearly providing information about the world to the other creatures around them, such as warnings of possible danger and so on.

You may have noticed that when talking to someone socially, you can sometimes feel a sensation like a mild glow within your heart—it feels good to talk. But when merely listening to the other person, this feeling is not there. It seems it is the action of *spreading information to others* that produces this effect, no matter what the information is. The act of simply talking to others appears to engage the heart function mentally, which then enhances the heart's physical function.

How this affects the health of the heart

As well as the heart function being enhanced in this way, the reverse is also possible. When the heart logic is used to process our thoughts but that logic is impeded or blocked by our conscious mind, this situation is duplicated in the heart which then behaves as though its *physical* function were being impeded. There are many situations in our daily lives where this scenario could apply.

Suppose you feel concern for someone (which may be an unfortunate person you see in the street, or a friend or work colleague who is in a difficult situation) but instead of acting on your concern and doing something to help them, you walk away. In this situation, your concern was produced by your heart's intention, which wanted to *reach out to those around you and spread nourishment to them*. And when your conscious mind overruled this emotion and you walked away, this impeded your heart's intention and hence also its physical function, which may have caused you to feel a physical pang in your heart as you walked away. That feeling was the physical discomfort your heart felt when its function was impeded. And if, after the event, you kept recalling that unfortunate person's plight, your heart would continue to feel the discomfort of having its function impeded. In this situation, you might sometimes be so aware of your heart's discomfort that this may cause you to finally do something to help the person, which would then remove this impediment to your heart function and bring relief.

Suppose that during the course of your work you were required to adopt a position you knew was morally wrong. You knew that the right thing to do was to reach out and assist a person in some way but your particular work role required you to overrule your emotions and do the opposite. Or suppose you decided to be dishonest towards a particular person, or in a particular situation. In all these types of situations, your heart's intention to *reach out to those around you and spread nourishment to them*, is impeded and consequently your heart's *physical* function would be impeded. You might feel "heavy in the heart", or as though a "dark cloud" were passing over your heart. Or with some people this impediment to their heart function would immediately affect their speech (due to the association between the heart and speech) and at the instant they started lying, or saying something they felt was morally wrong, or simply adopting a position they knew was morally wrong, they might start to stutter or stammer.

This happens with people who otherwise have no problem with their heart function (what we might call "normal" people in their everyday lives) but because they adopt this conduct that they know to be morally wrong, this impedes their heart's intention and they develop a mild stammer or stutter, which clears when they change the topic of conversation.

The heart also uses sight to communicate

When we consciously overrule the heart's intention in this way, we might also be unable to look the other person in the eye. This action of us looking the other person in the eye is another expression of the heart's intention to *reach out to them and spread nourishment to them*; but in this case the connection is made by using eyesight as the means of communication. But since our conscious mind has impeded the heart's intention (by us being dishonest, and so on), it also impedes our ability to look the other person in the eye.

The connection between the organ functions and our thoughts is immediate

These physical effects usually occur instantly; we feel the heaviness in our heart or the detriment to our speech or our inability to make eye contact, the moment our conscious mind chooses to overrule the heart's intention. This demonstrates just how direct the connection is between the heart's physical function and any of our thought processes that utilize the heart's logic.

These effects, though, would be felt to different degrees by different people. The more sensitive a person is, the more likely they would be to notice any impediments in their social connections, and therefore the more likely it would be for their speech to be affected by such things; or for the degree of their speech impediment to be greater.

Another example of an impediment in our connection to *those around us* is when we are involved in a dispute of any kind. Because our connection to those people is "faulty", this fault is duplicated in the heart function.

> **Patient example**
> Male, aged 49. This patient initially sought treatment following chest pains. He suffered a suspected heart attack and was found to have an inflamed pericardium. He was involved in a long-standing serious dispute with one of his neighbours, which had certainly caused a pain in the patient's jaw and probably also contributed to his heart problems. See the full case history on page 253.

Another obvious example of this phenomenon is when a relationship or friendship ends. This type of relationship is probably the most powerful mental and emotional expression of the heart's intention to *reach out to those around us and spread nourishment to them.* And we would have built a large part of our lives around that particular connection, which is then suddenly broken. Such a break is probably the greatest impediment that could be made to the mental application of the heart's intention, which impediment is duplicated in the physical heart, causing us to experience an intense pain in the heart and (with sensitive people) possibly even palpitations (see the case histories on pages 254-255, where palpitations and panic attacks were triggered by such a loss).

Loneliness weakens the heart

A similar situation is loneliness. This involves, in effect, a conscious suppressing of the heart's intention to *reach out to those around us.* This is a fundamental aspect of the heart's intention and when we mentally block it, or impede it, this impediment is duplicated in the physical heart which produces that feeling of "heaviness" in the heart—the physical pain of loneliness.

It is certainly possible to die of a "broken heart" or to eventually die from loneliness; such a death would usually occur due to a heart attack. Heart attacks have always been far more common amongst men than women. This may be because, socially, men have always been much more alone than women. In most societies it is the normal practice for women to talk to one another about their emotional concerns, or about anything that troubles them. But with men, such talk is usually discouraged and even socially frowned upon. This creates in them a great sense of loneliness. Ultimately, they have no-one to confide in and must cope alone with whatever troubles they have. Due to social pressures, their conscious mind suppresses their heart's intention to *reach out to those around them*, and in doing this they impede their heart's physical function. Eventually this could lead to a heart attack.

It is also notable that speech defects such as stammering or stuttering are much more common amongst men than women, which seems to reflect the fact that men are required by most societies to adopt a persona that is bad for their heart.

On page 190, I said that the circulatory system may have evolved due to the expression of the heart's intention. Its desire to *reach out to those around it and spread nourishment to them* may have resulted in the evolution of the arteries and other blood vessels—spreading out from the heart and feeding the other organs and every tissue in the body. In people who suffer heart attacks, they sometimes also have diseases of their blood vessels. Or some people may suffer serious arterial disease before any pronounced defect is noticed in their heart. In such people, their social connections with the people around them may have been severely impeded (or "faulty") for years. These social connections are the mental expression of the heart function, and any impediment in this mental expression is duplicated in the heart, producing poor heart function, but also—since the fault is in our *connection* with other people—producing faults in the arteries and veins (which are the heart's connections to the other organs and areas of the body). In other words, our social connections are diseased, so our physical blood vessels become diseased.

Simply talking, or helping others, improves the heart's health

On the other hand, when we do something that seems good or morally correct, such as helping others, this emphasizes the heart's intention within our thoughts, which emphasis is duplicated in the physical heart, strengthening its function and possibly producing that "warm glow" or a similar feeling in the heart. And any other action that is an expression of the heart's intention to *reach out to those around us and spread nourishment to them*, would also have a beneficial effect on the heart. Simply talking to other people socially will do this, as will sharing our knowledge in some way.

Other effects on speech

Our *connections with other people* are produced by the mental application of the heart's intention. And when a person has poor heart function, these connections would also tend to be poor, or "faulty". This could cause the person to have doubts about their position in society, or their worth in relation to other people, or to have other similar doubts or concerns. This may cause them to constantly try to please other people or to be inappropriately smiling and using an amused tone of voice.[16] And since speech is the main vehicle the heart uses to form these connections with other people, this could also cause "faults" in the person's speech, such as them speaking in inappropriate ways, making socially inept comments, or pouring out indiscriminate words—saying whatever words entered their head, to whoever would listen.

They would certainly be prone to talking too much, and could appear unable to stop talking, which may cause further social problems (further faults in their connections with other people), such as causing people to avoid their company. This would only fuel the person's insecurity, focussing their conscious mind on this "fault" in their connections with other people, causing the fault to be further duplicated in their heart's physical function, which would, in turn, only increase their tendency to adopt such behaviour—until the cycle is broken.

Poor heart function can cause dyslexia

Written words or numbers (and such things as written music) are another medium through which communication takes place, and just as with speech, written words or numbers must have originally been devised in response to the heart's intention to *reach out to those around us and spread nourishment to them.* In other words, they are yet another expression of the heart's intention.

In patients, the start of speech defects or dyslexia can sometimes be clearly linked to disruptions in their relationships. For example, when a child's parents split up, or the child loses a parent or sibling or close friend for some other reason, the child can sometimes develop such problems. This would certainly be more so with a sensitive child, since they would be more aware of their connections with other people and therefore more affected by any disruptions in them.

The same process that produces speech defects in us, can also be responsible for making it hard for us to smoothly read words, numbers or written music. Since these faculties are also an expression of our heart's intention, any awareness we have of "faults" in our social connections (particularly in childhood) would cause those faults to be duplicated in our heart function, which, in turn, could impede our ability to smoothly read words or numbers.

If such symptoms (and the underlying poor heart function) were caused by the person's "faulty" relationships, once the relationship issues were resolved, their poor heart function would tend to eventually rectify and the speech problems or dyslexia would clear. But treating the poor heart function with acupuncture helps the person's heart to more quickly and more fully recover from the damage caused to it by the relationship issues.

Heart transplants seem to confirm the heart's mental function

Experiences reported by many heart transplant patients seem to confirm the mental and emotional functions of the heart. After their transplant, many recipients reported having new memories that appear to have come from the donor. The memories concern the donor's connections with other people, or memories of the things they loved; in other words, their emotional attachments to the things in their lives. These include preferences inherited from the donor related to food, art, music, sexual and recreational activities, and even the name of the donor's partner. Some striking examples are a young girl who received a heart transplant from a murder victim and then had such vivid memories of the victim's interaction with their murderer that these were able to be used by the police to apprehend and convict the murderer. In another case, a militant lesbian who received a heart transplant from another woman, became straight. And a vegetarian, after a heart transplant, started having irresistible cravings for meat, and meat of the particular kind that was loved by the heart donor.

Experiences of this type are so commonly reported by heart transplant patients that serious studies have been conducted of the phenomenon.[17,18] In all cases, the memories contained in the implanted heart were related to the mental and emotional functions of the heart: *to reach out to other people and spread nourishment to them*; in other words, to interact with people, care for people (and things) and to form emotional attachments to them.

The other fascinating implication is that the heart itself may store our memories of these emotional attachments. This would seem to add strength to the argument that it is the organs themselves that process our thoughts, rather than this being done by a brain-matter copy of an organ's logic, or some similar arrangement (p.94). But on the other hand, this may only apply to the heart; or it may suggest that it is only the related memories that are stored by the organs themselves, while the processing of our thoughts *is* done by the brain-matter copy of each organ's logic. Again, this issue is largely of academic interest. However, such evidence from heart transplant patients *does* add even further weight to the argument that the abdominal organs produce most of our thoughts.

Improper function

Poor heart function

The *Nei Jing* authors (or their ancestors) noticed that when a patient had poor heart function (also called "Heart chi deficiency") they tended to have a selection of the signs and symptoms from list "A" below. The signs and symptoms included in lists "B" to "G" below are possible complications of poor heart function. Likewise, it was noticed that when a patient had poor heart function, they might also develop any of these extra signs and symptoms (along with those in list "A").

A. Palpitations[19,20]; shortness of breath on exertion[19,21]; spontaneous sweating[20]; lethargy; and a weak pulse.
B. Anxiety, panic attacks, restlessness, unease[19,20]; being easily startled by noises or anything unexpected in the immediate environment; speech defects such as stammering or stuttering[13]; dyslexia[22]; poor long-term memory[23]; dream-disturbed sleep[21]; insomnia.
C. Low grade fever during the day (hot flushes); night sweating[20]; feeling a sensation of heat on the soles of the feet and palms of the hands[24]; dry mouth, or feeling constantly thirsty.[20,25]
D. Stuffiness or stabbing pains in the chest, which may radiate to the left shoulder and arm[26,25]; and possibly also a blue-purple tinge to the face, lips and nails.
E. Muttering to oneself[27]; depression or mental dullness; introverted manner, unable to make eye contact[13,23]; incessant or incoherent talking[20]; violent behaviour (hitting or scolding people); laughing and crying without reason[16,27]; paranoia,[23] hysteria, mental confusion[20,27]; aphasia (partial loss of the ability to communicate with

words*); loss of consciousness (sudden collapse or coma).

F. Chills, cold limbs[20]; and a blue tinge to the lips.

G. Profuse sweating; feeble breathing; feeble and fading pulse; mental "cloudiness" or even coma.

Face colour, tone of voice, and food craving

It was noticed that when a patient had poor heart function, this would often produce a red complexion.[28]

Chapter 10 of the *Su Wen* states "If the complexion is generated by the heart, it resembles vermilion wrapped up in white silk."[29]

Such a patient would also tend to have an amused tone of voice, as though they were constantly about to laugh,[16] and they would tend to crave bitter food.[30]

Treatment

When a patient has poor heart function (has signs and symptoms from list "A" above), the following acupoints tend to become tender. When one of these acupoints is stimulated, this encourages the organ to cancel out the malfunction in itself that caused the tenderness (p.372), and the organ returns to normal function. In this way, the problem is corrected by the organ itself (p.78):

- Heart-7 (*Shenmen*),
- Pericardium-6 (*Neiguan*),
- Bladder-15 (*Xinshu*), and
- Ren-14 (*Juque*).

* There is a graphic example of this in the patient example on page 245.

The causes of poor heart function

This condition can be caused by the steadily declining heart function due to a prolonged illness (just as the function of all the organs would be affected) or, in a similar fashion, after a sudden severe disease; or it may be due to the general decline of organ functions in old age; or due to a similar weakness being inherited from our parents. It may also be caused by any of the mental or emotional factors mentioned from page 191 onwards, if these are present for a prolonged period.

In today's Chinese medicine, this condition is called "Heart chi deficiency", which is translated here as "poor heart function" (p.27). In contemporary medicine, this same condition may be described using various terms, including: arrhythmia, cardiac insufficiency, coronary arteriosclerosis, angina pectoris, or general weakness.[31]

Possible complications

The following conditions could be viewed as complications of poor heart function. In today's Chinese medicine these conditions are each given a specific term (described below), but it should be noted that none of these terms were used in the *Nei Jing* and have been adopted more recently (p.449).

Poor quality blood

When a patient has poor heart function, they might also have any of the symptoms included in list "B" on page 196 above. In today's Chinese medicine, it is recognised that such patients would also usually have poor quality blood (also called "Blood deficiency").

In this case, the condition would then be called "Heart blood deficiency".

When the quality of a patient's blood becomes poor, this would usually have occurred as a result of poor function of the digestive organs, particularly the pancreas,* possibly combined with a poor diet (which itself could be a result of poor pancreas function, which may produce a poor appetite and intolerances to some staple foods, such as wheat). The weakened digestive organs are then unable to manufacture blood of sufficient quality to nourish the body and organs, including the heart and the literal blood vessels.

Many of the symptoms in list "B" are of a mental or emotional nature. Using concepts from contemporary physiology, these could be accounted for as follows.

Since the patient's blood is of poor quality (and after a while, even the tissue of the heart and blood vessels may also be affected), the heart cannot properly carry out its intention to *reach out to those around it and spread nourishment to them.* In other words, it cannot properly nourish the other organs and tissues of the body. This heart intention is also used to process our thoughts—where it causes us to form relationships with the people around us. And since the intention of the heart is impeded in the heart organ itself (in that it cannot now properly nourish the body), the mental application of its intention would also be impeded. It is as though our connections to the people around us are impeded, but we may not be consciously aware of why; we just feel that our connections are "faulty". And this could produce the symptoms of anxiety (concern about these poor connections with the people around us, which may be of an unspecified nature), restlessness, being easily startled (by noises and anything unexpected in the surrounding environment—which we are now fundamentally uneasy about), dream disturbed sleep, poor long term memory (memory of our connections with the people in our lives, the events and so on).

Today's Chinese medicine term of "Heart blood deficiency" could be interpreted to mean: the effects that poor quality blood has on the heart. In contemporary medicine, this same condition may be described using various terms, such as: insomnia, anaemia, severe malnutrition, or depressive neuroses such as postnatal depression following haemorrhage during or after childbirth.[32]

Treatment

Since this condition usually develops due to poor pancreas function, the main pancreas acupoints would usually be tender (due to the association between the pancreas and these acupoints), which include Pancreas-6† (*Daheng*) and Bladder-20 (*Pishu*). As usual, needling these acupoints utilizes this same association but in reverse, so tends to normalize the pancreas function, which would improve the body's ability to manufacture blood. Bladder-17 (*Geshu*) is often also tender in patients with poor quality blood and is therefore also frequently used in the treatment.

Since poor heart function is also present, this would also be treated, as described on page 197 above.

To treat insomnia, there is a frequently used empirical acupoint called, in Chinese, *Anmian*, which translates as: "peaceful sleep".

* Also called the spleen in Chinese medicine.

† Also called Spleen-6.

Empirical acupoints are sometimes not located on the main meridians but were found through experimentation. *Anmian* was found to become tender in some patients who suffer from insomnia, so can sometimes effectively treat insomnia.

> **Patient example**
> Female, aged 29. This patient had a history of depression and panic attacks, going back 18 months, and also suffered a wide range of other symptoms. After a few treatments, all her symptoms improved markedly. See the full case history on page 245.

How poor quality blood is diagnosed

When a patient has a number of the signs and symptoms from the following list, Chinese medicine considers them to have poor quality blood (also called "Blood deficiency"), since, theoretically, all the following signs and symptoms may be accounted for due to the organs and tissues of the body not being properly nourished:

- pale complexion and lips;
- pale tongue;
- dry skin and hair, dry and withered nails, or brittle nails;
- seeing dark or light specks floating in the visual field; and
- dizziness and vertigo (due to the brain not being properly nourished).[33]

This is a good example of the holistic approach used in Chinese medicine. There is a wide range of signs and symptoms listed above, all of which are treated by normalizing the function of the pancreas (the underlying cause) which improves the quality of the blood, so that the signs and symptoms gradually clear by themselves. The alternative approach would be to try to treat each symptom individually (for example, the dizziness, insomnia, dry skin and hair, anxiety, and so on) while leaving the function of the pancreas unchanged (the underlying cause).

In today's Chinese medicine, this condition is called "Blood deficiency"; and when this affects the heart, the combined condition is known as "Heart blood deficiency". In contemporary medicine, this same condition may be described as anaemia or malnutrition.

Internal production of heat

When body tissue is stressed or damaged (such as when overworked, diseased, wounded, or deprived of nourishment for some other reason), it often produces heat. And this same principle applies to the internal organs. When these are stressed in some way, they may produce heat.

In the case of patients with poor heart function, the heat produced by the stressed tissue of their heart would be experienced in the form of some, or all, of the symptoms in list "C" on page 196:

- low grade fever during the day (hot flushes);
- night sweating;
- feeling a sensation of heat on the soles of the feet and palms of the hands; and
- dry mouth, or feeling constantly thirsty.

As well as these general symptoms, the person would also be likely to experience more pronounced mental or emotional disturbances than with mere poor heart function alone (the symptoms in list "B" on page 196 above), which can be explained as follows.

Since the tissue of the heart is stressed to the point where it is producing heat, this would more severely impede the heart's intention to *reach out to those around it and spread nourishment to them* (i.e. circulate blood to nourish the organs). And this increased impediment would also be duplicated in the mental application of the heart's intention, causing an increased impediment in our connection with the people around us, which could worsen the following symptoms:

- anxiety, panic attacks, unease, restlessness, being easily startled;
- insomnia; and
- dream-disturbed sleep.

The translation of "Yin deficiency"

In today's Chinese medicine, this condition is known as "Yin deficiency". And when the heart is affected in this way, this is known as "Heart yin deficiency". In this book, I have translated "Yin deficiency" as "internal production of heat".

But (hypothetically speaking) when the *Nei Jing* authors considered such symptoms, how might they have theoretically accounted for them?

In the minds of the *Nei Jing* authors, the organs were generally considered as "administrative centres" within a metaphorical system that resembled the organization of the state. These "centres" then mainly stored or processed the grain "brought in from the fields" (as it were). Each "centre", like any other phenomenon in nature, was considered to be made up of *yin* and *yang* forces, which interact to produce a state of equilibrium. The *yang* element, in this case, could be considered to be the activity of the "administrative centre", while the *yin* element could be the resources themselves that were being processed. When there is a lessening of the *yin*, this is usually accompanied by an increase in *yang*. *Yang* is comparatively hot in nature (more aggressive or active than *yin*; for example, fire is *yang* while water is *yin*), therefore an increase in *yang* produces heat. Therefore (their thinking might have been) when the resources have diminished (i.e. there is less nourishment to the heart), then the *yin* has diminished, therefore the *yang* would increase, which would explain the unusual warmth.

This (hypothetical) argument *could* be seen as analogous to the explanation I gave above using concepts from contemporary physiology (i.e. when an organ's tissue is stressed or damaged, this produces heat, just as damaged tissue does anywhere on the body). Yet, the *yin-yang* argument is still difficult for today's minds to grasp, since we do not think in that way about the body and health. But by instead describing a possible scenario using concepts from contemporary physiology which *could* account for this same phenomenon, this hopefully enables today's minds to understand the condition, and thus accept the validity of the *Nei Jing* practical observations of symptoms.

In contemporary medicine, this same condition (of "Heart yin deficiency") may be described using various terms, such as: arrhythmia, tachycardia, hypertension, hyperthyroidism, or anxiety neurosis.[34]

Treatment—the body's ability to self regulate

When patients have this condition, poor heart function and probably also poor quality blood would usually have been present for some time, and the condition would be addressed by treating those underlying causes.

However, the function of the other main organs is likely to also be affected (since their nourishment is impeded), producing a wide range of other signs and symptoms. But as a general rule, when the function of a single of the main organs is normalized by acupuncture treatment, the entire organ network appears to have an almost miraculous ability to self-regulate. The functions of all the organs are interrelated and therefore complex situations can sometimes develop between them, producing a wide range of signs and symptoms—on the physical, mental and emotional levels. But, perhaps due to this very interrelation, once a few of the key acupoints are needled, this appears to enable all the main organs to simply self-regulate. And after a few such treatments, patients often experience a dramatic improvement in their health, on every level. This principle applies when treating any of the main organs, not just the heart. And this self-regulatory ability tends to make the treatment of most patients straightforward*.

Stagnation of blood

When the heart function is poor, the blood may begin to stagnate. In other words the circulation may become too sluggish. In this case, the patient may experience a selection of the signs and symptoms of poor heart function (list "A" on page 196 above), but added to this would be the signs and symptoms from list "D".

In today's Chinese medicine, the condition is known as "Heart blood stagnation". In contemporary medicine, the same condition may be referred to as angina pectoris, or myocardial infarction (heart attack).[35]

Treatment

Since this condition is a complication of poor heart function, the treatment is the same as with poor heart function, only the following acupoints are often added:

- Bladder-17 (*Geshu*), or
- Pericardium-4 (*Ximen*).

These acupoints often become tender when the patient experiences blood stagnation. And, as with all acupoints, needling them encourages the body to clear the condition that caused the acupoints to become tender; in other words, to normalize the blood circulation.

As with all treatments, any other organs not functioning normally would usually be treated as well. In the case of "Heart blood stagnation" and poor quality blood, this may include the main digestive organs (the pancreas and stomach), since they would have usually been functioning poorly for some time in order for the quality of the blood to become poor—and there would be clear signs and symptoms related to the poor function of these organs.

* But see page 238, regarding the mind's ability to block acupuncture treatments; and page 258, regarding the tendency of pharmaceuticals to block all natural treatments.

Mental disorders

When describing the causes of poor heart function, I said that mental or emotional states (such as those described from page 191 onwards) could sometimes impede the function of the heart. This same principle works in both directions, and sometimes extreme mental problems can be caused by poor heart function. The *Nei Jing* authors observed that patients with poor heart function could sometimes develop any of the mental symptoms from list "E" on page 196 above.

The term "phlegm"

The mechanism responsible for causing these symptoms is similar to that described under the heading: "Poor quality blood" (p.197). The poor quality blood may impede the heart's intention to *reach out to those around it and spread nourishment to them* (i.e. prevents the heart from properly nourishing the other organs and tissues of the body), which would then correspondingly impede the mental application of this intention, causing problems in the patient's connections with the people around them, which is at the root of many of the symptoms in list "E".

However, with the present condition, the impediment is stronger than with mere poor quality blood. When poor quality blood is present, the digestive organs (particularly the pancreas) would have functioned poorly for some time, in which case the state of *dampness* would have existed for some time (p.76). In contemporary physiology, this state could be summarized as follows. The normal excess of glucose, fats and proteins that exists in the blood shortly after eating is not properly regulated (probably mainly due to poor pancreas function), which affects the supply of nutrition to all the organs and processes, which then produces a wide range of possible signs and symptoms.

When this *dampness* has existed for some time, the poor function of the organs and systems gradually worsens, producing an increase in the number or severity of the signs and symptoms.

In today's Chinese medicine, the *dampness* would now be regarded as having transformed into *phlegm*. Simplistically, this state could be visualized as a thickening of the "soup" of excess nutrients in the blood; and since this "soup" is regarded as pathogenic (in Chinese medicine), the pathogen would now be stronger.

Hence this current condition is known in today's Chinese medicine as "Phlegm misting the mind". The meaning of this poetic term can be understood as follows. The prolonged presence of *phlegm* impedes the heart's normal function of *reaching out to those around it* (the organs and tissues) *and spreading nourishment to them*, which also prevents it from performing this same function when processing our thoughts. In other words, it severely impedes our connections with the people around us, causing the symptoms in list "E" on page 196 above. That is, the phlegm "mists the mind".

In contemporary medicine, this same condition could be referred to using a variety of terms, including: hysteria, manic and depressive psychoses, stroke sequella, aphasia, epilepsy, and in children: speech or mental retardation.[36]

Treatment

As well as directly treating the poor heart function, the patient's main digestive organs would also be treated. When this state of *dampness* and *phlegm* exists, certain acupoints would be tender and these would usually be included in the treatment, such as Stomach-40 (*Fenglong*).

Apart from *one or two* of the main acupoints for treating the heart and improving the digestion—such as Bladder-15 (*Xinshu*), Heart-7 (*Shenmen*), Pericardium-5 (*Jianshi*), Ren-14 (*Juque*), Pancreas-6 * (*Daheng*), or Bladder-20 (*Pishu*)—one of the following, more targeted, acupoints would usually also be used in this case, to assist the patient to become more clear headed:

- Du-20 (*Baihui*),
- Kidney-9 (*Zhubin*), or
- Gallbladder-20 (*Fengchi*).

In clinic, I find that many mental and emotional conditions can clear within a few treatments, such as anxiety, panic attacks and depression, but the speed of recovery very much depends on the underlying health of each patient. And a further large determining factor can be whether or not the patient is using strong pharmaceutical remedies. If they are, this can notably slow down the recovery time, since the patient's body no longer has chemical autonomy, therefore the ability of their main organs to self-regulate is limited (p.258).

Worsening of poor heart function

When poor heart function has been present for some time, this may gradually worsen and eventually produce the signs and symptoms in list "F" on page 197 above.

In today's Chinese medicine, this condition is known as "Heart yang deficiency", which can be understood as meaning a more severe case of poor heart function. When applied to an organ, the term *yang* refers to the functioning of the organ, rather than the condition of its tissue (which would be the *yin* aspect). And when the *yang* aspect (the functioning) has diminished to this level, this implies that the heart functions are themselves starting to fail. And if the condition worsens still more and becomes critical, this may produce the signs and symptoms in list "F".

Treatment

The treatment is very similar to that for poor heart function, only the use of moxibustion would usually be added (p.175). It is very unlikely that a patient's heart could have become this unwell without the function of their other main organs also being affected, and those would also be treated.

The small intestine

In contemporary physiology, the small intestine is about five meters long. It lies between the exit of the stomach and the entry to the large intestine. It fills the abdominal cavity; and the large intestine, which is about 1.5 meters long, surrounds it. The first section of the small intestine, which is about twenty-five centimetres long, is called the *duodenum*. Food from the stomach is released into this section, and the pancreas and gallbladder secrete digestive juices into the duodenum, which are combined with intestinal juices to chemically digest the food. This takes place in the walls of the small intestine, where nutri-

* Also called Spleen-6.

ents are absorbed into the blood and lymph, which then circulate the nutrients to every part of the body (see p.205 below).

In Chinese medicine terms, the small intestine is described as follows.

Extract from *Su Wen*, Chapter 8

The small intestine is the official functioning as recipient of what has been perfected. The transformation of things originates in it.[37]

Wang Bing (in 762 AD) commented on the above

The small intestine takes orders from the stomach to receive and hold the waste. Once it has received the waste, it transforms them anew and transmits them into the large intestine.[38]

In other *Nei Jing* passages, the large and small intestines are simply described as the "intestines", with no distinction between them; or in some other passages the small intestine even appears to be omitted altogether.

Extract from *Ling Shu*, Chapter 18

The lower [section of the *san jiao* (i.e. the kidneys, intestines and bladder)] discharges into the curved intestine and pours out into the urinary bladder where its liquids seep in. The fact is: Water and grain are regularly present together in the stomach. There they are transformed to dregs and together they descend into the large intestine, where they constitute the lower [section of the *san jiao*], where its liquids seep in. A separate juice is secreted along the lower [section of the *san jiao*] and seeps into the urinary bladder.[39]

Here, it is unclear whether both intestines are considered to be a single entity, or the small intestine has been left out. It could be argued that the "curved intestine" might refer to the small intestine. However, anatomically the "curved intestine" might more closely describe the large intestine; and the two separate terms used here, the "curved intestine" and the "large intestine" do both seem to be referring to the same organ. Alternatively, "curved intestine" could be understood as referring to the small intestine, which, anatomically, does curl and twist in the torso. But then again, the *Nei Jing* authors' knowledge of the anatomy of the organs was limited; and this particular author's knowledge may even have been nonexistent.*

However, the important point is that the small intestine was theorized to only play a role in managing waste—*after* the digestive organs had extracted the influences from ingested food. This theory, like most *Nei Jing* theories on metabolism, is untrue (pp.40-48).

There was a range of contradictory theories on metabolism. It was theorized that nutrients were extracted from ingested food by the stomach, then passed directly to the "meridian" network; or, passed to the lungs, which then passed them to the "meridians"; or, passed to the pancreas, which then either passed them to the other organs or the "meridians", or to the lungs which then passed them to the "meridians"; or, that the stomach extracted the nutrients, then passed them to all the organs, which then passed them to the "meridians" (pp.40-47). These theories are

* No *Su Wen* chapter describes any knowledge of the body's internal anatomy; and such knowledge is only referred to in two *Ling Shu* chapters; see endnote 16 from this book's Chapter 1.

contradictory, and commentators have argued about them for millennia. But the fact is they are *all* untrue—which is understandable when considering the theories were not informed by any knowledge of the microscopic workings of the body. In reality (that is, in contemporary physiology), the small intestine plays a vital role in absorbing the digested nutrients into the blood. These are first processed by the stomach, then processed by the pancreas and gallbladder, then by the small intestine, which absorbs the nutrients into the blood, as follows.

The small intestine absorbs nutrients into the blood

The inner wall of the small intestine contains many *villi*, which are tiny finger-like structures which project from the inner wall of the small intestine. They are about one millimetre long, and the exposed wall of each villi is made up of many cells which contain blood and lymph capillaries. It is these capillaries that the nutrients are absorbed into.

The food is broken down by various chemical processes. Enzymes in the pancreatic juice are responsible for starting this process. These enzymes are mixed with intestinal juice secreted by the small intestine, and also with bile secreted by the gallbladder. Together these enzymes break down proteins and carbohydrates; and the components of these (*amino acids* and *mono-saccharides*) are then absorbed into the blood via the capillaries in the walls of the villi (p.387). Fats are also broken down into their components (*fatty acids* and *glycerol*) but these are absorbed into the lymph capillaries.

Fats are not soluble in water, which makes them difficult to absorb through the intestinal wall into the blood, so instead they are absorbed into lymph. It is the bile from the gallbladder that initially breaks down the fats to enable them to be more easily digested. The presence of fats in the lymph gives it a milky appearance, and for this reason the lymph capillaries are called *lacteals*.[40]

The "meridian" network was the only circulatory system known to the *Nei Jing* authors, so they theorized that all nutrients were circulated in the "meridians" (which was a system of, in effect, imaginary artery-like tubes that was thought to travel the same routes taken by the *pathways on the skin*—what we today call the meridians—p.29). In their theory, most of the nutrients took the form of a vapour, known as influence (*chi*). The blood was thought to be another form of nutrient which was also circulated within the "meridians". Hence, the blood circulatory system known today played no part in the *Nei Jing* theories. The blood was not considered to be used for communication (as in the circulation of hormones, etc.), nor for the transport of digested nutrients—as it is in contemporary physiology. It was simply a nourishing liquid in its own right, which was made from the liquids extracted from ingested food and drink—in a process *separate* from the extraction of other nutrients (p.42). And the small intestine was thought to play no part in any of these processes.

The small intestine as a "drainage ditch"

There are also conflicting ideas in Chinese medicine about the roles played by the small intestine, large intestine and bladder in the body's processing of water.

In the extract from Chapter 18 of the *Ling Shu* quoted on page 204 above, it states that the water and grain are "transformed to dregs" in the stomach; then they descend into the large intestine, where a "separate juice" is extracted, which seeps into the bladder. Hence, the urine was thought to pass from the large intestine, directly into the bladder.

Extract from *Nan Jing*, Section 31

The [*san jiao*] encompasses the passageways of water and grain in the body.... The lower [section of the *san jiao*] begins exactly at the upper opening* of the bladder and extends downward. It is responsible for separating the clear from the turbid portions. It masters discharge but not intake, and it serves as a transmitter. [41]

Li Chiung (in 1269) commented on the above

The lower section of the [*san jiao*] separates the water and the grains which were taken in through the upper section of the [*san jiao*]. The clear portions become urine; the turbid portions become faeces. They are then transmitted to the outside.[42]

And Hsü Ta-ch'un (in 1727) commented

The clear portions enter the bladder and become the urine; the turbid portions enter the large intestine and become the dregs.[43]

In this extract from the *Nan Jing*, and the quoted commentaries on it, the clear notion is conveyed that the "lower section of the *san jiao*" (in other words, the kidneys, intestines and bladder) excretes liquids and solids to the outside, rather than any portion of those liquids being circulated back into the body.

Yeh Lin (in 1895) also commented on the above extract

The lower section of the [*san jiao*] is located exactly at the upper opening of the bladder.... From there the clear portions enter the bladder where they become influences and urine. The turbid portions enter the large intestine where they become dregs and waste. Hence the lower section of the [*san jiao*] masters discharge but not intake; it serves as a transmitter.[44]

In the above commentary, it is now suggested that the "clear portions" (i.e. urine) enter the bladder and the "turbid portions" enter the large intestine—and they do this separately, rather than the large intestine separating out the "clear portions" and passing these to the bladder.

However, it is unclear whether Yeh Lin is theorizing that the *small intestine* first separates out the clear and turbid portions, then routes them to the large intestine and bladder respectively, or whether this separation is perhaps performed in the stomach.

Many of the *Nei Jing* theories on metabolism and organ physiology are contradictory, and the choice of which contradictory theory to follow tends to be academic, since they are all usually untrue anyway, as here—where all the above theories on the small intestine are untrue. So it is frustratingly unimportant which theory is chosen to adhere to. But to make matters worse, this muddle of conflicting (and incorrect) theories in the *Nei Jing* is only confused even further when some contemporary Chinese medicine textbooks add

* The terms "opening" and "hole" are usually used to refer to acupoints. Therefore, when interpreting such passages, it should be remembered that the description is not referring to the anatomy of the organs, but to the location of their related acupoints.

their own untrue theories, which are presented as though originating from the *Nei Jing*.

For example, Maciocia states that the small intestine separates "re-usable" liquid, which is then "transported by the [pancreas] to all parts of the body to nourish the tissues."[45] No such function is stated in any part of the *Nei Jing* or *Nan Jing*. To be fair, perhaps the author invented this extra function to attempt to make sense of the contradictory theories, but this added function is as untrue as most *Nei Jing* theories are, so it is difficult to see the reason for adding it. And in his following paragraph, Maciocia then adds a further new function, which appears to contradict the previous one—and is equally untrue anyway. He now states that

> After "dirty" fluids are passed down from the stomach, they are further separated by the small intestine into a "clean" part which goes to the large intestine for re-absorption, and a "dirty" part which goes to the bladder for excretion as urine.[46]

Again, these notions are alien to the *Nei Jing* and *Nan Jing*—and also to the two thousand years of Chinese commentaries that followed. It is clear that the *Nei Jing* and *Nan Jing* authors regarded the small intestine, large intestine and bladder as only serving the function of excreting waste from the body (as stated in the above extracts—p.204 onwards). And this is why Chapter 18 of the *Ling Shu* described the lower section of the *san jiao* as being "like a ditch".[47] There was no notion of these organs circulating substances back into the body. The large intestine function of absorbing liquids from the stool is derived from contemporary physiology alone (p.149). Yet it is presented as though deriving from the *Nei Jing*.

It is difficult to understand the purpose of adding this new, *true* function, while, at the same time, repeating *Nei Jing* theories that are clearly untrue. If the goal was to attempt to "correct" the wrong *Nei Jing* notions of physiology, why also repeat the clearly untrue theories?

It seems to me that this practice only compounds the difficulties of understanding Chinese medicine.

The roll of the small intestine in Chinese medicine treatments

Clinically, the small intestine is not considered to be significant, which is not to say that it suffers no problems. It is extremely common for people to experience a swollen, tender or clearly dysfunctional small intestine (what has become known as IBS in contemporary medicine). However, in Chinese medicine, this is regarded as a problem related to the pancreas.

The pancreas is responsible for enabling the completion of the digestive process. In contemporary physiology, it provides the enzymes which the small intestine then uses to enable it to absorb nutrients into circulation (p.63). When a person has poor pancreas function, the secretion of these enzymes could only be inadequate in some way, which may be what prevents the small intestine from functioning properly—and the person may develop symptoms of a swollen and tender abdomen, or even loose or runny stools. Therefore, when a person has poor pancreas function they also usually suffer intestinal problems; and once the poor pancreas function is treated, the small intestine function would usually also return to normal.

It is for this reason that Chinese medicine regards the symptoms of a tender and swollen abdomen, together with loose or runny stools, as symptoms of poor pancreas function—even though they are produced by the small intestine. And when a person has these symptoms, it is their pancreas that is treated.

It should also be noted that intestinal problems are only common because poor pancreas function is extremely common. Indeed, in developed countries poor pancreas function is epidemic (p.79).

The association with the heart

In Chinese medicine it is recognised that there are clear associations between various organs, which associations are demonstrated in their functional relationships, the effects of treatments, and also in the paths of the meridians. All the organs are thus paired in a *yin-yang* fashion—the *yin* being the "deeper" organ, and the *yang* being the more "superficial" organ (that is, it communicates more directly with the outside world than its coupled *yin* organ does—p.347). In this way, the heart is paired with the small intestine.

There is also a similar pairing between the lungs and large intestine. With both these pairs of organs, it is often commented that it is difficult to understand the reason for the pairings when considering the functions of the organs. With the other pairings (such as the liver and gallbladder, the kidneys and bladder, and the pancreas and stomach) the close functional association between the organs is obvious.

With *all* the paired organs, their meridians are consecutive. And since the other three organ pairings mentioned above appear to be due to their functional relationships, this suggests that evolution may have determined the paths of the meridians *based* on these functional relationships (pp.351-353). If this were the case, a similar functional relationship ought to exist between the heart and small intestine. But to identify this relationship it is necessary to compare the intentions of the two organs.

In contemporary physiology, the heart spreads nourishment to all the organs and tissues of the body via the blood vessels*, which all originate at the heart. But the small intestine is responsible for absorbing nutrients into the blood stream—which then *allows* the heart to spread that nourishment by circulating the blood. Therefore, both organs are intimately involved in the role of *spreading nourishment to those around them* (the other organs and the tissue of the body), and the two organs depend on one another to be able to perform this role.

Hence, the close functional relationship is between the blood vessels (in contemporary physiology) and the small intestine. But the blood vessels are merely the vehicle the heart uses to fulfil its intention, and, in evolutionary terms, are simply an extension of the heart (p.190). This suggests that this functional relationship is, in effect, between the small intestine and the heart.

The possible mental functions

The intention of the small intestine is the same as its physical function (in contempo-

* Here "blood vessels" refers to the literal system of arteries, veins and capillaries; and not to the "meridians" and collaterals, which is what the *Nei Jing* intended when referring to "blood vessels" (p.42).

rary physiology), which could be summarised as: *to complete the extraction of nutrients and incorporate them into circulation* (amongst those around it). As mentioned above—the physical function of the heart and small intestine are dependent on one another to be able to carry out this role. And this also applies when their functions are used to process our thoughts. But on top of this, the small intestine's close working relationship with the pancreas *also* applies in the processing of our thoughts.

The small intestine completes the digestion begun by the pancreas. The pancreas's function (and intention) is *to further break down food* (which process the stomach began) *to find any inherent nutrition and to control the body's uptake of the main nutrition* (p.93). When this function is used to process our thoughts, this means: looking for ideas about the world around us that may be "nourishing" (ideas which might be from the media, from other people's comments, or from our own observations). The small intestine then *completes the extraction of nutrients and incorporates them into circulation* (amongst those around it). In other words, it enables the heart to perform its function of *spreading this nourishment to the people around us.* After all, if we have no ideas (no "nourishment"), we cannot spread them to other people.

To summarize, when we read or hear another person's words (for example), the stomach *begins* the process of us mentally digesting the information; and the pancreas then looks for any "nourishing" ideas amongst the words—ideas that might be suggested or implied by them, as well as any that are immediately apparent. The pancreas then absorbs these into the body (the mental equivalent perhaps being to store them in memory). The small intestine assists the pancreas to do this, by completing the extraction of these "nutrients". And both the small intestine and heart are then able to circulate any nutrients we have found—to the other people around us. By working together, they can spread the nutrients to the "body tissue" (in other words, store them in memory), or to "the other organs" (in other words, the people around us). And they do this by urging us to use some means of communication, whether it be speech, written words, eye contact, or simply body language.

When looked at in this way, the interdependence between these organs in this aspect of the processing of our thoughts seems clear. Any impediment to the stomach or pancreas function, also impedes the small intestine function, which, in turn, impedes the heart function. And conversely, when the heart function is impeded (either physically or mentally), this *also* impedes the small intestine function, exacerbating any IBS symptoms. This is because the small intestine cannot properly absorb nutrients into the blood if the blood circulation is inadequate; and also, the same mental factors that impede the heart, also impede the small intestine—as shown in the following example, which also demonstrates this interdependence.

By far the most common cause of poor pancreas function is overthinking (trying to digest too many thoughts), which may produce in us the "small intestine" symptoms of feeling bloated and having a tender and swollen abdomen. Here, the small intestine has stopped working properly, so cannot complete the digestive process; the fabric of the organ may become inflamed, and because the food that normally passes through the small intestine cannot be processed properly by it, we may also develop loose stools. This symptom of a swollen abdomen seems to be just as common amongst men as women, only the swelling is often more severe in men. A possible explanation for this is that most societies encourage men to suppress their heart function. Men are encouraged not to share their deepest concerns, or to discuss emotional matters at all (ultimately, to live a lonely existence), which impedes their heart function (p.193). And due to the heart's interdependence with the small intestine, this would also tend to impede the small intestine function. Its function is impeded mentally—due to the reluctance to *spread nourishment to those around us*—and this impediment would be duplicated in the physical organ, weakening its function and thus exacerbating the small intestine symptoms.

The functions of all twelve organs are used to process our thoughts

It is most likely that the functions of *all* the abdominal organs are used to process our thoughts, and that the same interdependencies that exist between the physical functioning of all these organs, also exist between their functions when used to process our thoughts.

It is mainly the *yin* organs (*zang*) that Chinese medicine considers to have mental functions (the pancreas, liver, lungs, kidneys, and heart). They undoubtedly perform the most important roles in the processing of our thoughts, but there is no reason to think that the *yang* organs (*fu*) are not also utilized. With the functioning of the *physical* organs, the *yang* organs tend to service the *yin* organs in some way (they perform less important roles but roles that make it possible for the *yin* organs to perform *their* roles). And this same arrangement probably applies in the processing of our thoughts—that the functions of all twelve abdominal organs play roles which mirror the roles the organs play in the physical body—with each *yang* organ servicing its paired *yin* organ in some way.

It should be noted that all this book's arguments on the mental functions of the organs are theoretical. I have used concepts from contemporary physiology to suggest a possible explanation for this phenomena, which has always been a routine part of Chinese medicine, from the *Nei Jing* onwards. Today, the associations between our thoughts and organ functions are apparent in any Chinese acupuncture clinic, yet the concepts are alien to contemporary physiology. My suggested explanations are intended to enable today's minds to at least accept that the phenomenon may be possible.

Chapter 10. Pericardium and lymphatic system

Attribution of Chinese medicine organs

As with the "spleen" and pancreas, when the theoretical Chinese organs were attributed to anatomical organ masses, the Chinese organ *san jiao* 三焦 was another problematic organ. No organ could be identified that seemed to match its descriptions. Indeed, from the *Nei Jing* onwards, the organ was often considered to have no physical form. Yet at other times, it *was* considered to have a physical form, which confusion only added to the difficulty (p.214). The problem was solved by *not* attributing this particular theoretical organ to an anatomical organ. And in today's English texts on Chinese medicine, this organ is simply known by its Chinese name, *san jiao*, or this name itself is translated literally into English, as either the "triple burner", the "triple energizer" or the "triple heater".

However, it is clear from the descriptions of the organ's functions that these are referring to the lymphatic system (as described on page 214 below), and this book therefore translates the term *san jiao* as "lymphatic system". But you should be aware that when reading other books on Chinese medicine, what I call the lymphatic system (and the lymphatic-system meridian and acupoints) would be referred to as either the *san jiao*, the "triple burner", the "triple heater", or the "triple energizer". This may cause a little confusion when reading different texts, but I believe it is important to correct such attribution issues to remove yet one further obstacle that prevents contemporary readers from properly understanding Chinese medicine.

The pericardium

In contemporary physiology, the pericardium is the protective membrane that surrounds the heart.

In the *Nei Jing* and *Nan Jing*, the pericardium was called either the "heart master" or the "heart enclosing network". In *yin-yang* terms, it is coupled with the lymphatic system (*san jiao*), and there has been almost as much debate and controversy over the pericardium as there has been over the *san jiao*.

> ***Nan Jing*, Section 25**
>
> There are twelve [meridians], but the body's five [*yin* organs (*zang*)] and six [*yang* organs (*fu*)] add up to only eleven. Of what nature is the one missing [meridian]? It is like this. One of the [meridians] encompasses the [heart] and the [pericardium] as separate [meridians]. The [pericardium] and the [*san*

> *jiao*] represent outside and inside. Both have a name but no form. Hence one speaks of twelve meridians.[1]

Unschuld cites a range of commentaries on the above, which provide a snapshot of the debate over these issues.[2]

Lymphatic system

In contemporary physiology, the lymphatic system is a circulatory system. Lymph is the fluid that all body tissue is bathed in. While in the tissue, it is called *interstitial fluid*. This fluid originates mainly from the blood plasma (p.43 and 165), but the lymphatic system assists in the circulation of this fluid by transporting the components that are not easily absorbed directly into the plasma.[3] But as well as assisting in the circulation of this fluid, the lymphatic system also forms an important part of the immune system, since it is responsible for the production and growth of *lymphocytes*, which are the white blood cells that provide immunity.

Lymphocytes are produced in the bone marrow, and when released into the blood they are modified into either *T- or B-lymphocytes*. T-lymphocytes recognise a single type of pathogen (a particular virus, bacteria, and so on) and then destroy that pathogen when they encounter it, but *only* that pathogen. B-lymphocytes manufacture *antibodies*, which are proteins designed to recognise a specific pathogen, and the antibody then destroys that particular pathogen—and *only* that pathogen.[4]

The lymphatic system consists of:

- Lymph nodes. These filter the lymph, removing microbes (such as bacteria), worn out or damaged cells or inhaled particles, before returning the lymph to the blood plasma. And T- and B-lymphocytes also multiply in these nodes.
- The spleen, which may be considered a large lymph node. It filters lymph but also contains T- and B-lymphocytes and activates these in response to infection.
- The thymus gland, which also activates T-lymphocytes. The "activation" of lymphocytes is a process that switches them on, so that when in circulation they look for infecting microbes and then become sensitised to that particular microbe.[5]
- The tonsils. These consist of lymphoid tissue that destroys swallowed or inhaled pathogens ("pathogens" are any agents that cause disease, such as bacteria or viruses, but also pollen, or any cells that are foreign to the body).
- Peyer's patches. These are patches of lymphoid tissue on the inner wall of the small intestine, which also destroy swallowed pathogens.[6]
- Bone marrow. This is where lymphocytes are initially produced, before being released into the blood and converted by lymph nodes or organs to provide immunity.[7]

The similar purpose of both "organs"

Both the pericardium and lymphatic system have a defensive function. The pericardium specializes in defending the heart, while the lymphatic system defends the entire body.

There are twelve meridians in the body, each one associated with a particular organ. This means that from evolution's point of view, we have twelve distinct organs[8]. The pericardium and lymphatic system each have a specific meridian associated with them, so they are each regarded as one of these twelve organs. What is remarkable is that the heart has an entire, distinct organ dedicated to protecting it. It is also protected by the immune system, but on top of this, it has its own defender. No other organ's protection is taken so seriously by the body, which can only reflect how important the heart is to our survival.

The *yin-yang* organ pairing

The meridians associated with the pericardium and the lymphatic system are consecutive, and the two organs therefore form a *yin-yang* pair (p.347), the pericardium being relatively more *yin* (situated more deeply within the body), and the lymphatic system being relatively more *yang* (nearer to the surface of the body). With all the organs, each of the two organs in any *yin-yang* pair either have some similarity between their functions or some other close functional relationship. In this case, both organs are involved in the protection of the body.

The importance of these organs in the treatment of illness

In Chinese medicine, neither the pericardium nor the lymphatic system are usually treated directly, since any symptoms that *could* be associated with them are usually addressed by treating one of the other main organs.

For example, the symptom of a chest pain, which may radiate to the shoulders and upper arms (particularly the left arm), is considered in contemporary physiology to indicate a problem with the heart or pericardium; and indeed the symptom may be accompanied by a swollen pericardium, in which case the term *pericarditis* would be used, meaning, literally, swelling of the pericardium (see the patient example on page 253). However, in Chinese medicine, this symptom is considered to indicate a problem with the heart alone, and when the heart is treated, the symptom clears—including any swelling of the pericardium.

It is true that some pericardium acupoints, such as Pericardium-6 (*Neiguan*), are commonly used to treat heart conditions (as well as other conditions, such as stagnated liver function—p.113), but this healing effect is the result of the close relationship between the two organs, rather than being due to this acupoint treating the pericardium *only*. Indeed, when Pericardium-6 (*Neiguan*) is used to treat stagnated liver function, it is certainly not treating the pericardium but achieves its effect due to the meridian relationship between the pericardium and liver.[9]

Another factor in the above is that, since the pericardium's role is to defend the heart, the pericardium only usually becomes stressed once the heart is stressed—due to it being affected by a pathogen of some sort, either of mental, emotional or physical origin. Therefore, any condition in the pericardium usually indicates that the heart needs treating, and once the heart is treated, any signs in the pericardium would clear. It is for all these reasons that the pericardium is not usually separately treated in Chinese medicine; treatment of all heart-related signs and symptoms is usually directed towards the heart alone.

Likewise, any symptoms that *could* be attributed to a weakness in the lymphatic system would usually be addressed by treating the "kidneys". This is because such symptoms would usually indicate a constitutional weakness, which, in Chinese medicine, would indicate poor kidney function. But in contemporary physiology, how could this treatment be explained?

As said on page 153, when the "kidneys" are mentioned in Chinese medicine, this consists of three structures—the kidneys, adrenal glands and gonads; and the adrenal glands play an essential role in the development and maintenance of normal immunity (p.156). Therefore any symptoms indicating a poor constitution (or poor immune function) would be addressed by treating the "kidneys" which would normalize the function of the three kidney-related structures, including the hormonal activity of the adrenal glands, which would explain how the treatment addresses issues with the immune system (of which, the lymphatic system is a key part). This, for example, is how the acupuncture treatment for hay fever and other allergies works. People with such signs and symptoms usually have poor kidney function, which they have often had since childhood; and once their "kidneys" are treated, their sensitivity to pollen and other irritants (such as animal fur, perfumes, dust, and so on) disappears.

The above refers to the treatment of the organs. With both the pericardium and lymphatic system (as with all other organs), meridian "blockages" may occur at any location along their related meridians. In this case, acupoints on those meridians are usually used to treat the condition, which is often not regarded as a problem with the organ, but with the local tissue along the meridian (p.219). However, in my view a meridian "blockage" would usually also be able to affect the function of the related organ, particularly when the "blockage" had been present for a while. In this situation, it is as though the local trauma is "remembered" by the related organ and thereby incorporated into its function in some way (p.221). In this situation, by using local acupoints to treat the meridian "blockage", this would also amount to a treatment of the organ. If this is the case, this situation provides the exception to the above "rule". That is, when treating a meridian "blockage", this also treats the related organ—whether this be the lymphatic system, pericardium, or any other organ.

In Chinese medicine, what is the *san jiao* organ?

The *san jiao* has always been a controversial organ. From the *Nei Jing* to the present day, its form and function have been debated. Indeed, over this time, depending on which text or commentator you choose to follow, its location, form and function have varied widely.

The varying notions

Chapter 4 of the *Su Wen* lists it as one of the six *yang* organs (*fu*); and Chapter 8 states its function as "opener of channels" and that the "paths of water originate in it". This suggests it was considered to be a real organ concerned with containing and maintaining the flow of liquids (of some sort) in the body.[10]

Chapter 18 of the *Ling Shu* states that one of the *san jiao's* functions is to guide the passage of the constructive influence (*ying chi*), the defensive influence (*wei chi*), and the chest influence (*zong chi*) from their origin in the digestive organs, out to the meridians.[11]

Extract from *Nan Jing*, Section 25

One of the [pairs of meridians] encompasses the [*san jiao*] and the [pericardium] as separate vessels. The [pericardium] and the [*san jiao*] represent outside and inside. Both have a name but no form.[12]

Commenting on this passage, Ting Chin (in 1736) wrote

If the [*san jiao*] has no form, how can passageways of water emerge from it? How can it be thick or thin? How can it be like a mist or fog or foam or a ditch? How can it emit influences in order to supply warmth to the flesh?[13]

And, just as the pericardium encircles and protects the heart, Ting Chin went on to visualize the *san jiao* as being a large bag that supported the [organs collectively] from outside and holds them inside.[13]

Extract from *Nan Jing*, Section 31

The [*san jiao*] encompasses the passageways of water and grain in the body. It represents the conclusion and the start of the course of the influences. The upper [section]... is responsible for intake but not for discharge. The central [section]... is responsible for the spoiling and processing of water and grains. The lower [section]... is responsible for separating the clear from the turbid portions. It masters discharge but not intake.... Its influences are collected at [Stomach-30 *Qichong*].[14]

Extract from *Nan Jing*, Section 38

The [*san jiao*] represents an additional source of original influences [*yuan chi*]; it governs all the influences circulating in the body. It has a name but no form.[15]

Commenting on the above passage, Li Chiung (in 1269) wrote

The kidneys are the proper source of the original influences [*yuan chi*]; the [*san jiao*] represents an additional source. [Ren-17 *Shanzhong*] is a sea of influences; it is located in the upper section of the [*san jiao*]. Also, a sea-of-influences [acupoint] exists two inches below the navel [Ren-6 *Qihai*]; it is located in the lower section of the [*san jiao*]. Hence the [*san jiao*] controls the influences of the entire body.... The [*san jiao*] represents nothing but membranes attached to the upper, central, and lower opening of the stomach. It has a name, but no real form.[16]

Taking exception to this, Yeh Lin (in 1895) wrote

The [*san jiao*] has a form! That has already been discussed in sufficient detail in the commentaries on Section 25 [of the *Nan Jing*].... It can be proven that the [*san jiao*] has a material form. But the transformation of influence through the [*san jiao*] is difficult to perceive. Hence, the text [in Section 38 above] says, 'It has a name but no form'.[17]

Extract from *Nan Jing*, Section 66

The [*Shu-stream* acupoints] on the [meridians] associated with the five [*yin* organs (*zang*)] are the locations where the influences that are sent out by the [*san jiao*] stop and rest.... The influences moving below the naval and between the kidneys constitute man's life. They are the source and the basis of the twelve [meridians]. Hence they are called "original influences". The [*san jiao*] is the special envoy that transmits the original influences....[18]

Commenting on the above passage, Yang K'ang-hou (in 1098) wrote

The influences moving below the navel and between the kidneys are called [Ren-4 *Guanyuan*]. [Ren-4] is man's source and root. It is the depot of the essence and the spirit... In males the essence is stored here; in females [Ren-4] regulates the monthly period. It constitutes the gate where *yin* and *yang* influences unite to create posterity.... It is attached to the vessels of the spine and to the root of the kidneys.... The location between the two kidneys is called "great sea"; another name is "submerged in water".[19] Inside of it is the spirit-turtle. It exhales and inhales the original influences.... The two kidneys are distinguished by their storing of the essence... The essence consists of immaterial influences; it constitutes man's source and root.... Hence it is obvious that [Ren-4] is the basis of life. When the Taoists contemplate the spiritual, when the Buddhist monks meditate, they all cause the influences of their heart to move below the navel....[20]

And also commenting on this same passage, Liao Ping (in 1913) wrote

[The *Nan Jing*] emphasizes the importance of the kidneys. Here, in addition, it emphasizes the importance of the [*san jiao*]. Nothing of this appears in the *Nei Jing*. These are all doctrines fabricated by the author of [the *Nan Jing*].[21]

A recent textbook in China, *Essentials of Chinese Acupuncture*, 1980, merely states that the *san jiao* is divided into three parts and "is not a substantial organ, but a generalization of part of the functions of some of the organs located in different sections of [the torso]."[22] This textbook appears to support the position stated in the *Nei Jing*; in other words, there is no mention of the *san jiao* being a passageway for original influence (*yuan chi*), as stated in Section 66 of the *Nan Jing*.

Whereas *Chinese Acupuncture and Moxibustion*, 1987, which is an updated edition of the above 1980 book, now states that the *san jiao's* main function is "to govern various forms of [influence], and serve as the passage for the flow of [original influence (*yuan chi*)] and body fluid. [Original influence] originates in the kidney, but requires the [*san jiao*] as its pathway for distribution in order to stimulate and promote the functional activities of the... organs and tissues of the whole body." And it quotes Section 66 of the *Nan Jing*.[23]

Today's notion of the *san jiao*

Today, the *san jiao* is generally considered to have the functions described in the last paragraph above.

As with many theoretical areas of Chinese medicine, to properly understand the notion of the *san jiao*, you need to put out of your mind all knowledge of contemporary anatomy and physiology, and regard the notion as being metaphorical rather than literally true. Only in this way is it possible to understand the notion as the original authors meant it.

However, from a physiological point of view, it is also clear that the *san jiao* is a real organ, since it has its own meridian; and it is the effect of information from the related organ that is thought to create each meridian (p.355). Because the organ exists, it ought to be possible to describe it using contemporary anatomy and physiology.

Attribution of the *san jiao*

This book attributes the *san jiao* to the lymphatic system. In the *Nei Jing* and *Nan Jing* (as described above), the *san jiao* was variously described as follows:

- It is located inside the body but separately from the other organs, in that it does not have an identifiable organ mass. Instead it is spread throughout the three main areas of the body (in other words, it extends everywhere in the body).

And its main functions are that it serves

- as the passage for body liquids; and
- as the passage for original influence (*yuan chi*), which was described as "originating in the kidneys but requiring the *san jiao* as its path for distribution in order to stimulate and promote the functional activities of the organs and tissues of the whole body".[24]

These descriptions appear to relate to the lymphatic system for the following reasons. The description of the organ as not having a mass (like those of the other organs) and of it instead being distributed throughout the whole body, and also having the function of circulating body liquids, exactly matches the lymphatic system, which is a system that assists in the circulation and management of the body fluids (in cooperation with the blood circulatory system, whose plasma is the main source of body fluids). And as to the last bullet point above, to show that this relates to the lymphatic system, the following passages demonstrate that something akin to original influence (*yuan chi*) flows in the lymphatic system and has the same effect on the organs that original influence is said to have. But first, it is necessary to show why original influence corresponds to hormones (in contemporary physiology).

The parallels between original influence and hormones

Original influence is said to be stored in the "kidneys" (which includes the adrenal glands and gonads).

One of the main hormones secreted by the adrenal glands is cortisol. One of its many functions is to regulate the production and use of energy in the body (p.154). This energy is the vital force that brings the body to life, including all the organs and tissues, not only giving the organs their vitality (the condition of being alive and of remaining alive) but also allowing them to perform their many functions. Thus this particular hormone, which originates in one of the three kidney-related structures, stimulates and promotes the *functional activities* of the organs and tissues of the whole body—just as original influence (*yuan chi*) is said to do.

In Chapter 1 of the *Su Wen*, the "influence of the kidneys" (in other words, original influence), is described as regulating growth and sexual development. [25] In contemporary physiology, these roles are performed by the hormones originating in the gonads and also the adrenal glands (two of the three kidney-related structures), which again confirms that Chinese medicine references to original influence (or to essence influence, as it was called in the *Su Wen*—p.25) are references to hormones.

From the above, it is clear that original influence equates to the hormone cortisol (as well as to other hormones, such as testosterone or oestrogen—p.155); and that, in this one application of cortisol, it has the same effect on the organs that original influence is said to do. But does cortisol require the lymphatic system for its distribution?

The relation between original influence and the lymphatic system

In contemporary physiology, hormones are mainly transported in the blood. *Some* hormones are transported in lymph, but the lymphatic system is certainly not the path for *all* hormones in the body, not by a long way.

In this particular application of cortisol (regulating the production and usage of energy), it would be transported in the blood.

However, in another "kidney"-related application of cortisol, the lymphatic system *does* play a vital role. One function of original influence (*yuan chi*) was said to be to provide the constitution. In contemporary physiology, this would equate to immunity. And the "kidneys" (i.e. adrenal glands, which are one of the kidney-related structures) regulate the immune system via their use of cortisol (p.154). And a key part of the immune system is the lymphatic system (which could be regarded as the "factory" of the immune system—p.212).

Therefore, the provision of immunity is achieved through the lymphatic system; and in Chinese medicine, original influence and the "Kidneys" provide the constitution—a key functional part of which is the lymphatic system.

This does not demonstrate that something akin to original influence flows in the lymphatic system. But rather that the same effects in the body are achieved by something akin to original influence (cortisol), which uses the lymphatic system as a vital mechanism to achieve its effects (i.e. provide immunity, which equates to the constitution).

When theorizing about the nature and form of the *san jiao* and also the "kidneys", even though the ancient Chinese did not get all the detail correct (in terms of contemporary physiology), they *did* correctly work out that a hormonal-like substance was circulating in the body, which controlled all the vital functions of the body and originated in the three kidney-related structures. To have worked this out over two thousand years ago was an incredible achievement.

They also correctly worked out the existence of the lymphatic system (even though it could not then be found when dissecting a body) and that *part* of the activity of these hormonal-like substances was associated with the lymphatic system (in the part played by cortisol in the immune system—which, in Chinese medicine terms, would equate to the constitution).

For all the above reasons, it is clear that when the ancient Chinese used the term *san jiao*, they were referring to the lymphatic system.

Chapter 11. Meridian symptoms

Apart from the signs and symptoms directly related to the malfunction of the main organs (as described in Chapters 4 to 10), further, separate symptoms can also result, such as muscular and joint pains that occur along the path of a particular meridian. These may be caused by a physical trauma to that location, or by being exposed to an external pathogen, such as *wind* or *cold*.

In today's Chinese medicine, this condition is known as *painful obstruction syndrome* (or *bi*, in Chinese, pronounced "bee"). In the *Nei Jing*, the terms "blockage-illness", "obstruction-illness" or "impediment-illness" were used (see below). In contemporary medicine, this same condition may be called repetitive strain injury (RSI), tendonitis, carpel tunnel syndrome, tennis elbow, golfers elbow, sciatica, neuralgia, and so on. Other muscular conditions, such as a hernia, may also present with similar symptoms, and can sometimes be successfully treated in the same way.

> **Patient example**
> Male, aged 34. This patient initially sought treatment for a pain in his neck and shoulder, lumbar pain, and hay fever, which all cleared with treatment. Two years later he suffered a hernia, which also healed with treatment, this being confirmed with an ultrasound scan. See the full case history on page 257.

Extract from *Ling Shu*, Chapter 66

When a [harmful influence (i.e. wind or cold)] strikes a person, in the beginning it is in the skin. When the skin is relaxed, then the skin structures are open. When they are open, the [harmful influence] enters via the body hair. Once they have entered, they proceed into the depth. When they are in the depth, the body hair will rise. When the body hair has risen, then that person shivers. Hence the skin aches. When the [harmful influences] remain there for some time and are not removed, then they are transmitted further and they will settle in the [meridians]. While they are in the [meridians] the muscles and the flesh are in pain.[1]

This passage describes the theoretical penetration of the skin by external pathogens such as wind, which then lodge at the affected location, eventually producing pain in the "muscles and flesh". The following passages provide further *Nei Jing* theories on how such pathogens cause pain.

Extract from *Ling Shu*, Chapter 27

Circulation blockage-illnesses are inside the blood vessels.... How does this pain emerge? ... Wind, cold and dampness [influence] settle in the outer region, in the partings of the flesh. They exert pressure [on the body liquids] and this results in the generation of foam. When the foam is affected by cold, it will collect. When it has collected, then it will fill the partings of the flesh and the crevices. As a result the crevices will ache.[2]

Extract from *Ling Shu*, Chapter 81

In the blood vessels, the [constructive and defensive influences] flow without cease.... In the case of cold [influence] settling inside the [meridians] and [collaterals], the blood will cease to flow. When the blood ceases to flow, it fails to penetrate the [meridians and collaterals]. As soon as it fails to penetrate the [meridians and collaterals], the [constructive and defensive influence] will [accumulate] there. This cannot be reverted. Hence obstruction-illness with swelling results.[3]

The above passages provide examples of the *Nei Jing* theories on how this type of pain occurs. Essentially, pathogens such as *wind*, *cold* or *dampness* were thought to enter the "meridian" network and obstruct the flow of the influences (the constructive and defensive influences) and the blood, which then resulted in pain.

Note that the term "blood vessel" was usually used to refer to the collaterals and tertiary network vessels (i.e. the superficial veins that were used for bloodletting—p.31). These were then thought to flow more deeply into the muscle layer, flowing into the "meridians", which were imaginary artery-like tubes (p.29). And the same blood and influences were thought to flow in all these vessels. This may explain why it was theorized that the veins were affected first by pathogens from outside, and that the pathogen then progressed deeper and entered the "meridians".

Considering the *Nei Jing* theory

Could the above theories be literally true? Do they describe what is really happening?

The *Nei Jing* authors imagined influences (*chi*) to consist of vapour-like substances that flow through the "meridians" and elsewhere in the body. These vapours were thought to contain some essence of the original entity they were derived from—such as some essence of food, water, wine, wind, cold, dampness. Hence different vapours would be named "food influence", "cold influence", "wine influence" and so on. But these influences do not really flow in the "meridians" (pp.41-47). In effect, they are imaginary (though the illusion can often be convincing—p.55). And what the *Nei Jing* authors thought of as the "meridians", are also imaginary. These were thought to be deep, artery-like tubes that did not usually follow the same paths as the literal arteries but instead followed the same routes as the *pathways on the skin* (which is what we today call the meridians—p.29). Therefore, when the *Nei Jing* authors attributed this type of pain to the obstructed flow of either influences or blood in the "meridian" network, this, also, could not possibly be true—since these substances do not really flow in the "meridians" anyway, so it is impossible for their imaginary flow to be blocked.

How might such a theory have been formed?

Even though the theory is untrue, to the *Nei Jing* authors, it clearly seemed reasonable. What could explain this?

Two thousand years ago, when a person was exposed to external wind, cold or dampness, and this led to a painful condition in their muscles, it was imagined that the pathogens had penetrated their skin and lodged within them. At the time, this was the accepted way of explaining such things. Indeed, this *appeared* to be what was happening. When a person was exposed to external wind, their resultant symptoms could equally be described as a form of "wind" (sneezing; shivering—as though a wind were inside them and making them shake). And the same applies with coldness and dampness. Exposure to external dampness often produces in us a state that *resembles* dampness; the pulses become "slippery" (p.75), the blood and body fluids seem to become sluggish and thicker, and swellings can occur—which all resemble the state of natural materials when they become saturated with liquid. Hence, it was natural to regard this situation as being the result of the external pathogens passing into the body and lodging there. And, clinically, the treatments worked—and were usually explained in terms of expelling the pathogens from the body.

A possible contemporary explanation

There is no doubt that the pains are real, since they are routinely seen in clinic today. This suggests that they were originally noted through practical observation, and like most other *Nei Jing* practical observations, they were fact based (it is only their explanatory theories that tend to be untrue). And since the pains exist, it ought to be possible to account for them using contemporary anatomy and physiology.

From my own clinical experiences, it is also clear that (though the pain is real) there is usually no underlying "illness" in the tissue at the affected location, for the following reason. Chinese acupuncture can often successfully treat such conditions astonishingly quickly. It is not uncommon for a person to stand from the treatment couch at the end of their first treatment to find that such a pain has disappeared without trace and does not return, despite them having previously suffered it for many months. Though with other patients, the initial improvement may only be in the order of about seventy percent, and a follow-up treatment is necessary. The speed of these initial results rules out any underlying "illness" in the local tissue or structures, since such problems could not be rectified so quickly.

Even though there is no physical disease in the tissue (in contemporary terms), the following phenomenon may account for such muscular and joint pains, and also acupuncture's effect on them.

The organs "remember" incidental symptoms

Chapters 17-20 describe how information about the function and malfunction of a person's organs is superimposed upon the electrical current that is ubiquitous in the body; and that it is this information that creates the meridians and all phenomena related to them (p.355). It is clear that this information also includes details of symptoms that are *incidental* to the organ malfunctions, for the following reasons.

The acute symptoms of hay fever attacks demonstrate the principle well. Such symptoms (sore or itchy eyes, itchy throat, sneezing) are among the many that have been transferred to me from my patients via the information radiated to me from their organs (p.363 and pp.375-376). This suggests that these symptoms were *also* present among the patient's organ information.

The usual underlying cause of hay fever is poor kidney function (p.214), and information about this "kidney" malfunction would be present in the patient's radiated energy. In the above example (p.363 etc), this was transferred to me, which would have then made me prone to hay fever (had my own kidney function permanently adopted the same malfunction). But this alone could not account for the patient's acute hay fever symptoms being immediately transferred to me, since there would not have been enough time for any reduced immunity in myself (due to this "borrowed" poor kidney function) to produce the allergy symptoms. But further, I do not have poor kidney function and never have done, so such symptoms could not have been produced in me in the usual fashion anyway. Instead, it was clear that these acute symptoms *themselves* were transferred to me via the patient's radiated organ information.

Are such symptoms "remembered" by the local tissue or by the organs?

This radiated information probably originated at the patient's organs, rather than being transmitted directly from the site of the symptoms. This is suggested by the following facts.

A patient's historic symptoms are also frequently transferred to me (p.364 and pp.375-378). At the time this happens, the symptom itself is no longer usually present in the patient's body, but rather, the patient either recently experienced the symptom or had a history of being prone to it. But since they do not currently feel the symptom and it is therefore not active, it is probable that any information radiated from that local tissue would not contain details of the symptom.

If this is the case, it seems that such historic symptoms are transferred between people via the information originating from the patient's organs, which suggests that the information about such symptoms is somehow adopted by the fine detail of the related organ's function. In other words, that an organ "remembers" the incidental symptoms that occur along its related meridian.

Another way of looking at this is that all meridian symptoms are simply another facet of organ malfunction, and this is why the organ "remembers" such symptoms.[4]

It might be argued that the local tissue could radiate such information, even when the symptom was not present—due to the tissue somehow "remembering" the symptom. But when I read a patient's pulses, I often experience in myself some of the patient's distal symptoms related to the particular organ whose pulse I am reading (p.363, 247 and 376). This might be a muscular ache or pain on the related meridian, or sensations at a related acupoint. And these symptoms always clear from myself when I lift my finger from the patient's wrist. This suggests that the information about such distal symptoms is contained in the organ information, since the information that produces a particular pulse originates from one of the patient's organs (p.303), rather than from information radiated from their whole body.

Extract from *Su Wen*, Chapter 43

Each of the five [*yin* organs (*zang*)] has a specific correlate; when the disease in the bones, sinews, [flesh, vessels or skin] lasts for a long time and does not go away, it pro-

> ceeds to the interior and lodges in the [*yin* organ (*zang*)] that is the correlate of the bones, sinews, [flesh, vessels or skin] respectively.[5]

The above passage expresses (in effect) the following idea. When a "disease" occurs in the local tissue (which was perhaps the result of a local trauma of some sort—including exposure to wind and cold—rather than resulting due to an illness in one of the main organs) then, when this local "disease" has been present for some time, it "proceeds to the interior" (meaning, it travels along a particular "meridian") and "lodges" in the *yin* organ whose meridian the local symptom was located on. This idea, written over two thousand years ago, is, essentially, also saying that the organs tend to remember local (incidental) symptoms.

Acupuncture also clears incidental symptoms

The following may account for acupuncture's effect on such symptoms. Assuming that information about any such symptom is contained in the fine detail of an organ's function (or malfunction), then when this function is persuaded to return to normal by acupuncture, this normalized function may, in turn, persuade the local tissue at the organ's acupoints and along its meridian to also return to normal function.

This principle is demonstrated in the phenomenon of disappearing tenderness at acupoints when the associated organ malfunction has been corrected with acupuncture (p.369). This happens even when the tender acupoint was not stimulated. The local tissue returns to normal function in response to its associated organ returning to normal function; and this change is communicated to the local tissue via that organ's information.

In the same way, if information about a distal symptom is "remembered" by an organ (adopted into the fine detail of its malfunction), when acupoints on the organ's related meridian are stimulated, possibly including those at the site of the local symptom, this would tend to normalize the function of the organ, which would also tend to encourage the organ to "forget" the distal symptom it had remembered. This state would then be communicated back to the organ's associated meridian and acupoints, which would tend to normalize the function of the local tissue that produced the symptom—in the same way that the tenderness at an acupoint (which was also produced by a "malfunction" in the local tissue) is cleared immediately the related organ's function is corrected.

Such a mechanism would explain why the acute symptoms of a hay fever attack are usually cleared within seconds by acupuncture, and also why aches and pains situated anywhere along a meridian tend to clear when acupoints on that meridian are stimulated, or when the function of the associated organ is corrected by using acupoints at another location.

How does this explanation account for meridian sensations?

If no influences (*chi*) flow in a meridian, what explains the sensations that are sometimes felt along a meridian during an acupuncture treatment? The most common sensations include

- the "needling" sensation itself (known as "de chi" in Chinese medicine),

- a tingling sensation,
- a feeling of warmth, and
- a sensation akin to an electric shock, shooting along a meridian.

These sensations are all accounted for on page 55 onwards.

Why some people become ill and others do not

Different people may be exposed to the same external pathogens, and some will become ill (and develop aches and pains) while others may not; and this situation was also observed by the *Nei Jing* authors.

> **Extract from *Ling Shu*, Chapter 66**
> When wind, rain, cold and heat cannot avail themselves of a depletion, their [harmful influences] alone are unable to harm man. When someone suddenly encounters a swift wind and heavy rain and does not fall ill, the reason is that he did not have a depletion.[6]

A "depleted" person is a weak or frail person, such as most elderly or chronically unwell people. When such people are exposed to a cold wind or draft, dampness, or excessive heat and dryness, they will often develop painful muscles or joints. Whereas a strong and well person who was exposed to the same conditions may not develop any symptoms. In contemporary physiology, one possible explanation for this is as follows.

The muscles normally have the ability to function well and to also repair any damage that may occur to them, but in a weak or frail person, their body's ability to repair itself may already be inadequate, so that their body may be unable to repair the effect of the trauma quickly enough. Hence the person experiences pain, which often develops after a few hours and is slow to heal.

Inexplicably painful muscles or joints

The same mechanism that produces tender diagnostic acupoints (where the patient is not usually aware of the tenderness until an acupuncturist presses the acupoint) can sometimes produce tenderness that the patient *is* constantly aware of.

A common example is when the liver function becomes stagnated due to stress (p.113). This often produces such pains at certain acupoints on the gallbladder meridian. The function of these two organs is closely related, and a problem with one will often cause a problem in the other. Therefore, such stress felt by the liver can lead to a stiff neck, near the acupoint Gallbladder-20 (*Fengchi*), or pain anywhere along the gallbladder meridian, particularly at the hips, where Gallbladder-30 (*Huantiao*) tends to become painful, or down the outside of either leg. In contemporary medicine these conditions are often called arthritis or sciatica. Treatment of the organ—usually together with needling of the local, painful acupoint—usually clears such conditions in a single treatment (in the same way that it rapidly clears the tenderness of diagnostic acupoints—these pains being produced in the same way as that diagnostic tenderness).

A similar situation arises following a powerful disruption to an organ's function, such as when the patient experiences an emotional trauma. Once this is treated and the organ begins to recover, this may lead to pain anywhere along that organ's meridian; and as the healing continues, the location of the pain may move along the meridian, either towards the fingertips or toes, depending on the meridian's location (p.314).

A common example of this phenomenon is when the patient is recovering from a bereavement. Such a loss heavily impedes the lung function (p.136), and as the patient recovers from their grief, they may develop painful and weak wrists, along the lung meridian, often centred on the acupoint Lung-9 (*Taiyuan*), which seems to the patient to have no apparent cause.

Patient example
Female, aged 65. This patient's lung function was already weak, but then her son died in traumatic circumstances and a year later she devolved a pain on the lung meridian at her wrist. See the full case history on page 254.

Another example is where patients experience a persistent situation in their life that they find difficult to stomach—that is, a situation that they cannot even *begin* to mentally or emotionally digest. This can impede their stomach function and hence cause a pain along the stomach meridian, which would typically be around their jaw or on their neck. These locations trace the route that chewed food *would* take, assuming this initial stage of digestion was successful; but since this process is mentally blocked, this aspect of the stomach function (the very beginning of the process of digestion) is impeded, and this produces pain in these locations.

Patient example
Male, aged 49. This patient had a pain on his jaw which persisted for two years and was caused by a long-standing dispute with his neighbour. See the full case history on page 253.

Another example of this phenomenon is when there is a problem in the patient's life that they cannot resolve, which causes them to develop a pain in their neck. This is probably the origin of the expression "pain in the neck", referring to a difficult person or situation.

Patient example
Female, aged 28. This patient sought treatment for a shoulder and neck pain. Initially the treatments greatly improved her symptoms, but the pain returned. And as the treatments progressed, it transpired that her pain was caused by her inability to resolve a relationship problem. See the full case history on page 247.

Chapter 12. Mental and emotional factors in causing disease

From my own clinical experiences I believe it is not possible to overstate the significance of everyday mental and emotional factors in causing serious long-term disease, so I felt it worthwhile summarizing and expanding on them in this chapter.

At the time the *Nei Jing* was written, it seems that the same situation existed.

> **Extract from *Su Wen*, Chapter 13**
> People in antiquity lived among their animals. They moved and were active and this way they avoided the cold. They resided in the shade and this way they avoided the summer heat. Internally, they knew no entanglements resulting from sentimental attachments, externally, they [were not stressed by the demands of society and the workplace]. In this peaceful and tranquil world, [they did not become seriously ill].... The people of today are different. Anxiety and suffering encircle their interior; [working excessively hard] harms their exterior. Also, the people have lost the knowledge how to follow the four seasons and they oppose the requirements of [the seasons]. [And they are frequently ill, with every part of their body affected, including their *yin* organs (*zang*)]. This is why minor diseases inevitably develop into serious [problems].[1]

The same could be said of most people in devolved countries today. And Chapter 58 of the *Ling Shu* emphasizes that diseases may be created from within us (as well as being caused by external pathogens). Among the possible "internal" causes listed are the following:

> **Extract from *Ling Shu*, Chapter 58**
> When [a person] suddenly is subject to excessive joy or rage, or drinks and eats something inappropriate.... When someone has an aversion to, or excessively longs after something.... The origins [of such an illness] are quite subtle. One may look at them, but will see nothing. One may listen to them, but hears nothing.[2]

Just as is the case today, the *Nei Jing* authors were aware of the importance of paying attention to the patient's mental and emotional state when making a diagnosis.

> **Extract from *Su Wen*, Chapter 13**
> Huang Di: I have heard the essentials of prognosis and treatment from you, Sir. In

your statements, Sir, you have never left complexion and movement in the vessels. That I know.
Qi Bo: The utmost principle in treatment lies with the oneness.
Huang Di: What is that to say, the "oneness"?
Qi Bo: There is oneness, and therefore one gets it.
Huang Di: How?
Qi Bo: Close the door and shut the windows, tie yourself to the patient, repeatedly inquire about his feelings, adapt your treatment to his sentiments. If one gets a hold of the spirit, the patient will prosper.[3]

Zhang Jiebin (in 1957) commented on the above

Shut the door, close the windows, and tie yourself to the patient. See to it that the patient is quiet and is not disturbed. Then both sides are relaxed and one can enquire about his feelings. Undertake every effort to follow his sentiments. The reason is that it is essential to achieve a welcoming mood in the patient. As a result, the one who asks does not feel awkward and the patient does not harbour any dislike. Hence one is able to examine the causal links from begin to end and the treatment will be faultless.[4]

A peculiarly human problem

The abdominal organs function in relation to each other; and the relationships between them are delicately balanced. But as humans, our conscious mind is able to readily upset this balance. How is this possible?

Over millions of years, the organs evolved complex logic to enable them to carry out their functions and coordinate these with the other organs. And once our conscious mind started having complex thoughts about the world around us, it seems that this pre-existing organ logic may have been used to process such thoughts (p.92). This would explain the many similarities that exist today between the organ functions and our thoughts (p.92); and also explain the two-way causative relationships that exist between those thoughts and the signs and symptoms of malfunction in the corresponding organs, as follows.

When our mind uses an organ's logic to process our thoughts, and our conscious mind suppresses, overuses, or is aware of the impeding of particular thoughts, this situation is duplicated in the related physical organ, which causes that organ to act as though its physical functions had been suppressed, overused, or impeded. This stresses the organ, which causes it to produce the signs and symptoms of our illness.

The effect on the main organs

Pancreas and stomach

In contemporary physiology, the stomach starts the process of digestion, and the pancreas acts *to further break down food to find any inherent nutrition and to control the body's uptake of the main nutrition* (p.93). In our mental world, our thoughts take the place of physical food; and the functions of the stomach and pancreas are used to digest those thoughts.

In developed societies today, we tend to think all day long—in our work, studies, recreation, or in simply trying to understand the apparently puzzling people around us. Therefore our conscious mind overuses the pancreas and stomach, which become weakened through overuse.

Significantly, the thoughts we most often strive to digest are those that are hard to understand. The physical equivalent would be to choose the hardest to digest food and to eat this difficult food all day long. And when we are unable to properly digest any particular thought, this *failure to digest* is duplicated in the pancreas, causing it to tend to fail to digest physical food. It is as though normal physical food were transformed into hard-to-digest food by the action of our mind. And when our mind does this for most of the day, year after year, it eventually renders the pancreas no longer able to properly digest normal food.

To make matters worse, the pancreas function peaks at eleven a.m. (p.379), which is when the normal digestive ability is at its strongest. From this time onwards, the pancreas function weakens as the day progresses. Yet our conscious mind continues heavily using this digestive ability all day long, which only weakens it even further. With physical food, once we have eaten enough, we are "full" and we normally stop eating; yet because it is our mind doing the digesting, we think it is okay to push ourselves to "eat" more and more thoughts, even though we may have the same feeling of being "full", of having "eaten" enough thoughts for the moment. If we were to do this with physical food and push ourselves to go on eating all day long, no-one would be surprised at the resultant symptoms of ill health. But we consider our mind to be separate from the body, and so do not normally make the connection between thinking too much and suffering the symptoms that would inevitably result from eating hard-to-digest food and doing this all day long.

The usual physical symptoms are: feeling tired and bloated after eating, having a swollen and tender abdomen, loose stools, intolerances to foods such as dairy and wheat, a poor sense of taste, low energy in general, and a sluggish mind (p.74). All such symptoms tend to be common amongst students, in people whose work requires them to think intensively, and people who habitually worry. And the more a person becomes exhausted through overthinking, the more pronounced these symptoms become. In particular, their ability to think would worsen. This is because the relationship between an organ's physical and mental functions is reciprocal, and once a person has poor pancreas function, their ability to mentally digest information also becomes poor. They would tend to get stuck in endless cycles of thought, unable to reach a satisfactory conclusion (that is, become unable to properly digest thoughts), which would usually result in them working their digestion even harder.

Added to the above symptoms can sometimes be a feeling of indigestion; that is, a cramping feeling on the front, left side of the torso (the location of the stomach). Often, with people whose digestion is already weakened through overthinking, when they are unable to *begin* digesting a particular thought, they experience this cramping feeling in their stomach—as though they had swallowed some physical food that their stomach could not digest.

Liver

In contemporary physiology, the liver regulates the production and supply of energy and the circulation of blood and other resources to the organs and tissues of the body. This could be summarized as: *to monitor the flow of substances to the organs and tissues, and when this does not seem right, to regulate the flow* (p.107).

When this function is used to process our thoughts, it is those thoughts that become the mental equivalent of the energy and substances in the body, and it so happens that our conscious mind often notices things that *do not seem right* in our thoughts, which then obstructs the flow of our thoughts. When this happens, this causes the liver to act as though the flow of the energy and substances in the body had been obstructed, so it applies its regulatory ability to attempt to remove the obstruction. It does this creatively, and (just as it does in the body with the supply of energy and other resources) it rearranges our thoughts, swaps or compares them with our memories (our reserve resources) until it has transformed the thought so as to remove the problem that was obstructing its flow (p.108).

This creative ability causes the liver to produce countless "rules" about how things should be done, and is responsible for us being able to efficiently organize the world around us and also every aspect of our own and other people's behaviour (p.109). Indeed, much of the organization that makes society function would not be possible without the liver's creative ability—such as the ordering of every activity into an efficient process, right down to the smallest of the routine tasks we perform.

However, this causes a problem for us when other people, or other things, do not behave exactly as we would like them to (when they break our "rules"). This obstructs the flow of our thoughts, which causes the liver to behave as though the flow of the energy and substances in the body had been obstructed. In response, it usually resorts to its emergency measure of producing a powerful force to remove the obstruction—the emotion of anger (p.109). We might express this by sighing or we may simply suppress our anger. But after a while, this suppressed anger builds up until we can no longer contain it, when we might start shouting to attempt to force people to do what we want; or we may even resort to physical violence to get our will obeyed (and the obstruction removed), which accounts for such things as road rage attacks and most relationship hostility—be it at home, work, or socially.

In all of us, this process is responsible for the daily stress-related symptoms we suffer—when our train is late, traffic moves too slowly, a queue is too long, or our employer expects us to produce several hour's work in one hour, or do the job of three people all at once. All these situations obstruct the physical function of the liver, which could eventually produce symptoms such as: moodiness, depression, irritability, rage, migraines, insomnia; stiff neck, shoulders and other joints; muscular cramps and spasms; painful periods, premenstrual syndrome; and also many other possible symptoms related to poor circulation, poor energy and poor digestion—which are indirect effects of the liver function being obstructed (p.113).

Due to the reciprocal nature of the relationship between an organ's mental and physical functions, once a person develops stagnated liver function, the mental application of their liver function would tend to become overactive—reflecting the liver's desire to remove the stagnation. In our mental world, the liver does this by applying its creative ability; or enforcing the countess "rules" this ability previously worked out; or frequently resorting to its emergency measure of producing anger. The person would become over controlling and excessively organized, would angrily insist on other people strictly obeying all rules; and would also tend to be paranoid.

The production of paranoia

Since the liver's creative ability is the key method it uses to remove an obstruction, when our conscious mind sees obstructions everywhere (our "rules" not being obeyed by people), the liver's creative ability is over applied to social situations, which tends to produce paranoia, as follows.

The liver would use its creative ability to try to work out why a person was behaving in a strange way, or was doing something that *we* thought was wrong. And it so happens that when someone else's behaviour is analysed from *our* point of view, it is easy to interpret their words, actions, tone of voice or facial expressions as indicating malicious intent towards ourselves. And this is the solution the liver would usually come up with, which it then presents to our conscious mind—the idea that the person was behaving maliciously towards us. Hence the liver has removed the obstruction to the flow of our thoughts—since the person's behaviour now makes sense to us.

But this would then usually cause the liver to also create countermeasures for us to adopt against this person, to, again, remove this further (now self-created) obstruction—the new obstruction being the notion that this person was breaking the rules of social conduct by behaving maliciously towards us. Our creative countermeasure would be designed to harm the other person. This might be a scheme to undermine them in other people's eyes, with carefully planned actions; or simply the making of malicious comments of our own. Though our behaviour would make perfect sense to us, it would only seem puzzling to the other person, since this further obstruction was imaginary (they were *not* behaving maliciously, so our response would make no sense to them). And the more the liver perceives such obstructions to the flow of our thoughts, the more it strives to find such creative solutions (now perhaps trying to imagine an explanation for why the "malicious" person was denying behaving in that way), and the more tormented we become.

The downside of creative ability

The ability to produce creative thoughts is an accidental offshoot of the liver's regulatory function. When our mind uses this simple liver function, which was designed to regulate the flow of substances and energy in the body, the function is, in effect, transformed into a creative engine that shapes our mental world. When used to process our ever-present thoughts, this creative ability goes rampant (since our thoughts are such that the obstructions to their flow are rampant), and it creates countless "rules" which are stored in our memory and *only* apply to our own particular mental world.

This massive collection of rules then creates advantages for us—enabling us to organize, to invent, to learn many skills. But these same rules also create a massive potential for obstructing the function of our physical liver—since all these rules must be obeyed for our liver to act as though the substances and energy in our body were flowing correctly.

How does the liver know when something is not right in our thoughts?

In the body, when the flow of energy or other resources is impeded, this would usually be because one or more of the organs were not functioning properly—due to their own functions being impeded for some reason. When the liver function is used to process our thoughts, it follows that the same must be true. Our thoughts are present amongst the logic of all the organs (just as the energy and substances are present amongst all the physical organs), and the flow of these thoughts would usually be impeded when the logic (mental function) of any of the main organs becomes impeded, which would usually happen due to it being unable to process a particular thought.

For example, the pancreas may be unable to digest a particular thought, or the lungs unable to find quality in the thought, or the kidneys may notice that the thought threatens our survival or status (the thought may undermine us socially or at work, or suggest we participate in conduct or a venture that is financially or physically reckless), or the heart may notice that the thought demonstrates poor social connections (it may be treating someone unfairly, unjustly or inappropriately). Any such situation would cause the flow of our thoughts to be impeded, which is the cue for the liver to act to "regulate the flow", since "something does not seem right" in the flow. The liver's creative ability would then attempt to modify the thought to remove the obstruction. It may rely on remembered solutions or rearrange the thought while perhaps combining it with other remembered thoughts, so as to create a new thought that solved the problem—just as the liver creatively manages the body's resources and energy to remove physical obstructions: by interchanging them when necessary, calling on reserves to solve a shortfall, creating new energy, such as ATP, and so on. At this point the thought may be digested (since it now makes sense); or its quality may be improved (the process, action, or appearance of an object or person now seems right); or the thought may now reflect a proper social connection (the other person is now being treated justly, fairly, or appropriately); or the new thought may no longer be too risky for us. This would pacify the "complaining organ" and thus restore the flow of our thoughts. And the liver would no longer have reason to act as though the flow of energy and substances in the body were obstructed—so would no longer produce the emotion of irritation or anger. And, indeed, the energy and substances in the body *would* return to flowing properly.

Lungs

In contemporary physiology, the lungs extract oxygen from the air we breathe and expel the waste products of respiration, which could be summarized as: *to take in something intangible from outside us, sort the good from the bad, incorporate the precious and let go of the waste* (p.133). When this lung logic is used to process our thoughts it enables us to notice quality in the things around us, to incorporate this within ourselves—so we are enriched through the appreciation of quality—and to *let go of the waste*; that is, to stop caring about something that is harmful to us, to let go of it and move on.

When our mind applies this logic in a balanced way, this enables us to gain pleasure from such things as music, nature, architecture, fashion, or design in any area, such as in electronic gadgets, cars, furniture, and so on. This also applies to personalities; we gain pleasure from the quality we recognise in certain people, in the way they conduct themselves, morally, physically, verbally. And the other aspect of this mental activity of *sorting the good from the bad* is that it enables us to recognise poor quality in all these things—in music, fashion, architecture, design, and in personalities. In other words, to recognise the opposite of what *we* personally think of as "quality". And once this "waste" has been sorted, if the lung function is healthy, we are able to *let go of the waste*, which enables us to let go of something harmful to us. As well as general "poor quality" experiences, this could also include activities, tasks or relationships that we have begun but which have become harmful rather than rewarding.

Our appreciation of quality can clearly greatly enrich our lives. But further than this, each time we appreciate quality in something, this strengthens the lung function. When our conscious mind uses this lung logic, and something precious from the things we experience is successfully extracted, this success is duplicated in the lungs and enhances the lungs' ability to extract oxygen from the air we breathe. This is why, when we experience something we enjoy, such as a landscape, fine piece of music or good design in any area, we may feel we can breathe more easily and may even sigh with pleasure.

However, when our conscious mind overuses this lung function we become perfectionists and inevitably end up living in an almost constant state of disappointment. The more we focus on quality, the higher our standards become and the less we are able to find it. This constant failure to extract something precious from the things we experience is duplicated in the lungs; and the lungs' ability to extract oxygen from the air we breathe is impeded. In time, this tendency could weaken the lung function, producing such symptoms as: shortness of breath, a weak cough, a quiet and weak voice, poor energy, the tendency to suffer colds and flu, a poor sense of smell, a blocked nose and sinuses, and wheezing or asthma—where it is difficult to breathe out (p.143).

Once a person develops poor lung function (either through mental factors or physical disease), their lungs' mental functions would also be poor. Their lungs' ability to breathe out and expel the waste products of respiration (CO_2) would be poor, so that the person's mental ability to *let go of the waste* would also be poor and they would tend to continue with projects, activities, habits, relationships, long after they had become harmful to them. And their lungs' ability to extract the precious oxygen from the air they breathe would also be poor, so that their ability to mentally *sort the good from the bad* would be poor. They would find it harder to appreciate quality in the things they experience (things they might otherwise have been able to enjoy), which would only increase further their tendency to be a perfectionist; for the lungs' ability to extract oxygen from the air we breathe is an essential and urgent urge (if we cannot extract oxygen, we will die) and once this is impeded, this urgent urge would be duplicated in the mental aspect of the lung function, driving us all the more to seek quality—with the quiet desperation of an animal trying to breathe air that is starved of oxygen. But since our ability to appreciate quality would be weak, we would feel dissatisfied with most things and end up living in a constant state of sadness.

Heart

In contemporary physiology, the heart circulates nourishment to the other organs and to every tissue via the blood vessels, which could be summarized as: *reaching out to those around us and spreading nourishment to them* (p.190). When this function is used to process our thoughts, this produces in us the desire to share our knowledge with those around us, or to help or assist them, which is all done most readily by talking to them—which reflects the fact that speech, and our facility with language, is the sense associated with the heart. And whenever we act on these desires and help other people or simply talk to them, this successful application of the heart's intention is duplicated in the heart, which enhances its physical function—sometimes to the extent that it produces that "warm glow" feeling within it.

However, our mind can also impede the heart function. In most societies this happens most commonly in men, who are encouraged not to talk about personal matters or their feelings, and to deal with things alone, without complaining or seeking assistance from others. When thinking in such ways, the heart's intention is suppressed in our thoughts, which state is duplicated in the heart, suppressing its physical function and also undermining the circulatory system.

The heart function can also be impeded in other situations, such as whenever a social connection is broken, which happens whenever a friendship, association, or relationship ends. The physical pain we feel in the heart reflects the degree to which the heart function is impeded, which can happen to such a degree that people can sometimes literally die of a "broken heart". A long-term relationship ends, or a job they held and loved for many years ends, and the break in that particular social connection is so severe that their heart can no longer function and simply stops working; that is, they suffer a heart attack.

When the heart function is routinely impeded and becomes weakened, this can eventually produce symptoms such as: palpitations, shortness of breath on exertion, anxiety or panic attacks, restlessness, being easily startled, speech disorders or dyslexia, having a poor long term memory, dream-disturbed sleep, insomnia, spontaneous sweating, lethargy, stabbing pains or "stuffiness" in the chest, possibly culminating in a heart attack (p.196).

Once a person develops poor heart function (either due to mental factors or physical disease), their heart's mental functions would also be poor, or "faulty". And since the mental application of their heart function produces their connections with other people, these would also be "faulty". They may habitually make socially inappropriate comments, behave in socially unacceptable ways, be constantly trying to please other people or inappropriately smiling or laughing or using an amused tone of voice. Every aspect of their interaction with other people could seem inappropriate.

Kidneys

In contemporary physiology, our "kidneys" (which includes three structures: the kidneys, adrenal glands and gonads) are responsible for a wide range of functions concerned with ensuring our immediate and long-term survival. This includes assisting in the regulation of our energy, releasing reserves to cope with emergency situations (the adrenaline surge), supporting and enabling immunity, and all functions related to reproduction (p.168).

When this logic is used to process our thoughts, this produces in us motivations and ideas related to our long-term survival, which includes us setting goals in life, having the drive to pursue them, and also the will to go on living. And the kidneys also generate defensive thoughts (such as the protective lies that seem to spontaneously pop into our mind when we are threatened), and also opportunistic thoughts that favour us (such as the idea to commit an opportunistic theft, or to act in some way or say something that favours us in the eyes of our boss or a potential partner).

The kidney function is most often weakened by overuse of the reserves the kidneys call upon in times of emergency. In the modern world, instead of this being restricted to truly emergency situations, such as when our life is physically threatened, it is more usual for us to draw on these reserves merely to achieve demanding tasks, or to keep functioning when the body is tired, causing us to live in an almost constant state of "emergency". This is most common in the workplace, but it also happens socially, recreationally and in family life. We are driven to work too hard, often through fear or ambition, but also sometimes through sheer excitement—which is just as harmful for the kidneys. Living in an almost constant adrenalized state overuses this kidney function and eventually weakens the kidneys, producing various symptoms which could include: low back pain, shortness of breath, asthma (where it is hard to breathe in), the tendency to suffer hay fever and other allergies; migraines, feeling constantly fearful, having a poor short term memory and concentration, frequent urination, weak knees and stiff joints generally, poor hearing, low libido and decreased engagement in life (p.174).

The kidneys also regulate the production and use of energy, support immunity and provide us with the urge to want to be alive and continue living. Our hopes, ambitions, or our own awareness of our status are all ideas produced in us when the kidney logic is used to process our thoughts. When any of these ideas are dashed, this impedes this kidney logic, which impediment is duplicated in the physical kidneys. Apart from contributing to any of the above symptoms, this could also remove our will to live, greatly reduce our energy, immunity, and possibly cause a long term depression. It is as though the body's drive were switched off.

Another mental cause of poor kidney function is when a person routinely feels fearful, vulnerable or unsupported. These feelings undermine our long-term survival, and since the kidney logic produces our thoughts concerning our long-term survival, this undermines the kidneys' logic and hence also their physical function.

This mental state is common in the modern world. Concerns about being able to pay the bills, pay the rent or mortgage, or about remaining in employment, or in a relationship—are common preoccupations for many people. And such fears are epidemic amongst men. Indeed, the self-imposed loneliness that society encourages men to adopt, tends to foster a feeling of being unsupported, which would cause feelings of fearfulness and insecurity, leading to poor kidney function, with its related signs and symptoms. This would then tend to worsen the situation, since the fear and insecurity would only increase (one of the possible symptoms of poor kidney function is an increased tendency to feel fearful). And the more the kidney reserves were further drawn on—to combat this threat to our survival—the more the kidney function would be weakened.

The interdependence of the organs when processing our thoughts

Just as the functioning of the physical organs is interdependent, this also applies when the organ logic is used to process our thoughts, and many of the daily tasks we perform require the combined use of the logic of all the main organs.

For example, the single task of researching something on the internet or in a reference book would require us to digest information (a pancreas function), an element of creative thinking (a liver function), attention to quality and the discarding of "waste" (a lung function), processing of other people's words and composing some of our own, to be either written or spoken (a heart function), and the task may have been motivated by us wanting to enhance our value in the eyes of other people, either with a long- or short-term goal in mind (a kidney function).

We are so used to the experience of our mental daily lives that we take it for granted and simply assume all tasks are performed by the brain which is some sort of massive computer. It is not until each task is broken down, as in the above example, that it becomes clear that our mental world is, in fact, made up by combining the mental functions of all the abdominal organs.

The downside of this is that, since the functions of all the main organs are usually utilized when we perform many tasks, all the organs can be affected when a task becomes stressful.

For example, in many work-related scenarios, there is pressure for us to do tasks in too short a time. This would impede the liver function, since the situation would be seen by the liver's logic as the breaking of our "rules". This would produce stress-related symptoms within us, and in particular, irritation and anger. But the lung function would also be impeded, since our desire for quality was disappointed. It is the lungs that enable us to appreciate the quality in abstract things, such as doing a good job, and when we are conscious of such quality being sacrificed, this impedes the lung's logic and hence also its physical function. And the kidney function could also be weakened, since if we did not do our job well, we might fear losing our job and then not being able to survive, which would undermine the part of the kidneys' logic concerned with our long-term survival, and thus weaken the kidneys' physical function. And we might also be inclined to draw on our emergency reserves to counter this and meet the demands of our job, which would only further weaken the kidneys. And if we did not have good social bonds at work (with supervisors and others—perhaps as a result of the stress), the heart function would also be impeded—possibly producing in us that "sinking heart" feeling whenever we thought of our work environment. And in many jobs, the work itself may also be depleting for the pancreas (even without the stress), since it is the pancreas and stomach that enable us to mentally digest information. And since we were employed for eight hours a day, we would be expected to be mentally digesting information for this whole time, even though our ability to do this peaks at eleven a.m. and weakens from then onwards as the day progresses. This forced overuse would greatly weaken the pancreas function. But also, our work may involve us attempting to digest hard-to-understand thoughts (the equivalent of difficult-to-digest food), which would add a further strain on the pancreas.

In all, these common work-related stresses could eventually produce in us signs and symptoms related to the poor function of all the main organs.

Our personality choices can impede the organ functions

Living in a human society is a complex task, and usually we must each use our own initiative to solve the problem of how to be a human being. Through years of experimentation, we make many decisions about how we should conduct ourselves in our daily lives, and these choices may also suppress the function of the main organs.

For example, there may be complex reasons why many of us sometimes avoid giving to charity. The liver creates countless "rules" and insists they are obeyed (by ourselves as well as by others); the kidneys are concerned with safeguarding our own survival; and the lungs appreciate quality—in the conduct of other people as well as in ourselves. All these desires, when combined, might cause us to develop a whole range of reasons why we should not give to charity. If our rules were broken by the person in need (perhaps simply by the fact that they were begging), or by the advertising that sought help on their behalf (such as when advertisers use emotionally manipulative devices to prompt us to support their cause); or if helping the other person could in any way threaten our own survival, by reducing our already meagre income—all these factors could cause us to suppress the heart function of *reaching out to the other person and spreading nourishment to them.* And if we did this routinely, this would only impede our own heart function.

As another example—if we allowed the "concerns" of the lungs to dominate our mental world and tended to focus too much on quality, this may cause us to notice the poor quality in other people's responses when we talked to them. For example, when making a comment we might notice they usually misinterpreted it, or seemed incapable of understanding it in the way we meant it; or each time we started to say something, a particular person might always try to anticipate what we were saying (but clearly getting it wrong) and so would never let us finish what we started to say. When we notice such poor quality, we may stop trying to talk to people in general, which would suppress the heart's intention (to *reach out to them and spread nourishment to them*) and thus impede its physical function. And this situation may also cause us to give up on pursuits or goals in life, feeling there was no point attempting to interact with people, which would impede the kidney function (which produces our engagement with life, activities and people), and the resulting low spirits, sadness and melancholy would also impede all the other organs and bodily functions—all resulting from us focusing *too* much on quality.

As yet another example—we may have decided it was not appropriate to defend ourselves against certain injustices, perhaps in the workplace (injustices that the hierarchy demands we silently endure), or injustices in our daily interactions with friends and acquaintances—because it seemed to us unseemly to complain about such things. In all these instances, these types of injustice would be experienced by the liver as the breaking of its "rules" (because the people were not behaving towards us as *we* believed they should), and the liver would produce anger to attempt to remove these obstructions to the flow of our thoughts. But since we had decided not to respond, this decision would also suppress our anger, producing stagnated liver function and making us prone to outbursts of anger (when we could no longer contain it) and other powerful symptoms, such as a stiff neck, muscular cramps, sciatica, abdominal or back pains, migraines, paranoia, painful periods in women.

Some people may even adopt a general policy of not defending themselves, since it seems to them improper in some way; in effect, they have decided to adopt the role of the martyr and to silently endure injustices inflicted on them by other people, because this response (or lack of it) seems to them more noble or more worthy in some other way. In this situation, not only would their liver be affected as described above, but the function of their immune system could also be impeded, since their conscious mind had decided to suppress their defences—which could affect the function of their pericardium or lymphatic system, and possibly also the aspects of their "kidneys" and lungs involved in immunity.

Acupuncture normalizes the mental functions of the organs

Acupuncture treatment seems to "get under the radar" of our conscious mind and return the physical organ functions to normal, which then also tends to regulate the mental functions of those organs. In the first few weeks of treatments, new patients often tell me of the mental changes they have spontaneously made in their lives. They might say they are less affected by things, or do not let things get to them like they used to; that they have started standing up for themselves, which makes them feel good; or they make other such comments.

The mind can block treatment

But in these first few weeks of treatment, some patients sometimes re-establish their previous mental habits, and the symptoms they were suffering start to return. For example, if a patient's liver function was stagnated for years, once this was treated they would be less inclined to mentally over-control everything in their lives—since their liver would now be functioning normally and therefore the flow of energy and substances in their body would not be obstructed, so their liver would be less inclined to control those substances. And this relaxation of control would usually be duplicated in their mental world. But if they had a long-term habit of controlling and organizing themselves and others, they may simply continue the habit—even though their physical liver was no longer experiencing obstructions. And just as before, their attempts to control and organize would often be either resisted or unsuccessful, and this obstructed state would be duplicated in their physical liver, re-establishing its stagnated function. When this happens, all the related symptoms would return and the old pattern would be re-established.

In this situation, the person's mental habits would have blocked the acupuncture treatment. With such patients, they tend to initially respond to treatment, with their symptoms being alleviated, but then after a few treatments they re-establish their mental patterns; and each treatment from then onwards has little effect on their symptoms, or the effects only last for a day or two before the symptoms return. This type of mental factor makes it harder to treat some patients and is the biggest *natural* block to acupuncture treatment.[5] The only way for such patients to improve their health would be to find some way to persuade themselves to change their mental habits—or to resist re-establishing them after treatment.

Extract from *Ling Shu*, Chapter 29

Huang Di: ... Kings, dukes, and eminent personalities, persons eating bloody meat, they are arrogant, they follow only their own desires, and they look down upon the common people. Hence it is impossible to approach them with dietary prohibitions. If one were to prohibit them something, this would be against their mind. If one were to follow their desires, this would aggravate their disease. To ease their condition, how can this be done? To cure them, what is to be done first?

Qi Bo: The intrinsic nature of humans is such: there is no one who does not abhor death and enjoys life. Inform them of what will destroy them. Tell them what will be good for them. Guide them to what will ease their condition. Open their minds to everything that will bring suffering. Even if these are people who do not follow the WAY, why should they not listen?[6]

Extract from *Su Wen*, Chapter 77

When a physician is unable to severely reprove the patient and, hence, is unable to move the patient's spirit and when [the physician's] outer appearance is soft and weak, so that the patient behaves disorderly to a degree where he fails to [take treatments regularly], and his disease cannot be removed, then no therapeutic activities can be performed.[7]

Wang Bing (in 762 AD) commented on the above extract

When warnings are not sufficient to make someone avoid what is wrong, when moving a person's spirit is not sufficient to make someone follow orders so that he can be employed to shoulder tasks and if he is disorganized to a degree that he fails to carry out the daily routines and if the patient does not move, what medicine could there be to treat him![8]

Our mental world is produced by the abdominal organs

In humans, the functions of the abdominal organs are now used to process our thoughts, so that our "mental" world was made possible because of the existence of our abdominal organ functions. Therefore our mental world is a reflection, or ghost, of our "organ" world. And because of the association between each organ's logic and its physical function, what happens in our mental world is duplicated in our organ world—and vice versa—so that each has become a model of the other.

This gives our mind the ability to cause serious physical illness

The organs were designed to do particular physical tasks, and our mental world is produced (accidentally) by this same processing. Hence, the liver provides us with the capacity to control and organize; the lungs, the capacity to appreciate quality; the pancreas, the ability to digest information; and the heart, the desire to help others. Such activities can be intoxicating and it is all too easy to fall into the habit of overusing a particular organ's processing ability—and becoming too controlling, too much of a perfectionist, a heavy thinker, or being too giving. When we do this, this causes problems for that particular abdominal organ, which is also overused; and sometimes its function my become blocked (just as its associated mental processing often meets obstructions). When these types of problems occur, it is this that causes many of the signs and symptoms of our illness.

This situation has created one of the biggest hazards for our health. If our mental world were separate from our "organ world", there would be no problem, but the two cannot be separated; what happens in the one is duplicated in the other. This means that the human intellect is a mechanism that can easily and very effectively impede the function of any, or all, of the abdominal organs. We cannot *un*-invent our intellect (that is what makes us human), so to achieve a healthy and happy life, we need to apply that intellect to regulate our own mental world, so that we do not undermine our very foundations—the functioning of our organs.

Avoiding thought patterns that impede our organ functions

On page 236 above, an example was given of the stresses we encounter in a typical work-related scenario, where there was pressure to do tasks in too short a time, and our response to that stress affected the five main organs. This is a situation many of us frequently find ourselves in. Indeed this type of scenario is almost unavoidable; these situations may draw us in, unsuspecting, until we find ourselves trapped into adopting such self-destructive mental habits.

One approach to avoiding the build up of such stress is to make adjustments in small steps. For example, many liver-related issues could be summarized as us trying to control too many things. In the tasks we routinely perform at home or at work, the liver would have worked out the most efficient process to do each task, and the liver produces in us the feeling of irritation or anger when we watch someone else doing it differently or if someone presses *us* to do it differently. Once our conscious mind is in the habit of overusing this liver function, it is easy to fill our days with endless things that must be organized or done in a very specific way, and to become entrapped into impeding our own liver function—which happens each time any of these tasks is *not* performed exactly as we would like. The particular way we would like each task performed is a "rule" our liver has created. If we could persuade ourselves to not care about such "rules" (particularly the ones other people routinely break), then the rules would go away and there would be less opportunities for the liver function to be impeded. With each such task, you could try asking yourself: is this really necessary? Can it be left out? What would happen if I did not do this at all, or in this particular way?

It is also easy to develop the habit of overusing the lung function of appreciating quality and to become entrapped into seeking ever higher standards in every aspect of our life, causing us to work excessively hard to meet our own high standards and to reject many things we might otherwise have been able to enjoy. One solution may be to try focusing on the good aspects of anything we encounter, rather than the bad; and each time we are able to appreciate something we might otherwise have rejected, the experience becomes enjoyable and our lung function is reinforced, rather than being impeded due to us failing to perceive "quality" in the things around us.

Our need to digest information will always be present, but the depleting effect on the pancreas could best be reduced by, where possible, reducing the amount of thinking (or worrying) we do and only processing the thoughts that are really "necessary". And when heavy thinking *is* necessary, if this were restricted to the morning, before about midday (the digestion peaks at eleven a.m.), this would reduce the depleting effect.

The best way to avoid weakening the kidney function would usually be to adjust our work-life balance. It is okay (and even desirable) to sometimes work hard, but this should be balanced by rest and relaxation. There should be an equal balance of activities in our life between work and play (activities that are purely enjoyable and have no element of stress). And of course the most relaxing activity we can perform is sleep. This is necessary to allow the body to repair itself. If you find yourself working hard too often and not allowing enough time each day for relaxation, or purely enjoyable activities, then you could try asking yourself what would happen if you did less. If you work hard to buy particular possessions or holidays, would you have a better overall quality of life if you modified those ambitions? If you were currently driven by the fear of unemployment or the loss of your current status, would you really be worse off if you changed your job, or might that lead to an improvement in your quality of life? And another important factor concerning kidney health is to ensure that our goals and ambitions are appropriate and achievable.

To enhance the health of our heart, we need to avoid thoughts that weaken our connections with other people; or find ways to strengthen those connections. The heart's intention is to *reach out to those around us and spread nourishment to them*. There are complex reasons why men (for example) tend to impeded this heart function. Peer pressure may inhibit men from being open about their feelings or from asking for assistance from other people. In such situations, for us to allow ourselves to share or express our opinions or feelings, it may be necessary to question the validity of the pressures that restrict us. These pressures are always self-created; it is our own response to the people around us (or our response to our own perceptions) that produces the pressure within us to keep silent, which only damages our own heart. But these types of issue are complex, and some experimentation may be required for each person to find the approach that works best for them—when every factor of their life is considered. It is often not easy to be a human being and it can take many years into adulthood (or sometimes decades) before we have become reasonably skilful at it.

Achieving the right balance in life

In our mental world, there should be a certain amount of organization, of us setting and following rules, seeking quality, thinking, having regard for others, and also watching out for our own security. The key is to get the balance right, to do each thing in proportion—to the right amount and at the right time.

A person who achieves this would always be able to "sort the good from the bad" and "let go of the waste", so they appreciate the good qualities in people (including themselves) and in all other things, without paying undue attention to minor flaws. They would also not fall into the trap of becoming *too* organized and regimented, would be able to relax rules when appropriate and allow things to happen in their own way, rather than trying to control all people and all things around them. They would not think *too* much and end up constantly mulling over every detail of their lives, the people in it, and every activity, object or idea they encountered. They would not seek too high a quality in all things and all people, so they ended up rejecting much they would otherwise benefit from. They would be able to form social connections appropriately and provide support and "nourishment" to others when appropriate, while not falling into the trap of doing this excessively. They would have formed long- and short-term goals that were achievable, rather than destroying themselves in the pursuit of goals that were not realistically achievable. And they would feel the appropriate amount of fear and excitement and sadness and anger in the appropriate situations, but not feel any of these excessively.

Observing seasonal changes

Another important element in the mental causes of disease is the disharmony with the seasons that life in today's devolved countries tends to encourage. The human body is still very much synchronized with nature. As one season changes to another, the functional balance between the organs also naturally changes. The organs find this transition demanding, which is why there tends to be epidemics of colds and influenza as each season changes. Leading up to the change, people are often drained due to driving themselves too hard; and as the season changes, this places even more demands on their organs, to the point where they are unable to maintain normal immunity and they succumb to colds and influenza. Epidemics at these times are mainly due to this effect, which is why they occur at *every* seasonal change, not only the change between Autumn and Winter—though this particular change is most demanding on our immunity, since the change is from lung-dominant to kidney-dominant, so that both the organs involved in our immunity are taxed. This explains why even more people tend to succumb at this time, and particularly the elderly, whose kidney function is often poor anyway.

Chapter 2 of the *Su Wen* advocates living in accord with the seasons, then goes on to say

> **Extract from *Su Wen*, Chapter 2**
>
> Only the sages follow the Way; hence, their bodies have no strange diseases.... To op-

pose one's root, is to attack one's basis and to spoil one's true [influences].... Opposing [the natural activities of the seasons] results in catastrophe and harms life. If one follows them, severe diseases will not emerge. This is called 'to achieve the Way'.[9]

Extract from *Su Wen*, Chapter 3

The fact is, the wind is the origin of the one hundred diseases. In case a person is clear and calm, the flesh and the interstice structures are firmly closed up and resist. Even though there is a strong wind which is a violent poison, it will be unable to harm that person. This is so because one follows the sequence of the seasons.[10]

When people have acupuncture treatment routinely (even if only once or twice a season), this tends to make them much more aware of their body and they can usually clearly feel the effect on themselves as the functional balance between their organs changes to prepare them for each new season. Usually they describe feeling a dramatic drop in their energy, with no apparent cause, which lasts for one or two days before their energy returns to normal and they feel subtly different. For all the above reasons, it is important to properly relax in the week when each season changes (see the tables below).

The body's resources also vary with the seasons. The Spring and Summer are the times of maximum energy, when new projects should be started and we can work hard at achieving our goals. In the Autumn and Winter our energy is naturally declining, and we should not expect to be able to work so hard. In the Winter our productivity may be about half of that in the Summer, or even less. The Winter is a time of hibernation, when our working day should be much shorter (even if present in the workplace, our productivity should be much less) and we should not start new, demanding projects. Only by living in harmony with these seasonal changes can we expect to maintain good health. And conversely, if we fail to observe the seasonal changes at all, we should expect our health to suffer.

When referring to the dates in the following tables (on page 244), it should be noted that not all people adjust to each new season on the same day. With each person, the exact day their body adjusts could occur several days (or even more than a week) on either side of the following dates.

The seasonal cycle of organ activity

Table 1. The seasons in the Northern hemisphere[11]

Approximate dates	Season	Dominant organ
21 Mar (vernal equinox) to 20 Jun	Spring	liver
21 Jun (summer solstice) to 21 Sep	Summer	heart
22 Sep (autumnal equinox) to 21 Dec	Autumn (Fall)	lungs
22 Dec (winter solstice) to 20 Mar	Winter	"kidneys"

The pancreas is not included in the above table, since the season in which its function dominates is unclear. From my own experience, it seems that the last three to four weeks of each season acts as a transitional period and that the pancreas is the dominant organ in each of these transitional periods. Also note that the body adjusts to this transitional period, just as it does to the start of each new season.

In Chapter 29 of the *Su Wen*, this transitional period is given as the last eighteen days of each season,[12] though with myself the length of this period can vary from anywhere between nineteen to twenty-nine days, depending on various factors.

Table 2. The seasons in the Southern hemisphere

Approximate dates	Season	Dominant organ
21 Mar (autumnal equinox) to 20 Jun	Autumn (Fall)	lungs
21 Jun (winter solstice) to 21 Sep	Winter	"kidneys"
22 Sep (vernal equinox) to 21 Dec	Spring	liver
22 Dec (summer solstice) to 20 Mar	Summer	heart

Chapter 13. Detailed case histories

With many patients it is common for them to have signs and symptoms relating to all five of their main organs (as in most of the following case histories). This probably reflects the fact that the organs are interdependent, so that once a problem exists in one for any length of time, the other main organs are inevitably affected.

In the case histories, I mention which organ malfunctions are responsible for causing the various signs and symptoms, but do not usually state which acupoints were used in the treatments and instead only record the general progress of the treatments. The typical acupoints used to treat each organ can be found in the chapters related to those organs.

Depression and panic attacks

Female, aged 29. This patient initially sought treatment for depression and panic attacks. She had a history of depression and mild panic attacks, going back 18 months, and recently suffered a severe panic attack. Following an argument with her boyfriend, she started to feel panicky in the street; she was hyperventilating, started to feel faint, felt cramp in the fingers of both hands, but more so on her left, and also cramp around her jaw and she was unable to speak. Apart from these attacks, she also had the following symptoms.

She generally felt anxious, was easily startled and had vivid dreams (all due to poor heart function). She had a weak low back, poor short term memory, mild hay fever in recent years and low libido (due to poor kidney function). Her emotions were variable, she felt a lump in her throat when stressed, and suffered period cramps, clots in her menstrual blood, and usually one week of PMS, feeling irritable, moody and more anxious (all due to stagnated liver function). She had a poor appetite, felt tired and bloated after eating, had food intolerances, was easily bruised, was always thinking and often humming or singing to herself (all related to poor pancreas function). Her energy became very low at three p.m., she suffered lots of colds each year, felt the cold a lot, had sensitive skin and dry hands (due to poor lung function).

Over the first few treatments all these symptoms gradually improved; she eventually felt calm and had a good appetite and energy. After six weeks, she split up with her boyfriend (of two years); her mood remained stable and she coped well with the split up. This is a common pattern with acupuncture treatments. After a few sessions, patients often tell me of big changes in their lives. It seems the treatment enables people to clarify issues in their lives and provides them with the courage to make positive changes.

This patient continued coming for maintenance treatments for years (sometimes once a month, sometimes every few months), through which time she continuously thrived, despite the stresses of a professional career. Her periods became symptom free; she was clear of hay fever, had good memory, concentration, sleep, energy, and had no low back problems.

Energy, sleep, and help to give up smoking

Male, aged 56. This patient initially sought treatment to help him give up smoking and to improve his energy and sleep. He was divorced twenty years ago and now lived alone. He had a stressful job and smoked to relieve the stress.

He also had a small appetite, felt tired after eating, had a poor sense of taste, sweet cravings, tended to worry and think a lot, found it hard to think after midday, and his stools were usually soft or runny (all due to poor pancreas function). His nose ran all day, was worse in the morning but became blocked at night; he was wheezy, for years had felt very sleepy between three and four p.m., was made very tired if he talked a lot, had dry skin, felt the cold, and suffered three to four colds a year (all due to poor lung function). He had palpitations, was easily startled, found it hard to get to sleep, but once asleep had vivid dreams two or three times a week (due to poor heart function). He was hard of hearing in his right ear, had frequent and urgent urination, shortness of breath, poor short term memory when stressed, and felt hot at night (due to poor kidney function). His moods swung high and low and he had dry eyes and high pitch tinnitus (due to stagnated liver function).

It was clear that his poor energy was due to the weakness in the function of both his pancreas and lungs. And he had clearly been driving himself hard for years, which had weakened his kidney function.

By the fifth treatment, his energy was normal (he no longer felt sleepy in the afternoon, nor at any other time of day), his stools were normal, he had no sweet cravings, his nose no longer ran, and he had cut down greatly on the amount he smoked each day. And after a few further treatments he stopped smoking, now regarded himself as a non-smoker and hated the smell of tobacco smoke; his sleep was greatly improved and he often slept solidly; the palpitations had stopped; his sinuses felt clear, and the morning cough which he developed as he started to give up smoking was also greatly improving.

Throat pulsations and general stress

Female, aged 29. This patient initially came for treatment concerning serious throat pulsations, whose cause could not be diagnosed. Her parents were in their late forties when she was conceived and both drove themselves very hard and were exhausted at that time. When born, the patient was deaf in her right ear and had only partial hearing in her left. She now had a stiff low back, frequent and urgent urination, and suffered hay fever for the past two years. She was in a very stressful job and often ran on adrenaline.

These symptoms were all caused by poor kidney function, which she inherited from her parents. This was at the root of her health problems and was exacerbated by her stressful lifestyle. But by this stage in her life, her pancreas, liver and heart were also affected. She had a small appetite, sweet cravings, felt bloated after eating and had excess gas (all due to poor pancreas function). Her emotions were up and down, she had pain on her front and back at the level of her liver, frequent cramps in her calves and feet, sighed a lot, felt a constant lump in her throat, and had painful and heavy periods with one week of PMS, in which she felt frustrated and emotional and had tender and swollen breasts (all due to stagnated liver function). She also had palpitations (due to poor heart function).

Over the first few treatments, all her symptoms (apart from her poor hearing) improved, including the throat pulsations; she said everyone was commenting on how transformed she was. She had taken the contraceptive pill for twelve years and decided to stop. This, combined with the continuing acupuncture treatments, produced a further dramatic improvement in her health (in my experience the contraceptive pill usually weakens the "kidney" function, and stopping this accelerated her improvement).

When taking this patient's heart pulse in one session, I felt a constriction around my throat, and the patient told me that as soon as my finger touched her wrist, her throat started pulsing. This appeared to confirm that her throat pulsations were produced by her heart (which is very often affected by poor kidney function). However, in Chinese medicine, we would normally associate throat-related symptoms with stagnated liver function (which is always exacerbated by stress, if not *caused* by it), so that there appeared to be no clear-cut physiological explanation for the symptom—beyond my insight that the heart produced it. All that could be concluded was that when the function of her main organs was normalized with acupuncture, the symptom stopped, therefore it must have been the improper function of one or more of those organs that caused it.

Neck pain caused by emotional factors

Female, aged 28. This patient sought treatment for a shoulder and neck pain. She had always had tension and tenderness in her neck, but in the last two to three months it became much worse and she was now getting shooting pains.

She also had food intolerances (to wheat and dairy), felt bloated after eating, with excess gas; her stools were soft and sometimes runny with undigested food in them; she was always thinking and could not accept compliments—in other words, was mentally reluctant to nourish herself (all related to poor pancreas function). She had a poor short term memory, asthma as a child and she used to get hay fever (which stopped two years ago) but was still allergic to cat fur; she felt hot at night; her back was stiff in the mornings; she had weak knees and stiff hips, frequent and urgent urination, shortness of breath when running up stairs, was hard of hearing, and recently felt fearful (all due to poor kidney function). She recently had vivid dreams and was easily startled (due to poor heart function). She was usually emotional and sensitive and tended to feel low, sighed often, recently had mild dizziness, had dry and itchy eyes and saw floaters (which in her case were light, transparent shapes); her menstrual cycle had a variable length, between 33-35 days, with seven days of PMS in which she felt irritable, depressed, angry, and had swollen and tender breasts; and her menstrual blood was dark with clots (all due to stagnated liver function).

This young patient had pronounced poor kidney function, which she clearly inherited from her parents (since she had asthma and hay fever as a child), and this gave her a weak constitution, which meant that the routine stresses of life affected her more deeply than they would most other people.

However, after the first two sessions her neck and shoulder were fine and she felt great, but her neck pain then returned and she started going through emotional turmoil. After the fifth treatment she told me she had a long talk with her boyfriend about many issues and felt much better; she also started "observing herself" at work and managed to relax when she became upset. Her digestion and sleep were now much better, though her energy was still low. For the next two weeks her neck pain got worse again and she said she noticed she was always analysing things and worrying about her insecurities with her boyfriend. The following week she felt good after the treatment, felt more clear and positive and was thinking less; she spoke to her boyfriend about the issues, which improved things; and her neck pain cleared. Her "inner turmoil" was much less and also less intense. The following week, she broke up with her boyfriend. For two weeks after this, her emotions and digestion were up and down but she was feeling much more clear. Her neck and shoulder pain then cleared and generally she felt good; her digestion was good and she started meditation.

This case is a clear illustration of how our physical problems are often directly caused by mental and emotional factors. Her neck pain and digestive problems initially cleared and she felt euphoric after the first session, but then the problems returned since the problems in her relationship with her boyfriend were all unchanged.

Problems with the people or situations in our life can often result in us experiencing a pain in the neck, which is certainly the origin of the expression "pain in the neck". Such pains are usually produced by stagnated liver function, which in this instance was made very much worse by the problem in the patient's life which she could not resolve. This amounted to an obstruction to the flow of her thoughts, which caused stagnated liver function (p.107), which then caused the strong pain and stiffness in the gallbladder meridian at her neck and shoulder. It is probably not a coincidence that the gallbladder provides us with the mental ability to make decisions (p.121) and that our inability to make this type of decision results in dysfunctional tissue along the gallbladder meridian as it leaves the head (the location of the obstructed thoughts).

But with the current patient, the continuing treatments gave her the confidence to face the problems in her life and deal with them, and once she resolved the problems for good, her health issues were able to clear. This is a familiar pattern; patients often tell me of the positive changes they have made in their lives, or that appear to have happened spontaneously since they started treatments.

There is another common pattern that occurs. Some patients (usually particularly strong willed and principled people) are so entrenched in the particular thought patterns that gave rise to most of their physical symptoms, that they cannot escape them. As they start acupuncture treatment, their symptoms initially improve, but then the symptoms return because the patient resumes their previous mental patterns, which reinforces the particular organ malfunctions that produced their symptoms in the first place (p.238).

Migraine

Male, aged 24. This patient had a ten-year history of migraines. They improved for about six months but had recently been much worse. He was working as a newly qualified teacher.

The migraines now only started at work; they tended to start at about three p.m. on the right side of his head (around the gallbladder meridian) with a dull sensation which gradually got stronger. He also felt pain behind his right eye, had blurred vision and nausea, and the right side of his neck and his right shoulder would stiffen. Apart from the migraines, he also sighed and suffered hiccups frequently, had cramps in his left leg, saw floaters (specks of light), had a loud voice and was a very structured and organized person (all due to stagnated liver function). He also had a poor short term memory (which was worse in recent years), tended to have a stiff low back, was slightly hard of hearing, had shortness of breath on exertion, mild hay fever (which he had since childhood) and was allergic to dog fur (all due to poor kidney function). He also had vivid dreams, was easily startled, had anxiety, and a slight speech problem (due to poor heart function). He had a small appetite, felt tired after eating, had food allergies, low energy (at work he "kept going on adrenaline" and was very tired in the evening), had sweet cravings, and was always thinking (all related to poor pancreas function).

By the fourth treatment, his headaches were less frequent and also less severe and did not last as long; he was calmer but still slightly anxious. He continued treatments, but with varying gaps between them. He could sometimes go for weeks with no migraines at all, but when the stress of his work was high this tended to trigger a migraine. With a treatment every two weeks, he was generally well and able to cope with the stress of his job, even having periods with no symptoms at all, including the digestive and allergy-related symptoms. He had clearly inherited poor kidney function from his parents (since he had hay fever as a child), which left him with poor stamina; on top of this, his work was extremely demanding and even a person with a strong constitution would have struggled to remain totally healthy while doing the job.

This is a dilemma that many people face and must solve in their own way. If your work is so demanding that your body's resources cannot cope, then if you want to remain healthy (or want to *regain* your health), you would need to either support your health with a system like Chinese acupuncture, change your work, or change the way you respond to your work. The advantage of acupuncture treatment is that it often clarifies all these issues for each person which then enables them to pick the path that is right for them.

Energy, focus, and direction in life

Male, aged 57. This patient sought treatment to improve his energy and "focus" (his sense of direction in life). He ran his own business and previously had two operations on his lower back (fifteen and eight years ago); his discs lumbar-4 and lumbar-5 had "broken up", as he put it. He now experienced back ache and shooting pains down his leg.

In holistic medicine, it is recognised that patients who do not feel supported will often develop a low back problem. In this case, he was used to running a business as a sole trader, and (when viewed metaphorically) his low back vertebra having "broken up" (as he described it) could be likened to the foundations of a bridge crumbling under the strain—the strain of him single-handedly holding up the responsibilities he took on. Any fear concerning our long-term survival would impede our kidney function, which, in turn, would account for the weak spine in the region of the kidneys.

As well as the low back problem, he also had shortness of breath on exertion and an allergy to dust (also due to poor kidney function). He was also easily startled, had palpitations, anxiety attacks, a slight stammer, and had very vivid and strange dreams (all due to poor heart function). He had a quiet voice, and his energy was drained when he talked a lot; he usually felt tired each day around two p.m. onwards; he felt at his best in Autumn (when the lungs are the dominant organ—p.244); his sinuses usually felt blocked; he would sweat at night but without feeling hot, and he usually felt "distant" or "not connected" and sad (all related to poor lung function). He had low energy generally, lots of gas, his stools were often very loose, he was always thinking, and had sweet cravings (due to poor pancreas function). He sighed frequently (people were always telling him this), got cramps in his legs and often felt irritated or emotional (due to stagnated liver function).

During the week after his first treatment, he felt very well, alert, had some deep sleeps, and he only felt the afternoon energy lag on one day. By the second week, his energy was up and down, but he felt mentally clearer (he said he did not get stuck in "thinking loops" anymore), and he no longer had the feeling of not being connected. And after a few more treatments, he felt very well, his energy was good, he was feeling more positive and focused and slept solidly with very few dreams.

Although this patient clearly had poor kidney function and poor heart function, which produced significant symptoms, it seems most likely he developed these over a long period of driving himself too hard in life. However, it was clear to me (as a healer) that his personality was dominated by his lungs, and this lung-dominance would have therefore existed *prior* to this. This would have made him a perfectionist, and it was probably this that caused him to drive himself so hard which, in the long run, caused all the other problems.

Abdominal pain and digestive signs (Liver invading stomach)

Male, aged 14. The patient's parents split up when he was aged ten, and a year later he developed stomach cramps. His elder brother then left home to attend university, which he also found hard to accept. His stomach cramps persisted for a further two years, when he was brought for treatment.

The pains were almost continuous but were very bad for about two days out of every two weeks. Over the previous two years he was taken to a range of medical practitioners, prescribed an anti-spasmodic drug (*dicyclomine*) which had no effect, and no reason could be found for the pain. The pain consisted mainly of an aching sensation on the centre of his abdomen between the acupoints Ren-8 (*Shenque*) and Ren-14 (*Juque*), sometimes accompanied by stabbing pains at Stomach-25 (*Tianshu*), and the pain was usually worse between seven and eight a.m. and between six and twelve p.m. (these morning hours being when the stomach function was at its strongest and the pericardium at its weakest; and the evening hours being when the large intestine, stomach and pancreas function were at their weakest—p.379). These pains had come to dominate his life and led to his exclusion from many activities.

The acupoints the pains were located on clearly indicated poor function of the stomach, large intestine and heart[*], and suggested a clear emotional cause in the split up of his parents—he had difficulty stomaching the situation (that is, he could not even *begin* to digest it), which impeded his stomach function; he had difficulty mentally *sorting the good from the bad and letting go of the waste*, which impeded his large intestine function; and his deeply felt social connections had been broken, which impeded his heart function.

He also had a poor appetite, frequent loose stools, felt bloated and tired after eating, but his general energy was ok (all due to poor pancreas function). He often experienced a lump in his throat at night, around eleven p.m., and a strong headache on his temples about four times a week, which usually started between six and seven p.m. (due to stagnated liver function). He had hay fever, a stiff low back in the mornings, weak knees which ached after sport, dizziness, and his head usually felt empty after he experienced the pain centred on the acupoint Ren-14, all due to poor kidney function. He experienced vivid dreams about four times a week, and "palpitations" (the pain centred on Ren-14), due to poor heart function. It should be noted that the heart and kidney function are very closely coordinated, which may explain why he felt empty headed (a kidney-related symptom) after experiencing the pain on Ren-14, which is a strong heart-related acupoint.[1]

After the first treatment, his mother said he seemed different, had more energy, more "spark", and the abdominal pains were much less for a few days. After a few more treatments his appetite had improved, his stools were variable, but the aching that was centred on Ren-12 (*Zhongwan*) was still there each morning and evening. He had weekly treatments over the following four months, with all his symptoms gradually improving, and even being completely absent from time to time. By the end of this course of treatments, he only experienced the pain occasionally, very mildly and for a short time. His energy was good and he was fully engaged in life and (in the words of his mother) was now a healthy thriving teenager.

---

[*] The acupoints Ren-12 (*Zhongwan*), Ren-14 (*Juque*) and Stomach-25 (*Tianshu*) are the most powerful acupoints on the front of the body associated with the stomach, heart and large intestine respectively.

A classic illustration of Liver invading stomach

At one point in this course of treatments, he felt strong cramping pains at Ren-12 for a few days, with loose stools, and felt tired and sick. His mother said he always felt bad at the start of May, and two of his family members said he often seemed "green around the gills" in this period. It was mid-Spring, which is the time of year that the liver function dominates (p.244). And his liver function was also stagnated, his stomach function was weak, and also, *all* his pulses were very "wiry" (indicating that the function of *all* his organs were stagnated due to the influence of his stagnated liver function). His particular pain and the other signs and symptoms were a graphic, textbook illustration of the Chinese medicine syndrome of "Liver invading stomach" (where his liver stagnation impeded the function of his stomach—p.104). But what I found most striking was that his family noticed his green hue, since it was so strong. Green is the colour associated with the liver. The hues on a person's face can often be used diagnostically. Without knowing it, his family had thus diagnosed that his stomach pain was caused by his liver and was due to "Liver invading stomach".

An element of stagnated liver function may also have been caused, or contributed to, by the original emotional traumas in this case. He was clearly a sensitive boy and the loss of his parents and cherished brother, perhaps together with the loss of his previous life (since his pains excluded him from much of that) may have been interpreted by him as the breaking of rules (it was "not fair" that all this was happening to him), which would have obstructed his liver function (p.109). Hence, this case also serves as a further demonstration of the interdependence of the organs when processing our thoughts (p.236).

Menstrual issues, acne, digestive problems and thrush (*damp heat*)

Female, aged 32. This patient sought treatment for issues related to her menstrual cycle—primarily acne but also PMS and painful periods; and she also had recurring thrush. For two to three years she was taking an antibiotic acne medication (*tetracycline*) which she also wanted to stop using.

Her menstrual cycle was 35 days long with one week of PMS, in which the acne around her jaw would flare up, and she was also anxious, moody, emotionally up and down and had tender and swollen breasts. On day one of her period she experienced painful cramps with a heavy flow of dark blood with clots (all due to stagnated liver function). One week after her period ended she would experience burning on urination and itching (thrush). She also had a small appetite, felt bloated after eating, had food intolerances, excess gas, loose stools which were sometimes runny and she was always thinking (due to poor pancreas function). Her energy lagged between four and five p.m., she felt the cold, had patches of dry skin, and used her voice heavily in her work (all related to poor lung function). She had poor short term memory, mild hay fever since the age of 21, felt hot at night, was generally very thirsty, and had a frequent headache on her occiput (due to poor kidney function).

She stopped taking the medication immediately and there was a mild flare up of her acne, which is to be expected when any such medication is stopped. However, the flare up was a lot less severe than she anticipated. By the fourth treatment, she had a period and the thrush symptoms were now completely clear and did not return. And after three further months of fortnightly treatments, she was generally feeling well, her digestion was greatly improved, her menstrual cycle had now reverted to 30 days, her period-related symptoms were all reduced, and her acne was greatly improved and not really an issue any more.

Damp heat, and Liver invading the stomach

She was taking the antibiotic for two to three years. Antibiotics deplete the pancreas function.[2] In Chinese medicine terms, this probably contributed to her thrush symptoms, which were *damp heat* in the bladder (p.181), the *dampness* being exacerbated by the depleting effect on her pancreas function of the antibiotic. The acne appeared along the stomach meridian on her face and neck and reflected "Stomach heat" (p.457), which was probably being produced by the stagnated liver function (since each flare up of acne coincided with her PMS phase). The stagnated liver function caused her liver to fail to properly regulate the flow of energy to the stomach, exacerbating the already poor stomach function, which produced the "Stomach heat". In other words the liver "invaded" the stomach (p.104).

Migraines, IBS, sleep, anxiety

Male, aged 49. This patient had a suspected heart attack four months prior to treatment. He was found to have a swollen pericardium (*pericarditis*). He had smoked for many years but immediately gave up when he went into hospital. He worked in a stressful, competitive environment and after a hard day at work, he used to work hard at the gym to help get rid of the stress. He sought acupuncture treatment to address his IBS, migraines, sleep, and stress.

He had a small appetite, poor sense of taste, felt tired and bloated after eating, had loose stools, sweet cravings, and was always thinking (all related to poor pancreas function). He usually had blocked sinuses, suffered frequent colds, a sharp energy lag between two and three p.m., was a perfectionist, tended to bear grudges for a long time and found it hard to "let go of things" (all related to poor lung function).

He suffered migraines since childhood. They usually started with very specific visual disturbances, which cleared for about thirty minutes, then the headache started and lasted for about two days. The pain was centred on the temples, was often a dull, background pain but could become intense. This was sometimes accompanied by nausea, a feeling of being detached, and a sensation of pins and needles or numbness in his fingers. He got the migraines about once every two months. When he worked a lot and was very tired, particularly after a period of stress, this usually triggered a migraine. Apart from his migraines, his emotions were unstable, with frequent irritability; he described himself as a control freak with a dislike of impolite people, and of rules being broken (all related to stagnated liver function).

He had vivid dreams for the last ten years and would often shout and jump out of bed in his sleep; he used to suffer frequent panic attacks about twenty years ago, which started again after his father died a few years ago (all these symptoms being due to poor heart function).

He suffered insomnia for many years. He could fall asleep ok, but then always woke around four a.m. with his mind thinking "all sorts of rubbish" related to work and other things, and he was unable to get back to sleep. He felt hot at night, had poor short term memory, poor concentration, an urgent need to urinate when he woke around four a.m.; his ears were often congested, and he had been running on adrenaline for years (all related to poor kidney function).

After the first treatment he felt calmer, had more energy, and did not need to urinate when he woke in the mornings. After the second treatment his concentration was better and he no longer felt the energy lag in the afternoon. After a few more weekly treatments his IBS symptoms had cleared, he was "not worrying about stuff", no longer felt hot at night and slept solidly. He continued to have regular treatments, at two or three weekly intervals, and only had an occasional migraine, which was usually less severe than previously—he often experienced the same visual disturbances but these did not usually develop into the migraine. He was a "driven" person who continued to work and play hard, and the regular treatments were required to counter the depleting effects of this, particularly on his kidney function.

Jaw pain caused by life issues the patient could not stomach

This patient was clearly a very sensitive person. In the second treatment session, he also told me about a deep aching pain around his jaw which he had for about two years. I asked if there was any situation in his life over this time that he could not stomach. He described a serious conflict with his neighbour which had built up for years; recently it progressed to the stage where he physically assaulted the neighbour. Every other neighbour had similar problems with this same person. The problem was so bad, the patient considered moving house. Along with addressing the other issues mentioned above, I also treated the jaw pain directly, needling the acupoints Stomach-6 (*Jiache*) and Stomach-12 (*Quepen*), which was also tender. The jaw pain cleared immediately and did not return. As mentioned above, he felt calmer and said he did not let things bother him anymore. It was clear that this jaw pain, on the stomach meridian, was caused by the fact that he could not stomach the situation in his life. In other words, his mental inability to even *begin* digesting the situation impeded his stomach function, which is what produced the pain on the stomach meridian—specifically, as it passed over his jaw. In this way, the body's symptoms are often metaphorical.

Extreme stress and grief

Female, aged 65. When this patient first sought treatment, a close friend of hers had died two days before. She was also retiring from a professional career, and was under great stress due to her son's substance abuse.

She smoked since the age of 16 and had no wish to give up smoking, only saying that she felt a bit croaky in the mornings. She also had shadows under her eyes from her late forties, had weak knees, tended to get achy knees and hips in Winter or if walking for about five miles; she had a stiff lumbar region and had problems with her low back for most of her life; she had frequent and urgent urination which started in recent years, very bad short-term memory, was slightly hard of hearing, got headaches at her occiput every two weeks, felt hot at night, thirsty during the day, and experienced hot flushes in the day about once a week, particularly when she was upset or anxious (all due to poor kidney function). When stressed, she felt a "hollow" feeling in her throat, like an uncomfortable space; she was irritable, got low when she worried about things (she felt she "could not cope with what the world was throwing at her"); she would often wake with a pain behind her eyes; she got cramp in her toes, and her nails had ridges. Her periods stopped at age fifty, but before this she would get PMS for three to four days and had bad pains on day one of her period (all related to stagnated liver function). She had palpitations, was easily startled, which started when her son was having drug and alcohol problems (due to poor heart function*). She felt the cold, which had always been the same, would get sneezing fits, and her energy was low in the afternoon (due to poor lung function).

After her first treatment, she initially felt very tired, which lasted for two days, but following this she felt greatly energized and positive. In the weeks that followed, she described herself as being under a lot of strain related to problems with her son, but was coping well with the stress and was sleeping well. She was feeling calmer, and found it easier to emotionally detach herself from the problems with her son, and was thinking clearly. After three months of fortnightly treatments, her hot flushes had cleared, the eye shadows greatly improved, and her low back felt better. Six weeks later, her son died of an overdose. After a few weekly treatments, she was coping well with her loss and increased the interval between treatments to one month.

Wrist pain due to a previous bereavement

About one year later, having mainly recovered from her loss, she developed a pain in her left wrist, along the lung meridian. There was no injury and the pain appeared to start spontaneously. When I told her my diagnosis (that this represented the emotional pain related to her bereavement, which her lungs were now recovering from), this made perfect sense to her. She told me she had been cradling her wrist in the last few days, like you would a baby.

Panic attacks and hay fever

Male, aged 45. This patient sought treatment for panic attacks. His father died three months previously and since then he suffered panic attacks, which were usually triggered by stress at work.

He had palpitations (awareness of his heartbeat), vivid dreams and nightmares, anxiety (which triggered nausea and pins and needles in his hands), panic attacks, after which he felt lightheaded (all due to poor heart function). He also had hay fever, which he had since childhood, with sinus pain, a runny nose, tightness in the chest and itching in his throat; he was allergic to dust and animal fur, had poor short term memory (which had always been the same), was hot at night, and heard a low pitch buzzing sound during

---

* It is significant that her heart function was clearly impeded due to the difficulties in her emotional connections, which highlights the mental/emotional functions of the heart, and how difficulties in these areas can physically weaken the heart (p.193).

the panic attacks (all due to poor kidney function).

It transpired that the patient's father was aged 48 when the patient was conceived, which probably explains why the patient was born with poor kidney function.

He also felt bloated after eating, had loose stools; his head felt muzzy each morning, but cleared after he was up for an hour or so—which had also always been the same; he had sweet cravings and was always thinking (all related to poor pancreas function). He had heartburn about once a week, which he felt as a hot sensation rising up the centre of his chest (due to poor stomach function). He was also quickly irritated, with fluctuating emotions, often got depressed, felt a lump in his throat, had cramp in his feet about twice a month (on the liver meridian), frequently had red and dry eyes; had frequent headaches on the temples and behind the eyes and at night had visual disturbances (all due to stagnated liver function).

All his symptoms gradually improved over the first seven weekly treatments, and by that time he had no hay fever symptoms whatsoever, despite it being hay fever season. The previous year, his hay fever symptoms were the worse they had ever been and he said the acupuncture treatment seemed like a miracle cure. After one of the early treatments, he returned the following week and told me his sinuses were clear and his sense of smell was dramatically improved; he was now noticing the smells everywhere which he was previously unaware of and complained of the world seeming almost *too* smelly.

His digestive signs were all improved (including his muzzy head in the morning, which was now gone completely); his energy was good; he was sleeping well with only an occasional dream, and had no nightmares; he felt calm and his anxiety was only mild and occasional.

He continued treatment, gradually increasing the interval between treatments from three weeks to six weeks. He clearly inherited poor kidney function from his parents (since he had hay fever from childhood), which left him with a weak constitution, but the monthly acupuncture treatments enabled him to cope with the stresses of life and remain healthy and largely symptom free. He now ran his own successful business which he set up a few weeks after starting the acupuncture treatments. This, as I have said elsewhere, is a very familiar pattern—after a few weeks of starting the treatments, patients often tell me of big changes they have made in their lives, or of significant opportunities that appear to have spontaneously come their way.

As with the previous case history, this case also serves as a clear illustration of the effect on the heart of emotional factors. The patient already had lifelong poor kidney function, and when his father died, the break in this strong social connection impeded his heart function (p.193), which caused his panic attacks (a heart-related symptom). Incidentally, if he had not also had the underlying poor kidney function, the impediment to his heart function would probably not have been sufficient to produce the panic attacks. But since his kidney function was already poor, this lessened the "stamina" of his heart—due to the "six channel theory" association between the heart and kidney (p.397).

Hernia treated with acupuncture

Male, aged 34. This patient initially sought treatment for a pain in his neck and shoulder, and a frequent lumbar pain. He also had a long history of hay fever, starting in childhood, and had other clear signs of poor kidney function (shortness of breath when running up stairs, wheezing when exercising, poor hearing in one ear, feeling hot at night). He ran his own business and was a sporty person.

After the initial treatments, which cleared all his significant symptoms, he came for routine maintenance treatments every month or two, for a period of around six years.

About two years after he started treatments with me, he reported feeling a "hernia" type pain, which had been developing for a few weeks. He thought it started due to an injury while canoeing. The pain was on the right of his abdomen, at the acupoint Stomach-26 (*Wailing*), and the pain radiated down the inside of his leg, on the liver meridian.

Apart from acupoints for his general treatment, I also needled Stomach-26.

Four weeks later he returned for another routine maintenance treatment. The hernia pain was still a problem. When getting out of bed in the morning, he felt a stabbing pain; and when canoeing, he felt a shooting pain.

Apart from general constitutional acupoints, I also needled *ashi* points on his right side, from Stomach-26 (*Wailing*) downwards, and also three acupoints on the liver meridian, Liver-12 (*Jimai*) to Liver-10 (*Zuwuli*).

Three weeks later he returned. The hernia pain was completely clear for a few days after the last treatment. The following week he went canoeing, and experienced no pain, but over the following few days, the pain returned and got worse; and he described himself as being in agony. He consulted his doctor, who said she could feel a tear in the muscle, so she referred him to a specialist at the hospital for surgery. But the initial consultation with the surgeon was three to four weeks away. He then had another canoeing session and there was no hernia pain during the session, but he still felt the pain every morning when getting out of bed. He asked if I could focus on treating the hernia, since, even if there was only a chance I could heal it before he saw the surgeon, then he could avoid having surgery.

I needled the same acupoints as in the previous treatment, only this time I added moxibustion as well (p.175).

One week later he returned. The day after the last treatment the hernia pain was worse, and was now worse along the whole line, from around Stomach-26 down to Liver-10. He had avoided canoeing this week.

I repeated the previous treatment.

Six days later he returned. This time, the pain was not worse after the previous treatment; and he now felt a dull ache around Liver-10 to Liver-11 (*Yinlian*), and a stabbing pain at Stomach-26. Again, he had avoided canoeing.

I needled ashi points again, but the locations had moved slightly. I needled four acupoints near to Stomach-26, and two acupoints about two *cun* below Liver-10.

Three weeks later he returned. Since the last treatment, he did one whole day of canoeing, and afterwards a bruise developed near to Stomach-26 which was the size of a tennis ball and he felt sick and bloated. He attended his appointment at the hospital, and the surgeon performed an ultrasound scan. The surgeon reported that at the exact location where the hernia was, there was a slight bulge in the muscle, as if a previous injury had healed. But otherwise, there was no problem and he was discharged. Since then, the patient had not experienced the hernia pain, though there was a slight ache in that same location.

In this session, I only treated him constitutionally and avoided using any of the acupoints related to the previous hernia treatments.

Three weeks later he returned for a routine maintenance treatment. The hernia was now completely clear and remained so for the following few years that I treated him.

The findings of the patient's doctor and also the surgeon provided compelling evidence that the acupuncture had healed this patient's hernia. However, even more compelling evidence would have been provided if an ultrasound scan had been performed *before* my treatments, as well as after, since there was only the experience of the patient's family doctor to confirm that a hernia was definitely present before my treatments. The patient confirmed he had never experienced a hernia before in that location and had certainly never had surgery there. But I suspect that even if an ultrasound scan *had* been performed before my treatments, sceptics would still choose to disbelieve the treatment outcome, simply claiming that the hernia must have got better by itself. And to be fair to the sceptics, when there is nothing in their own knowledge that could possibly account for the treatment outcome, what other choice would be open to them?

Note on the general "symptom picture" of a patient

None of the above patients were taking strong pharmaceutical remedies, hence their "symptom picture" was clear and made perfect sense from the Chinese medicine point of view—and their response to treatment was exactly as expected. I deliberately selected such case studies since this best illustrates the effects of Chinese acupuncture. With these patients, their main organs functioned (and also malfunctioned) just as human organs had always done; and the patterns of organ malfunction identified by Chinese physicians over the last two thousand years were clearly identifiable in these patients today.

When I take the case history of a new patient and they describe their symptoms, it quickly becomes obvious whether or not a patient is taking strong pharmaceutical remedies. With those that *are*, their symptoms fail to make sense, and certainly do not fall into any of these historical Chinese medicine patterns of organ malfunction. Yet with those who are *not* taking such remedies, their symptom picture always makes perfect sense. In fact, sometimes I have wondered if such patients had read a textbook on Chinese medicine and were simply reciting the symptoms from a list they had read. Of course they were not doing this. But the nature and pattern of their symptoms were often so textbook "Chinese medicine" that it was uncanny.

The chemistry of the body is extremely complex and changes from second to second. All the organs send chemical messages through the blood to coordinate their function with that of the other organs and systems in the body. However, most strong pharmaceutical remedies are designed to attempt to take control of a particular aspect of the body's chemistry. And since the normal function of the organs relies on their ability to constantly vary the complex chemistry of the body, any measures that diminish the chemical autonomy of the organs will, inevitably, ultimately prevent the organs from functioning normally. Hence, the symptoms and patterns of malfunction which have been present through history, no longer occur, so that the symptom picture is muddled and makes little sense when compared to the patterns identified by Chinese medicine (as relayed in this book).

Treating such patients is often challenging. Sometimes only small improvements are possible, which may only last for a day or two before the undesirable symptoms reappear. When the body no longer enjoys its chemical autonomy, this also tends to prevent natural healing systems like Chinese acupuncture from working. Such systems achieve their results by using some natural method to prompt the organs to resume their normal function. The healing therefore relies on the body's command of its own chemistry to effect the healing, but because the organs no longer have chemical autonomy, they cannot make the necessary adjustments—at least not permanently. However, acupuncture can still be used to give temporary relief from the undesirable effects of such remedies. And further, acupuncture is probably one of the most effective systems for providing this relief, since it corrects organ malfunction directly, without attempting to interact with the chemical or hormonal control systems—the very systems that pharmaceutical remedies act upon. This last fact probably also explains why such relief is only temporary—the organ functions are initially normalized by acupuncture, but they adopt the same malfunctions again, since the organs no longer have chemical autonomy and so cannot sustain normal function.

Chapter 14. Should the *Nei Jing* be interpreted literally?

The *Nei Jing* was compiled around the 2nd century BC (p.14) and is the foundation text that most of Chinese acupuncture is based on. It is clear that certain of its content is fact based, since the same facts are still routinely seen in clinic today. Some examples are

- the details of the meridians and acupoints;
- the organs they relate to;
- the signs and symptoms produced when a particular organ is stressed (as referenced throughout the organ chapters of this book);
- the tone of voice, face colour and scent also produced when each organ is stressed;
- the mental and emotional factors that impede the organ functions; and
- the lifestyle factors that promote either good or ill health.

All this knowledge was acquired over two thousand years ago and remains valid today. Therefore, these facts were probably discovered through practical observation, which would explain their veracity. However, the *Nei Jing* authors then began forming theories to attempt to explain their observations. They theorized about how the organs functioned, processed ingested food to produce useful resources, how those resources were transported and used, what the pathogens were that affected us, and how the organs became ill. Unfortunately they had no *useful* knowledge of the body's internal anatomy. Consequently most of their theories turned out to be untrue.

This does not detract in any way from the validity of the original observations, but it is important to separate the fact-based observations from any incorrect theories that attempt to explain them, lest those misguided theories discredit the valuable fact-based elements of Chinese medicine.

The chronology of discovery

How can we be sure that the factual observations came before the theories? Firstly, this is how it works. We only tend to theorize when there is something to explain, so if the practical observations were not made first, there would be nothing to theorize about. But secondly, since many of the theories are untrue (see the many examples below), *if* the practical observations (of signs and symptoms and so on) did not already exist, it is unlikely that incorrect theories could have been used to predict them.

The misconceptions about metabolism and physiology

Chapter 2 (p.23) describes the *Nei Jing* theories on metabolism and physiology, which were often contradictory. It was theorized

- that the stomach extracted a vapour from ingested food ("food influence", *gu chi*) which was then either passed directly to the "meridian" network, or passed to the lungs which then passed it to the "meridians", or was passed to the other organs which then passed it to the "meridians" (depending on the author);
- that another type of vapour was extracted from this food influence ("constructive influence", *ying chi*), which was circulated within the "meridians" to nourish the body;
- that a further type of vapour was also similarly extracted ("defensive influence", *wei chi*) and circulated via the "meridians" to warm the skin and muscles, which warmth then protected us from attack by external pathogens;
- that "meridians" consisted of imaginary artery-like tubes, which did not follow the paths of the literal arteries (known today) but instead existed deep beneath the *pathways on the skin* (which is what we today call meridians), and that the superficial veins and arterioles (which they called collaterals), branched off from these imaginary "meridians";
- that both the blood and these various vapours flowed through every branch of this circuit of "meridians" and superficial veins (collaterals);
- that blood was manufactured from the liquids extracted from ingested food, the manufacture either taking place in the stomach or the "meridians" (depending on the author);
- that blood and "constructive influence" were sometimes the same thing (depending on the author);
- that *wind*, *cold* and *dampness* penetrated the body from outside, resided in the veins (collaterals) and "meridians", and, if not expelled, travelled along the "meridians" to lodge in the *yin* organs (*zang*), which was one of the main ways that serious illness developed;
- that oxygen (or its equivalent, *qing chi*) was only needed by the lungs and heart and was not circulated to every part of the body;
- that the small intestine was only concerned with the passage of waste, and played no part in the extraction of nutrients;
- that urine originated from digested food and was extracted by the large intestine, which passed it to the bladder; and
- that the constitution was determined by the physical qualities of the organs we were born with, so that their location, size, texture, shape, whether standing upright or inclined (which all

varied from person to person), determined how well or badly the organs functioned.

All these theories were untrue (pp.40-48, and p.156). This, together with the fact that different *Nei Jing* authors often made contradictory statements, creates a considerable challenge for today's students when attempting to make sense of *Nei Jing* passages, such as those quoted between pages 33 and 40. But when reading the commentaries in Unschuld's translations (or elsewhere), it is clear that even Chinese scholars of the past two millennia experienced the same difficulties.

The fact that the original authors often made contradictory statements, and that subsequent scholars often produced contradictory interpretations of the same passages, suggests that in *some* passages, there *is* no nugget of truth to be extracted. This is only to be expected when such passages were often the product of an incorrect theory. However, it is still necessary to carefully read every *Nei Jing* passage, so that the genuine nuggets of truth *can* be rooted out.

The five phase doctrine

Prior to the compilation of the *Nei Jing*, Chinese sages were concerned with trying to understand the natural world. Around the same time, two doctrines were formed, one was the *yin-yang* doctrine, and another was the five phase doctrine. Its creator is thought to be Tsou Yen (circa 350-270 BC),[1] who arranged natural phenomena into five categories, rather than the two categories of *yin* and *yang*. According to Tsou's doctrine, all phenomena may exist in any one of five states, and these five states (or phases of existence) may transform into one another in an organized cycle, with the progress determined by one of several relationships that exist between the five phases. To name the phases, Tsou chose five natural substances: wood, fire, earth, metal, and water.

This doctrine was then applied to Chinese medicine. For each class of phenomena (such as organs, colours, seasons, directions, etc.), five examples were chosen that appeared to represent each of the phases. And the theory predicted that the same relationships ought to exist between each of the examples within any class, so that the relationship between fire and metal (for example) was the same as between heart and lungs, red and white, Summer and Autumn, South and West, and so on. And these theoretical relationships were used to explain and predict the interactions between the organs, and between the body as a whole and such things as the seasons and climates.

Table 3 on page 265 below shows the correspondences for each of the five phases. These are derived from Chapters 4 and 5 of the *Su Wen* (the italic entries being from Chapter 5).[2] If five phase theory is correct, then the relationships between all the examples in any class should obey the theory.

The "domination" or "control" relationship

The cycle of phases progresses from left to right in Table 3 (p.265), from Wood, to Fire, to Earth, to Metal, to Water, to Wood, etc. And each phase is said to "dominate" (or "control", "subdue", "overact on" or "attack") the phase two places in front of it, so that Wood dominates Earth, Earth dominates Water, Water dominates Fire, and so on. However, in these relationships, if the phase that normally dominates, is weak and fails to dominate the phase two places in front of it, then the normally subservient phase is said to be able to "insult" the phase two places behind it and dominate *it* instead—so that the "domination" relationship is then reversed. This is known as the "insulting" sequence.

If this theory is correct, this would mean that

- chicken dominates ox, sheep dominates horse (but is not able to dominate chicken), and horse dominates chicken, except if horse is weak and fails to dominate chicken, in which case chicken can then dominate horse—as well as being able to dominate ox.
- Red dominates white (but is unable to dominate yellow, green-blue or black), and black dominates red (but is unable to dominate white, yellow, or green-blue).
- West dominates East, and East dominates the centre—except if East is weak and fails to dominate the centre, when the centre is then able to dominate East.
- Venus dominates Jupiter (the largest planet) but is not able to dominate Mercury (the second smallest planet).
- Weeping dominates shouting (but does not dominate laughing, singing or groaning), except if weeping is weak and fails to dominate shouting, in which case shouting can dominate weeping. But shouting is unable to dominate laughing or groaning under any circumstances.
- Pancreas dominates kidneys (but cannot normally dominate lungs, heart or liver), except if pancreas is weak and fails to dominate kidneys, in which case kidneys dominate pancreas. However, if liver is weak, pancreas can also dominate liver.

It is difficult to see the sense in any of these relationships. How can a sheep dominate a horse but not dominate a chicken? How can Venus dominate Jupiter (the biggest planet) but dominate no other planet? How can any direction (such as East or the "centre") dominate another single direction but no other? And how does one direction dominate another anyway?

The whole notion of the five phase "domination" relationship seems imaginary and hence untrue. Yet it is frequently applied to the five *yin* organs (*zang*) to make a diagnosis. It is true that in clinic, there can appear to be "control" relationships related to the liver, where the liver "dominates" the pancreas and stomach (p.103), and the lungs "control" the liver (p.145), but the same is not true of the other organs. And in the same way, it is easy to imagine how a horse may dominate a chicken, yet it is difficult to see why it could not also dominate the other animals. If the correspondences in the above table were determined randomly, it would be expected that some isolated relationships could be found that would seem to make sense. But when all the other relationships do not also make sense, this certainly cannot be taken as proof of the theory.

Table 3. The five phase correspondences

	Wood	Fire	Earth	Metal	Water
Season	Spring	Summer	late Summer	Autumn	Winter
Direction	East	South	centre	West	North
Organ	liver	heart	[pancreas]	lungs	kidneys
Colour	green-blue	red	yellow	white	black
Climate	*wind*	*heat*	*dampness*	*dryness*	*cold*
Orifice	eyes	*tongue* (or ears)	mouth	nose	*ears* (or urethra and anus)
Disease location	*sinews*	*blood* (or vessels)	*flesh*	*skin and body hair*	*bones and marrow*
Disease it brings forth	shock	in the *yin* organs	base of tongue	back	where water flows and stagnates
Flavour	sour	bitter	sweet	acrid	salty
Odour	fetid	burnt	aromatic	fishy	foul
Domestic animal	chicken	sheep	ox	horse	swine
Grain	wheat	glutinous millet	panicled millet	rice	bean
Planet	Jupiter	Mars	Saturn	Venus	Mercury
Number	eight	seven	five	nine	six
Voice	*shouting*	*laughing*	*singing*	*weeping*	*groaning*
Movements indicating changes	*grasping*	*anxiety*	*"hiccup" (or belch)*	*coughing*	*shivering*
States of mind	*anger*	*joy*	*pensiveness*	*anxiety*	*fear*

The sequence of numbers

It is sometimes said that the numbers were assigned to the phases in the following way. The order of the phases was assumed to be entirely different to the order in the five phase doctrine, as follows.

1. Water (6)
2. Fire (7)
3. Wood (8)
4. Metal (9)
5. Earth

And to obtain the number assigned to each phase, *five* was added to the first four phases in the above list, so that Water becomes six, Fire seven, and so on.[3] When the phases are then ordered as in five phase theory, which is cyclic, this provides the following pattern.

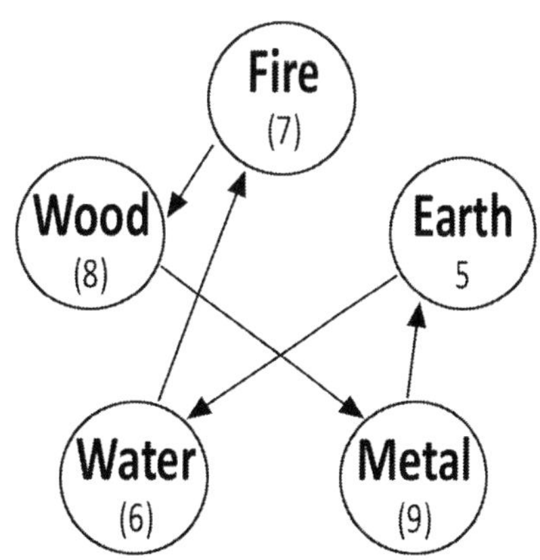

Figure 1. Five phase number sequence

As can be seen in Figure 1 above, the progression of the numbers through the phases now appears to stagger drunkenly between them, so that there is no apparent relationship between this numbering system and five phase theory.

Firstly, the numbers were assigned in a linear progression from one phase to another, but five phase theory is a cyclic progression, not a linear one, so that, mathematically, the one scheme could not be expected to match the other. And secondly, the choice of which phase to begin the sequence on (Water, in this case) could only be regarded as an arbitrary choice. Why start at Water and not Metal, or Earth, or Wood? And to make matters worse, the order was then jumbled up, apparently at random, and applied to the progression of phases in the five phase cycle. How could a linear progression, of successive integers, when then jumbled up, be expected to make mathematical sense in a cyclic pattern? Numbers were chosen, therefore any relationship between the phases ought to be definable mathematically. This includes in a stepwise fashion, around the cycle (the "generation" cycle—described below), but also in the pattern of the "domination" relationship described above. And whatever mathematical equations were devised to express these relationships, it is supposed that the results for each phase would always be an integer in the range of five to nine. This is mathematical nonsense, and it could only be concluded that, in effect, these numbers were assigned to the five phases arbitrarily.

In other words, if a mathematical equation were devised that predicted that *eight* (the Wood phase) dominates *five* (the Earth phase), and the same equation were applied to the numbers of the other four phases, the outcomes would not match the numbers specified in the five phase correspondences. For example, if the equation were applied to *seven*, the result would not be *nine*; and if applied to *five*, the result would not be *six*; and so on. Therefore, no such "domination rule" behaviour could be said to exist between the numbers that correspond to each of the phases.

The "generation" cycle

In the cycle of phases, it is theorized that each phase generates the following phase, so that Wood generates Fire, Fire generates Earth, and so on. In this relationship, the generating phase was known as the "mother", and the phase it generated was known as the "child", so that Wood is the mother of Fire, and Fire is the child of Wood. If this theory were correct, this would mean that

- Jupiter generates Mars, Mercury generates Jupiter;
- groaning generates shouting, singing generates weeping (even assuming the singing is in tune);
- dampness generates dryness, cold generates wind;
- chicken generates sheep, horse generates swine, swine generates chicken;
- yellow generates white, black generates green-blue, red generates yellow;
- liver generates heart, lungs generate kidneys; and
- East generates South, South generates centre, North generates East.

Again, it is difficult to imagine the sense in any of these relationships. How does one animal generate another animal of a completely different size and nature? How does dampness generate dryness? How does yellow generate white; or black generate green-blue? How does one particular direction generate another? How do the lungs generate the kidneys?

This five phase theoretical notion, if correct, ought to be correct for every phenomena in every class in Table 3 above. Again, it might be possible to find a few single examples where it might be said to apply (such as blood generates flesh, or anxiety generates fear) but such rare successes would be expected even if the phenomena in the table were assigned randomly. This suggests that the theory is simply untrue.

However, these five phase relationships have been applied extensively throughout the *Nei Jing*, the *Nan Jing* and beyond, to produce further medical theories.

Dissenting voices of the past

In the *Nei Jing*, the five phase doctrine only had limited applications, but in the *Nan Jing*, its use was greatly extended, causing some commentators to complain that five phase theory was now being inappropriately applied and that this had reduced medicine to something akin to demonology.

Section 53 of the *Nan Jing* expresses a theory concerning illnesses being transmitted through the organs. That is, once one organ becomes ill, then it was theorized that the illness tends to pass to another organ and then another, in the exact order predicted by the five phase domination relationship, so that a disease that starts in the heart, would pass to the lungs, then the liver, the pancreas, the kidneys, then back to the heart. But since (according to the theory) one organ cannot be harmed twice, if the progression reaches this stage (returning to the organ it began in), the patient would die. Whereas, if the progression is transmitted via the "generation" cycle (i.e. from heart, to the pancreas, lungs, kidneys, liver, then to the heart again, and so on), then (according to the theory) the cycle will go on indefinitely and the patient will not die.[4]

Commenting on the above, Liao P'ing (in 1913) wrote:

The medical classics focus on the [*yin* and *yang* organs], on the [meridians and collaterals]; they seek truth through facts. If one speculates on the basis of the Five Phases, it is as if one drew a picture of demons and spirits. The medical classics are concerned with the concrete; the theories of the Five Phases are but empty talk. The medical classics are difficult, the theories of the Five Phases are easy to comprehend. Because the physicians have set aside the [*yin* and *yang* organs], the [meridians and collaterals], and because they have focused on the Five Phases, medicine has deteriorated day by day. In its discourse on general laws, the *Nei Jing* frequently refers to the Five Phases. But in those [chapters] that deal with illness, it does not refer to the Five Phases. In the medical literature of later generations—just as in the writings of the astrologers—one finds detailed discussions of the Five Phases as they generate and overcome, control and transform each other. The *Nan Jing* has originated this.[5]

And the following section of the *Nan Jing*, continues the theme:

Nan Jing, Section 54

Illnesses in the [*yin* organs (*zang*)] are difficult to cure; illness in the [*yang* organs (*fu*)] are easy to cure. What does this mean? It is like this. Illnesses in the [*yin* organs] are difficult to cure because they are transmitted to [*yin* organs] that can be overcome. Illnesses in the [*yang* organs] are easy to cure because they are transmitted to the respective child. This pattern coincides with that of the "transmission through seven [*yin* organs]" and with that of the "transmission skipping one [*yin* organ]" outlined in [Section 53 of the *Nan Jing*].[6]

Hua Shou (in 1361) commented on the above passage. He clearly disagreed with the theory offered and suggested the real reason why such illnesses are difficult or easy to cure, quoting an earlier physician:

> Mr. Ch'en from Ssu-ming, states: As long as the five [*yin* organs] are guarded internally by the seven spirits, evil influences of minor significance will not be transmitted easily. However, if major evil influences enter the [*yin* organs], the spirits will lose their guarding function and the illness will penetrate deeply into the body. Hence illnesses in the [*yin* organs] are difficult to cure; they may even result in death. The function of the six [*yang* organs] is to revolve and transport, to transmit and transform their contents. It is quite normal that influences pass through them. Also, the gall is the place of clarity and purity. Even if evil influences were to enter it, it would be difficult for them to penetrate deeply and to stay. Hence illnesses in the [*yang* organs] are easy to cure.[7]

Hsü Ta-ch'un (in 1727) also commented on the above *Nan Jing* passage

This paragraph certainly does not agree with the text of the *Nei Jing*; also, it contradicts the preceding paragraph. [Chapter 42 of the *Ling Shu*] states that the liver transmits an illness to the [pancreas], the [pancreas] transmits it to the stomach, the stomach transmits it to the kidneys, the kidneys transmit it to the bladder, and so on. That is to say, the [*yin* organs] and the [*yang* organs] do transmit illnesses among each other. [Section 53 of the *Nan Jing*] states: "The [pancreas] transmits the illness to the lung; the lung transmits it to the kidneys." That is to say, the transmission among the [*yin* organs] can also proceed from the mother to the child. Here it is stated: "illnesses in the [*yin* organs] are transmitted to the [*yin* organ] that can be overcome" and "illnesses in the [*yang* organs] are transmitted to the child." How could that make any sense? Now, illnesses in the [*yin* organs] are located in the depth; illnesses in the [*yang* organs] are located below the surface. It would make perfect sense if one distinguished, on this basis, between illnesses that are difficult and others that are easy to cure. Everything else is irrelevant.[8]

And Liao P'ing (in 1913), also commented on the same passage

How could anybody distinguish between [*yin* organs] and [*yang* organs] on the basis of such criteria? To read this is sufficient to make it clear that the authors of the *Nan Jing* have not penetrated the meaning of the text of the *Nei Jing*. For details see Hsü Ta-ch'un's critique [above].[9]

Hence these commentators suggest that the *yin* organs (*zang*) are difficult to treat simply because they are the deeper, more important organs (which seems to be common sense), and they reject the explanations offered by five phase theory.

Application within Chinese medicine

Five phase prediction of organ peaks

The following extract states which times of day diseases in each organ ought to be eased or exacerbated. In other words, it states which times of day each organ's function is strongest and weakest.

> **Extract from *Su Wen*, Chapter 22**
>
> In the case of liver diseases, the patient feels better at dawn. The disease becomes serious in late afternoon. At midnight the disease calms down. In the case of heart diseases, the patient feels better at noon. The disease becomes serious at midnight. At dawn it calms down. In the case of [pancreas] diseases, the patient feels better when the sun begins to decline westwards. The disease becomes serious at sunrise. In the late afternoon it calms down. In the case of lung diseases, the patient feels better in the late afternoon. The disease becomes serious at noon. At midnight it calms down. In the case of kidney diseases, the patient feels better at midnight. These diseases are severe during the final thirds of all four quarters of a day. In the late afternoon they calm down.[10]

Many centuries after the *Nei Jing* was compiled, the theory of "midnight to noon, ebb and flow" was described, which also states the times of day when each organ's activity is at its highest and lowest (p.379). From clinical experiences today, it is clear that these "ebb and flow" times are accurate, and therefore must have been deduced from practical observation, rather than theoretically calculated. What is notable is that the times stated in the *Su Wen* quote above are completely different, often make no sense when compared to clinical experiences, and that they were clearly calculated using five phase theory, as described below.

The predicted times for Kidney peaks and troughs are notably bizarre. The organ function is predicted to peak at midnight ("the patient feels better at midnight"), to be at a low point *four* times a day ("during the final thirds of all four quarters of a day") and to be somewhere between these two states in late afternoon. This bizarre rise and fall in organ activity seems particularly implausible. But in the "ebb and flow" theory, the kidney function peak is said to be between five and seven p.m. and its trough between five and seven a.m., which corresponds exactly with clinical experiences today, since kidney conditions are usually at their worst between five and seven a.m., when its function is said to be at its weakest (p.381).

The commentaries on this *Su Wen* passage make it clear how the times were calculated. In 762 AD, Wang Bing commented on the kidney-related part of the quoted *Su Wen* extract, saying "At the time of the day when water rules, the patient feels better. At the time of the day when the soil rules, the disease becomes more serious. At the time of the day when metal rules, the disease calms down."[11] And in 1957, Zhang Jiebin also commented on this same passage, saying "Water rules at midnight; hence the turn to the better. The soil ruling through all four periods dominates the water; hence kidney diseases are serious throughout the final thirds of the four quarters of a day."[12]

It is clear that the times for each organ's peaks and troughs were calculated using five phase theory, which explains why the times are incorrect, and sometimes bizarre (five phase theory itself being untrue—or, at best, misapplied to medical matters).

Of the other organ peaks and troughs predicted in the *Su Wen* extract

- the heart's is most accurate (high at noon and low at midnight, though "at dawn it calms down" makes no sense);
- the pancreas's are wildly inaccurate (high "when the sun begins to decline westwards", yet the actual high is between nine and eleven a.m.; and low at sunrise, yet the actual low is at nine and eleven p.m.);
- the lungs' low point is only three hours out, but its high point is wildly inaccurate (low at noon, yet the actual low is between three and five p.m.; and high in late afternoon, yet the actual high is between three and five a.m.); and
- the liver's low point is one or two hours out, but its high point is wildly inaccurate (low in late afternoon, yet the actual low is between one and three p.m.; and high at dawn, yet the actual high is between one and three a.m.).

Abdominal diagnosis

In the following extract, it is suggested that one form of diagnosis is to palpate various areas of the abdomen, which were said to correspond to various organs.

Extract from *Nan Jing*, Section 16

Consider feeling a movement in the vessels that is associated with an illness in the liver.... Internal evidence of such an illness is the presence of moving influences to the left of the navel which, if pressed, respond with firmness and pain.[13]

Lü Kuang (in the 3rd century AD) commented on this passage

The "internal evidence" is the evidence provided by the liver itself. The liver is associated with the eastern region; it represents the virid dragon. It is located on the left side. Hence, internal evidence of an illness in the liver appears to the left of the navel.[14]

It is clear from this commentary that these diagnostic areas were calculated using five phase theory, rather than being discovered through practical observation. The (five phase) idea is that the liver correlates to East, which corresponds to left, therefore the liver is on the left of the abdomen, which means that when the liver is distressed, this region would produce "firmness and pain" when pressed.

What makes it absolutely certain that this diagnostic notion is fictional is that the liver is on the right, not the left. This not only means that by applying five phase theory, the *Nan Jing* author calculated a fictitious diagnostic method, but that the mistake also highlights further inaccuracies in five phase theory itself, since the theory predicts the liver is on the left. The fact that we do not use this diagnostic method today is a further reflection of its inaccuracy.

In Lü Kuang's commentaries on the remainder of Section 16 of the *Nan Jing*, he stated that the pancreas is "located in the centre. Hence, internal evidence of its illness appears exactly in the navel". But in fact, the pancreas is located on the left, not in the centre (in the five phase correspondences, Earth is said to correspond to "pancreas" and "centre"; hence it was theorized that the pancreas was located in the centre of the abdomen). He also stated that "the lung is located in the Western region. This is the region of the white tiger. It rules the right side. Hence, the evidence appears to the right of the navel."[15] But in fact, the lungs are placed centrally in the chest, not on the right (though it could be argued that the right lung is slightly larger than the left, since the heart is situated to the left of the midline, consequently the left lung is slightly smaller to accommodate the heart[16]).

Inaccuracies of the above type occur in the *Nei Jing* and *Nan Jing* where the content was not discovered through practical observation but was instead theoretically calculated—usually using five phase theory, as here.

Problems then result when such passages are later taken to be factual and even applied in clinic. In practice today this is less of a problem though, since practitioners soon discover for themselves which ideas work and which do not. But when studying the ancient Chinese medical classics academically, it is important to be aware of this issue and to be able to separate fact from fiction.

How the correspondences may have been chosen

The table on page 265 above, lists the five phase correspondences, as defined in *Su Wen* Chapters 4 and 5. But if some (or many) aspects of the five phase doctrine are untrue, how were these correspondences determined?

It is clear that some of the associations in each column are fact based, simply because, over two thousand years later, these same associations are evident in clinic on a daily basis. Primarily, these are the associations between each organ and a particular season and "orifice"; and also the states produced in the person when that organ is stressed—such as the colour of their complexion; the bodily "location" affected; the flavour the person craves; the odour produced by the organ; and the person's tone of voice and state of mind.

For example, when the liver is stressed, this often produces signs and symptoms related to the eyes (its associated "orifice") such as red or sore eyes and disturbed vision. This might include seeing bright specs of light, wavy lines; the colours being dim; having blurred vision; or seeing the visual disturbances associated with migraine. And other signs and symptoms often include a green-blue complexion, cramp or stiffness in the muscles (the "sinews"), cravings for sour food, a fetid body odour, a loud voice, as though continuously shouting, and the tendency to be angry. And all these factors would usually be more prominent in Spring.

As with the other fact-based content of the *Nei Jing*, such signs and symptoms were most likely discovered through practical observation, rather than being calculated theoretically (p.261). And such practical observations were probably mainly made by the ancestors of the *Nei Jing* authors. In the surviving texts, it is clear that Chinese medicine, in one form or another, was practiced from at least 1800 BC (p.13), which is well over a millennium before the *Nei Jing* was compiled. It is difficult to imagine that over all that time, certain aspects of the above knowledge (the signs and symptoms related to "disease" in a particular organ, for example) had not gradually built up (whatever the theoretical explanations for the illness were, including possession by demons). If this is the case, then all these particular associations with each organ would have been discovered well before the five phase doctrine existed.

In the *Nei Jing* texts, there was then the desire to explain illness with one of the new theories. The five phase doctrine theorized that all things in nature could be explained by the cycle of five interdependent phases, Wood, Fire, Earth, Metal, and Water. Therefore, the task was to fit these already-known medical facts into the theory.

There were too many organs to fit the theory

The known facts were a series of associations with each of the five main *yin* organs, so the problem could be solved by associating each of those organs with a phase, and all the organ's associated signs and symptoms would then also fall under that same phase.

The first difficulty may have been the fact that there were six *yin* organs and not five. The pericardium is also a *yin* organ. However, there was controversy over this organ, as to whether it was a real organ or not (just as there was over its *yin-yang* paired organ, the lymphatic system, or *san jiao*—p.211). This was perhaps sufficient justification to simply leave out the pericardium, which then reduced the number of *yin* organs to five, and solved the problem of there being too many organs to accommodate the five phase doctrine.

How the organs were ordered

The next difficulty was what order to place the cycle of organs in. Today, the association of each organ with a particular phase is well-known, so that to us it seems obvious which phase each organ belongs to, simply because we are used to the knowledge. But if we imagine the time *before* these associations were decided upon, the associations are far from clear.

I can think of no inherent quality in most of the organs that suggests they should be associated with a particular phase. In the body, there is no wood, earth, or metal. There is certainly water. And there is no literal fire, but there is perhaps metaphorical fire, in the "spark" that drives all organs, or the warmth of the body. Water is processed by the stomach, pancreas and kidneys, so it is not clear which single of these organs should be associated with water. It was decided to associate the kidneys with water. The physical qualities of the kidneys are that they are solid and more dense than the other organs. Of the phases, metal seems closest to these qualities. Functionally, the kidneys are seen as the root of life, as the place where the seed from our parents is stored, and from where the product of that seed "grows". These qualities seem to match both earth and wood.

Fire, in a metaphorical sense, could also be seen as being present within us. This metaphorical fire is associated with the kidneys (in that they are seen as providing the "spark" that enables the other organs to function, the *yuan chi*), so that the kidneys could also be associated with fire. But the warmth of the body is provided most directly from the digestive processes, so that the pancreas could also be associated with fire. However, it was decided that the heart should be associated with fire. This decision may have been influenced by the fact that the heart produces a red facial hue, and that there is an association between red and fire, in that fire often makes things glow red. However, the flames of fire are mainly yellow in colour, so that the pancreas could also be associated with fire (since the pancreas produces a yellow facial hue).

It could also be said that the heart is associated with blood (in contemporary physiology), and blood is red, which seems to confirm the association; but blood is produced by the digestive processes (in contemporary physiology), so that the pancreas could be said to be more closely associated with blood than the heart is.

It is difficult to see an association between fire or water and any one organ, which is not capable of contradiction. And these ought to be the easiest two of the five phases to associate with an organ.

Could each organ's existing associations be matched to a particular phase?

Some of the associations may have seemed to fit one phase more than the others. For example, the facial tone of "red" seems to fit fire (provided that only the red glow produced by fire is considered, rather than the colour of fire's flames—which would then fit "yellow"), but the other colours are less easy to match with a particular phase. Either black or green-blue *could* fit the colour of metal, particularly when it is being forged. But there are no other obvious matches. It is only by thinking tangentially that the other colours could be reconciled with particular phases. For example, with the phase of Wood, if the leaves of trees and bushes are imagined, rather than the wood itself, then the green-blue colour now seems to obviously match Wood.

As for the various signs and symptoms associated with each organ, it must have seemed impossible to directly match each of those with one particular phase. For example, how could the disease location (sinews, flesh, blood, skin, bone) be matched to one particular phase over the others? There seems to be no inherent character in each that has a direct similarity with any of the phases, so that metaphor must be used to attempt to invent an association, but the problem with this is that the association could then be challenged by adopting a different metaphor. And the same is true of the voices, odours, flavours, and orifices.

The organs were ordered according to the seasons

In terms of placing the organs in a particular order, there is only one class of associations that has an inherent order, and that is the seasons. In each season, the function of a particular organ tends to be prominent—the liver in Spring, the heart in Summer, the lungs in Autumn, the kidneys in Winter. In five-phase terms, this suggests the order that the organs ought to progress in—from liver, to heart, to lungs, to kidneys.

But there are only four seasons and five (or six) organs. The pericardium had already been set aside, to leave five *yin* organs; so to be able to solve this "five-phase riddle", the pancreas also needed to be somehow associated with a season. The solution was, for more or less arbitrary reasons, to place the pancreas in the centre of the year, which is the sixth month. This comes in the last month of summer, so its associated month was named "late summer".[17] This may have been justified with arguments along the lines of any of the following: digestion is at the centre of our existence because the pancreas produces the resources that enable the other organs to function; or, in the middle of the year is harvest time, when most grain can be ingested, whose digestion the pancreas is responsible for, so it could be imagined that the pancreas function is prominent in the middle of the year.

It was decided to consider the pancreas as being prominent in "late Summer", the sixth month of the year, so that the (assumed) five *yin* organs could be reconciled with five phase theory. However, in practice it is clear that the pancreas function is dominant at the end of every one of the four seasons (p.244), so that in order to artificially create a sequence of organs that matched five phase theory, it was wrongly assumed the pancreas was dominant only at the end of Summer.

Matching the organs to the phases

With the order of the organs now decided (based on seasonal activity), it only remained to now match the organs to the phases.

As mentioned above, with most of the classes of organ associations (the voices, sounds, orifices, and so on), it is difficult to find clear-cut matches of the associations to the phases. However, it seems the only clear match can be made in the category of "colours", where "red" seems to match Fire. But this only works if thinking tangentially and considering the red glow that fire often produces; if considering the colour of fire's flames, then "yellow" would more closely match Fire. However, we know that "red" was the choice made, so that it appears that tangential thinking was adopted for the sake of solving the problem.

The remaining four colours cannot be definitively matched to the other four phases (that is, if you clear from your mind the associations we are accustomed to from the *Nei Jing*, and start again from scratch). However, you only need to match a single colour to a single phase, and because the order of the organs is now established (using the seasonal association), all the organs would then fall into place.

The facial colour of red is associated with the heart, therefore this implies that the heart ought to be associated with the phase of Fire. If this is the case, then the next organ along in the sequence of organs would be associated with the next phase in the sequence of phases. In this way the pancreas is associated with Earth, the lungs with Metal, the kidneys with Water, and the liver with Wood.

The above process is so full of weaknesses that it seems tenuous at best, but perhaps "arbitrary" would be a more fitting description. However, after carefully considering how the "riddle" might have been solved, I could come up with nothing better. The above is therefore one possible example of the thought processes that *could* have been used to solve the problem. The other, non-medical associations (directions, climates, domestic animals, grains, planets, and numbers) were probably more or less arbitrarily assigned to the phases, perhaps using similar tangential thinking or metaphor to make the assignments; and, as demonstrated on page 263 above, these associations do not stand up to scrutiny when using five phase theory's "domination" and "generation" relationships to test them.

The fact-based associations

When all the arbitrary content is removed from the table on page 265 above, this leaves the following table of associations. The phases have been left out, since their associations with particular organs has no real meaning and is, in effect, arbitrary; and the columns have been ordered alphabetically based on the organ names. This is to avoid the suggestion that there is any sort of natural cycle existing between the organs, including any assumed five-phase relationship.

Table 4. The fact-based organ associations

	Heart	Kidneys	Liver	Lungs	Pancreas
Season	Summer	Winter	Spring	Autumn	none*
[Facial] colour	red	black	green-blue	white	yellow
[Sense]	[speech]	[hearing]	eyes	nose	[taste]
Disease location	blood (or vessels†)	bones and marrow	sinews	skin and body hair	flesh
Flavour	bitter	salty	sour	acrid	sweet
Odour	burnt	foul	fetid	fishy	aromatic
Voice	laughing	groaning	shouting	weeping	singing
States of mind	joy	fear	anger	anxiety‡	pensiveness

* Since the pancreas is associated with all the seasons, it cannot be said to be associated with any one in particular, hence its seasonal association is "none" (p.244).

† "Vessels" is meant in the *Nei Jing* sense, which means all the "meridians" and collaterals (p.42).

‡ In today's Chinese medicine the recognised association for the lungs is "sadness".

Applying five phase theory to the organs

Such passages as the following have elements of truth in them (as long as your thinking is flexible), but also elements that are plainly untrue. And it is not difficult to see how such passages were constructed.

> **Extract from *Su Wen*, Chapter 5**
>
> The liver generates the sinews; the sinews generate the heart.... The heart generates the blood; the blood generates the [pancreas].... The [pancreas] generates the flesh; the flesh generates the lung.... The lung generates skin and body hair; skin and body hair generate the kidneys.... The kidneys generate the bones and the marrow; the marrow generates the liver.[18]

When reading such passages in the *Nei Jing*, it is clear from the commentaries that every word is understood (and quoted) as though it were literally true.

Is it true that "the liver generates the sinews"? Well, not literally. Of course the liver does not "generate" the sinews. But this statement is based on practical observations that certainly *are* true. When the liver is stressed, the patient may experience muscular cramps, or tightness in the muscles along the liver and gallbladder meridians (particularly over the neck, hips, and the sides of the legs—p.113). These are routinely seen in clinic today, so we can assume that, over two thousand years ago, this knowledge was probably discovered by making similar practical observations of the signs and symptoms that occur when the organ is stressed—and such observations were almost certainly made by the ancestors of the *Nei Jing* authors (p.261). In the *Nei Jing*, "sinews" refers to the movement of the muscles, rather than to tendons, which is the meaning understood in this term today. Hence, when it is said that "the liver generates the sinews", this is understood to mean that there is an association between the liver and the smooth movement of the muscles, which is certainly true.

Is it true that "the sinews generate the heart" and "the blood generates the [pancreas]" and "the flesh generates the lung" and "skin and body hair generate the kidneys" and "the marrow generates the liver"? Of course not. All these statements are untrue. And this is because they are not based on practical observation, but were calculated using five phase theory.

The sinews are associated with the liver, which is assigned to the Wood phase. In five phase theory, it is assumed that each phase "generates" the phase that follows it. So, if the theory is applied literally, Wood generates Fire, and Fire is assigned to the heart; therefore it is stated that the sinews (which belong to Wood) "generate" the heart (which belongs to Fire). And in the same way, the marrow, which is associated with the kidneys (which are assigned to Water) "generate" the liver (which is assigned to the next phase along, Wood), and so on for the other three *yin* organs.

You may attempt to perform intellectual gymnastics to find some tangential or metaphorical justification for how the marrow may generate the liver, but it would be easier to accept that the statement is simply untrue, since the five phase theory which produced it, is also untrue. Or to put it a little more politely—when applied literally, five phase theory has few reliable practical applications.

Applying five phase theory to explain the correlates

The following extract describes the correlates of each of the *yin* organs. It is clear that these were discovered through practical observation, since the associations are still seen in clinic today. Hence, the correlates are true. However, in his commentaries, the famous 8th century practitioner, Wang Bing, then uses five phase theory to explain *why* each organ is correlated with the tissue it is, and his theories are all transparently *untrue*, even though the correlates themselves are fact based.

> **Extract from *Su Wen*, Chapter 10**
> The correlate of the lung is the skin; its splendour appears in the body hair.... The correlate of the liver are the sinews; its splendour appears in the nails.... The correlate of the [pancreas] is the flesh; its splendour appears in the lips.... The correlate of the kidneys are the bones; their splendour is the hair on the head.[19]

To explain why "the correlate of the lung is the skin" Wang Bing states "The [influence] of metal is firm and fixed. The appearance of the skin is so, too. The lung [organ] corresponds to the metal. Hence it is a correlate of the skin."[20]

The reason why the skin is often affected when the lungs are stressed would be due to some physiological association between the two (whatever that might be, in contemporary physiology), and is certainly not because metal is "firm and fixed" and the skin also appears to be "firm and fixed", though I can not imagine an interpretation of "firm and fixed" that *could* apply to the skin but not to any other part of our anatomy. The association of "metal" with the lungs appears to be arbitrary anyway, but then Wang Bing has searched for some similarity between metal and the skin to provide a theory to explain why the two are associated in the body. In his own mind, he may have been able to persuade himself that he had succeeded, though any similarity between "metal" and the skin has to be viewed as invented, for the sake of satisfying his theory.

Likewise, to explain why "the correlate of the liver are the sinews" Wang Bing states "The nature of wood includes being bent or straight. The physical appearance of the sinews is identical. The liver [organ] corresponds to the wood. Hence it is a correlate of the sinews."[21]

Again, the fact that "wood" may be bent and straight, and the "sinews" (i.e. the muscles) expand and contract, is not the reason why the muscles may cramp and stiffen when the liver is stressed. There would be an explanation for this in contemporary anatomy and physiology. Any similarity between "wood" and the muscles is an invented one, clearly inspired by the arbitrary assignment of the Wood phase to the liver, and invented in an attempt to create a theory to explain the association of liver with the muscles.

Similarly, Wang Bing theorized that "The nature of the soil is soft and thick. The physical appearance of the flesh is identical. The [pancreas organ] corresponds to the soil. Hence it is a correlate of the flesh." And "The nature of water is to flow and be moist. The essence [influence] is identical. Bones are penetrated by essence marrow. Hence the kidneys are linked to the bones." And "The brain is the sea of marrow; it is ruled by the [influence] of the kidneys. Hence the hair on the head is where the splendour of the kidneys appears externally."[22]

Though the correlates are fact based, Wang Bing has used five phase theory to attempt to explain them, which has produced theories that are clearly untrue. This demonstrates further pitfalls when attempting to apply five phase theory to reality.

Other notions that do not appear to be fact based

The remainder of this chapter features other *Nei Jing* notions and theories that are not fact based. And there are also further examples of five-phase theory being used to produce explanations that do not stand up to scrutiny.

The progress of pathogens through the body

The following type of passage was discussed in Chapter 2, in the section that analysed the *Nei Jing* notion of defence against pathogens (p.44).

> **Extract from *Su Wen*, Chapter 63**
> When a [harmful wind] settles in the [body], it will first lodge in the skin and its hair. It stays there for a while and does not leave.

> Then it enters more deeply and lodges in the tertiary vessels*. It stays there for a while and does not leave. Then it enters further and lodges in the [collaterals]. It stays there for a while and does not leave. Then it enters further and lodges in the [meridians]. It links up with the five [*yin* organs (*zang*)] internally and spreads into the intestines and the stomach. With both the *yin* and the *yang* regions being affected, the five [*yin* organs] will be harmed. That is the sequence whereby a [harmful wind] enters through the skin and its hair and finally reaches the five [*yin* organs]. In such cases, then, treat the respective [meridians].[23]

This, and similar *Nei Jing* theories about the processes through which pathogens affect us are untrue. It is true that when we are weak or depleted and are exposed to a cold wind, we will often develop aching or painful muscles, and if the problem is not remedied (by whichever method), the *yin* organs could eventually be affected, producing a serious illness. This knowledge, of course, was based on practical observation, and is therefore fact based. But the above *Nei Jing* theory that explains this is untrue. *Wind* (or a vapour which contains some essence of the *wind*) does not enter the body through the skin at all, and it certainly does not lodge in the spaces between the muscles and then travel through the "meridians". All this is untrue.

Even though a *Nei Jing* theory is untrue, this does not mean that there is no real clinical condition that the theory is attempting to describe. In such cases (when there *is* a real condition), there would usually be a fact based explanation for the condition or symptom (see pp.44-47, pp.221-224 and 308-310).

Movement contrary to the normal course

Chapter 34 of the *Su Wen* discusses the notion of influences "moving contrary to their normal course" which is said to explain the signs and symptoms of a person's condition.

> **Extract from *Su Wen*, Chapter 34**
> When someone rises and rests as usual, with his breathing being accompanied by noises, this is a case of a movement contrary to its regular course in the [collaterals] of the lung. The [influence] in the [collaterals] cannot rise or descend following the [meridian]. Hence, it stays in the [meridian] and does not move. Diseases of the network vessels affect a person only slightly. Hence, rising and resting are as usual, but the breathing is accompanied by noises.[24]

In this extract, it is theorized that the influences in the lung "meridian" (or in the veins inside the lung itself—i.e. the collaterals) are not moving as usual, and it is this that causes the person's breathing to be noisy (that is, affects the lungs).

The theory is untrue, if only because "influences" do not flow in the "meridians" and collaterals anyway (pp.41-47). In fact, the whole notion of the metabolism consisting of various types of vapour flowing through the "meridians" and collaterals and thus producing all the effects needed to sustain us, such as generating the blood, nourishing the tissue of

* The "tertiary vessels" branch off from the collaterals. And both these refer to the superficial veins that were used for bleeding patients, and which were thought to branch off from the "meridians", which were thought to be artery-like tubes that ran more deeply beneath the skin (p.29).

the organs and body, and producing the resistance to attack by external pathogens—this whole notion is untrue (pp.40-47), so any theories that rely on these facts can also only be untrue.

This does not mean that the person does not have a lung condition. But the theory that the condition is caused due to imaginary vapours ceasing to flow properly in the lung-related "meridians" and veins is untrue.

Likewise, the theory that the condition should thus be corrected by needling an acupoint on the lung meridian, which would then return the flow of influences in the "meridian" to normal and hence heal the lung condition—this theory is also untrue. But, again, this does not mean that needling an acupoint on the lung meridian will *not* heal the lung condition. In most cases it will. But there is a different explanation for how the treatment works (p.145).

The explanation for hiccup

The following passage theorizes about how hiccups are caused.

> **Extract from *Ling Shu*, Chapter 28**
> The grains enter the stomach. The stomach [influences] ascend and pour into the lung. Here now old cold* [influence] and new [food influence (*gu chi*)] together turn into the stomach. New and cold come into conflict with each other; [stomach influence] and [cold influence] attack each other. The influence meet in mutual counterblow and leave the stomach again. Hence this results in hiccup.[25]

* "Cold influence" may refer to influence that neither transmits further nor disperses. See Unschuld, 2016, p.330, fn.6.

Intuitively, this seems to me to be nonsense. But it can only be untrue anyway, since "food influence" does not literally ascend to the lungs. Indeed, nothing resembling "food influence" literally exists; that is, a vapour which was somehow extracted from ingested food by the stomach and then flows (albeit in the form of further vapours which are themselves derived from "food influence") through the "meridians". This substance itself does not exist, and it certainly does not ascend to the lungs. These are misconceptions of *Nei Jing* metabolism; and any theory based on these can only therefore be untrue.

Liquids flowing via the meridians

Chapter 35 of the *Ling Shu* states "The [Ren-23 (*Lianquan*)] and [Ren-18 (*Yutang*)] openings are the paths taken by the *jin* and *ye* liquids." In 1670, Zhang Yin'an commented on this line, stating "The liquids spilling over into the lower [section of the *san jiao*] proceed via the [Ren meridian], from where they exit via the [Ren-23] and [Ren-18] openings to supply dampness to the upper orifices."[26]

In the *Nei Jing* texts, acupoints were usually referred to as "openings" or "holes", since it was believed, firstly, that influences flowed through the "meridians", and, secondly, that the influences (including "harmful influences" such as "evil wind") could be let out of the "meridians" via these "holes", or that the influences within the "meridians" could be affected through these "holes", so as to remove blockages, reduce a repletion (excess), or counter a depletion (deficiency). But both these beliefs are untrue. Vapours (influences) containing the essence of food or cold or *wind*, and so on, do not flow through the "meridians" (pp.42-47), and hence, these imaginary vapours cannot be either released through a meridian's acupoints or affected in any way via the acupoints—since they do not exist in the first place.

But further, the above passage also states that the body liquids flow through the "meridians". The *Nei Jing* notion of a "meridian" is that they consisted of artery-like tubes, but these tubes were imaginary, since they were thought to follow the same paths as the *pathways on the skin*, rather than the paths of the literal arteries (p.29). Even though body fluids *are* transported in the literal arteries (and also in the lymph), these arteries do not equate to the *Nei Jing* "meridians", therefore it cannot be considered true that body liquids flow in the "meridians".

The acupoints Ren-18 (*Yutang*) and Ren-23 (*Lianquan*) are located at the top of the neck and on the upper chest respectively,[27] which may be the origin of the belief that liquids could be released from the Ren meridian to "supply dampness to the upper orifices."

It is true that Ren-23 (*Lianquan*) is noted for its effect on the voice and tongue and to regulate the production of fluids in the mouth,[28] but I am certain these effects are not produced by supplying liquids which are released from the Ren "meridian" via these acupoints.[29]

In the absence of any meaningful anatomical knowledge, these were the types of explanations the *Nei Jing* authors used to describe such effects. They are certainly interesting to study, and such ideas can often be helpful in clinic, in that they can guide the practitioner on the choice of an acupoint to achieve a particular effect. But it should be remembered that such descriptions are not literally true.

Explanations for dizziness, double vision, and insomnia

Extract from *Ling Shu*, Chapter 80

When [harmful wind (*xie chi*)] strike the nape, they will connect with the body's regions of depletion. When they enter deeply, then they follow the eye connection and enter the brain. When they have entered the brain, the brain will rotate. When the brain rotates it pulls the eye connection which will become tense. When the eye connection is tense, the eyes will be dizzy and one feels as if they were rotating. When the [wind influence] strike the essence, the essence is unable to remain concentrated where it was struck. Hence the essence dissipates. When the essence dissipates, one's vision separates into two directions. When the vision has separated into two directions, one sees the items twice....[30]

It is doubtless the case that after some people (particularly if depleted) are exposed to a cold wind, they may sometimes develop symptoms of dizziness and double vision. But no detail of the above explanation is literally true. Firstly, harmful wind does not literally enter the body through the skin, and no "wind influence" circulates in the "meridians" as a result (p.44), nor does it enter the brain, and the brain certainly does not rotate (in response to this imaginary "wind influence", or in response to anything else). And the supposedly rotating brain does not pull the "eye connection", which then becomes tense and thus causes the dizziness. And the same applies to the explanation for double vision.

Though the symptoms are real and the original cause (exposure to a cold wind) is true, the theoretical explanation of how the body's physiology then produces the symptoms is untrue—and is *so* untrue, it is difficult to even regard the explanation as being either metaphorical or an analogy.

The same chapter includes the following passage.

Extract from *Ling Shu*, Chapter 80

Huang Di: When someone has a disease of being unable to sleep, which [influence] cause that?

Qi Bo: The [defensive influence (*wei chi*)] are unable to enter the *yin* realms; they permanently remain in the *yang* realm. When they remain in the *yang* realm, then the *yang* realm is filled with [influence]. When the *yang* realm is filled with [influence], then the [influence] in the *yang* walker [meridian]* abound. Because they are unable to enter the *yin* realm, the [influence] in the *yin* realm are depleted. Hence the eyes cannot be closed.[31]

Zhang Jingyue (in 1624) commented on the above

The [defensive influence] flow through the *yang* realm during the day and they flow [through] the *yin* realm during the night. As long as they flow through the *yang* realm, one is awake. While they flow through the *yin* realm one sleeps. This is the normal situation. In the case of disease, this normality is left and the [defensive influence] remain either in the *yin* [or] in the *yang* realm. When they remain in one of these realms, a unilateral dominance results in the *yin* or *yang* realm. Unilateral dominance is associated with unilateral depletion. Hence being awake and sleeping lose their normal rhythm.[32]

Again, the symptoms are real; there are often situations when, due to a particular organ being stressed, it is hard to sleep. However, the above theory that attempts to explain how this symptom is produced, is untrue. In Chapter 2 of this book, it was explained why there is nothing resembling "defensive influence" (*wei chi*) circulating in the "meridian" network (p.44). Therefore any theory that relies on the existence and circulation of "defensive influence" cannot be true. But is it possible to interpret the above passage either metaphorically or as an analogy of some actual mechanism in the body?

"Defensive influence" could be regarded as being analogous to the active components of the immune system (p.46). So, the question is, is there any malfunction in the immune system (or in the organs that enable and regulate it) that could produce insomnia? In contemporary physiology, the "kidneys" (i.e. adrenal glands) secrete hormones that are necessary for the development and maintenance of normal immunity (p.154). When the "kidneys" function poorly, this certainly produces low immunity (possibly resulting in hay fever and other allergies, and rendering the person susceptible to colds and influenza) and also sometimes insomnia (p.174). So, could the explanation in the above passage be understood as being analogous to poor kidney function? In other words, as being a tangential reference to poor kidney function? It does not seem to fit. The passage would have to be understood as suggesting that it would be (the

* In today's Chinese medicine, this meridian would usually be called the "*yang* motility vessel" (Deadman, p.21).

equivalent of) the malfunction in the immune system (i.e. the "defensive influence" not circulating where it was supposed to) that was directly responsible for somehow producing the insomnia. I cannot imagine this.

Or another approach might be this. When looking for an analogy, the passage could be seen as suggesting the notion that the immune system usually behaves differently at night than at day, but that (in this diseased state) it is stuck in its daytime mode, which then produces the insomnia. In contemporary physiology, I do not believe that the immune system does function differently during either day or night—not substantially anyway. So, again, it is difficult to perform the intellectual gymnastics necessary to rescue the passage from the realm of make-believe. It would certainly be easier to simply accept that the passage is untrue.

The same could be said of the following passages.

Explanation for why we yawn

> **Extract from *Ling Shu*, Chapter 28**
> When the *yin* [influence] gather below, and as long as the *yang* [influence] have not been exhausted completely, the *yang* [meridians] pull the [influence] upward, and the *yin* [meridians] pull them downward. When the *yin* and the *yang* [meridians] pull each other, one frequently yawns as a result.[33]

Explanation for how tears are produced

> **Extract from *Ling Shu*, Chapter 28**
> When someone is mournful and grievous, then his heart will be excited. When the heart is excited, then all the five [*yin* organs] and six [*yang* organs] will sway. This swaying affects the stem vessels.[*] When the stem vessels are affected, the pathways of the liquids will open. When the pathways of the liquids are open, tears will leave there.[34]

Explanation for why we sweat after eating hot food

> **Extract from *Ling Shu*, Chapter 18**
> Huang Di: When a person has *heat* in his body and ingests beverages and food that move down into the stomach, and before the [influences] are stabilized this results in sweating, sometimes in the face, sometimes on the back, sometimes involving half of the body[;] that is, the sweat does not follow the paths of the [defensive influence (*wei chi*)] and leaves the body, why is that?
> Qi Bo: This is a harm caused by wind from the outside. Internally the skin structures open. The body hair is steamed with heat, and the skin structures experience outflow. The [defensive influence] proceed there. Hence they are unable to follow their regular paths. These [influences] are wild, smooth and fast. When they see that the skin structures have opened they leave from there. Hence they are unable to follow their regular paths. Hence that is called "leakage outflow".[35]

Is left, *yin* or *yang*?

In today's Chinese medicine, it is usually stated that left is *yang*, but this is based on

[*] In this context, it is not clear what the term "stem vessels" 宗脈 was intended to refer to. When the term "vessel" was used, this always referred to some level of the "meridian" system. Hence it is possible the reference was to the heart and lung "meridians". That is, those that were thought to carry the "chest influence" 宗氣 (*zong chi*).

theory alone, rather than on practical observation.

From practical observations, it is clear that left is *yin*, and right is *yang*. The left of the tongue relates to the liver and the right to the gallbladder (p.383), making left *yin* and right *yang*—since the liver is clearly more *yin* than the gallbladder. Most people are right handed, making their right side more active and therefore more *yang* than their left. And rather than this being a conscious choice, it is the body itself that considers the right side to be more *yang*—and the body is not swayed by any theoretical considerations.

The pulse positions (which are also naturally determined) also confirm this polarity. They are shown in Figure 2 on page 301. The main pulses at the left wrist are all the *yin* pulses (heart, liver, kidney) while those at the right are relatively more *yang* (lungs, pancreas, kidney *yang*), though the evidence is not entirely clear cut, as follows.

In the first position, the heart is certainly more *yin* than the lungs, making the left *yin*.

The middle position is unclear though. Table 6 on page 348 shows the *yin-yang* hierarchy of the organs. The liver is listed as more *yin* than the pancreas, but with a caveat. The hierarchy between these two organs is variable, depending on which criterion is used to determine it (p.393), which is why (uniquely) their meridians cross one another at three different locations on the body. Therefore it is not possible to state definitively which organ is the more *yin*.

In the third position, the kidney is clearly more *yin* than the kidney *yang*. In the *Nan Jing*, this third position was regarded as reflecting the kidneys on the left and the pericardium on the right (p.305). However, the kidneys are still clearly more *yin* than the pericardium, so that this still confirms that left is *yin* and *right* is yang.

On balance, these practical observations overwhelmingly indicate that the left of the body is *yin* while the right is *yang*.

There is now also experimental data that demonstrates that left is *yin*. In an experiment where the subject drank chilled water,[36] the immediate effect of this was notable in the impedance at his left ST-36 acupoint, while there was hardly any effect at right ST-36. Since the chilled water would have mainly affected the inner wall of the stomach (i.e. the stomach's fabric, rather than its function), its effect would have been on the stomach's *yin* (its fabric), rather than on its *yang* (its function). And since the effect registered mainly at the left instance of ST-36, this confirmed that the left of the body is *yin* while the right is *yang*.

The Nei Jing theories

On page 270 the *Nan Jing* notion of abdominal diagnosis was discussed. As demonstrated in the commentary on Section 16 of the *Nan Jing*, the five phase directional correspondences were used to predict the location of the main organs in the body. Because the liver was said to correspond to East, and East was considered left, five phase theory predicts that the liver is on the left of the body, while the pancreas is in the centre and the lungs on the right (p.270).

This does support the above notion that the left is the *yin* side, since the liver is clearly more *yin* than the lungs. However, the theory is incorrect, since, in reality, the liver is on the right, the pancreas on the left and the lungs in the centre. Therefore the predictions of this particular *Nan Jing* theory have to be discounted. However, the theory does help to clear up another related matter, since it demonstrates that the five phase directional correspondences are incorrect, which can only mean that they were, in effect, arbitrarily determined in the first place. This means that, either East does not correspond to the liver, or that East does not correspond to left.

In the following extract from Chapter 5 of the *Su Wen*, the nature of *yin* and *yang* and left and right are discussed. The reasoning is based on the five phase directional correspondences. And it was theorized that when a person faces South, East would then be left, and West right. Apart from other issues (discussed below), this in itself is arbitrary, since if we happen to face East instead, then North is left and South right, and the same for each direction. But what about if a person faced Southwest? Then, East-south would be left and Northwest right. If left and right were based on the compass bearing of which direction we happened to face, there would seem to be endless possible assignments of left and right.

However, this aside, if we assume that our facing South always determines the assignment of left and right (so that East is always left), the theory still does not work. This was seen above, in the *Nan Jing* application of this "East is left" notion to abdominal diagnosis, which predicted the location of the organs incorrectly, indicating that either East is not left, or that these directional associations were incorrectly attributed to the phases (or that the organs were incorrectly attributed—so that East and the liver do not correspond to the same phase).

Extract from *Su Wen*, Chapter 5

As for left and right, they are the paths of *yin* and *yang*. Heaven is not sufficiently present in the North-West. Hence the North-West is *yin*, and the ears and the eyes of man on the right are not as clear as on the left. The earth is incomplete in the South-East. Hence the South-East is *yang*, and the hands and feet of man on the left are not as strong as on the right.

Huang Di: Why is this so?

Qi Bo: The East is *yang*. As for the *yang*, its essence collects above. When it collects above, then the above is brilliant and there is depletion below. Hence, this lets the ears and eyes be clear, while the hands and feet do not move comfortably. The West is *yin*. As for the *yin*, its essence collects below. When it collects below, then there is abundance below and there is depletion above. Hence, the ears and eyes are not clear, while the hands and feet move comfortably.[37]

Hu Tianxiong (in 1991) commented on the above

If one stands facing South, after midnight, the sun rises from one's left. After noon, the sun descends on one's right. When it rises, the *yang* [influence] gradually gains force; when it descends, the *yin* [influence] gradually gains force. The [influence] in man corresponds to this. Hence, in the morning the *yang* [influence] emerges; in the evening the *yang* [influence] is depleted. This is meant by "left and right are the passageways of *yin* and *yang*".[38]

The above *Su Wen* passage relies on the notions that left is *yang*, since it corresponds to East, and that the distribution of resources in the body correlates to the distribution of the planet's resources, which, in any location on the planet, are determined by where the sun rises and sets. Using these notions, the passage theorizes that on the right, the hands and feet are stronger, while on the left, the ears and eyes are stronger. There are several problems with this.

It is true that with right-handed people, the limbs on their right are usually stronger than those on their left, and there can be no doubt that this assertion in the *Su Wen* passage was based on practical observation. And this may have been the starting point of the above theory. In other words, starting with this fact-based observation, a theory was perhaps devised that agreed with the observation, but the theory then predicted that (with all people) the left ears and eyes ought to be stronger than the right ones. However, this is untrue. Around two-thirds of people are right-eye dominant and this is unrelated to whether they are right or left handed.[39,40] This is contrary to the theory's predictions. And it appears that the hearing on the left or right varies only in that each side is more sensitive to different types of sound,[41] which again bears no resemblance to the theory's predictions.

Another problem is with the notion that the distribution of resources in the body corresponds with the distribution of the planet's resources. The exact location that the sun rises and sets varies enormously, depending on the time of year and our location on the planet. If the above theory were correct, it would predict that the differences in strength between the right and left limbs and senses would vary depending on the time of year and our location on the planet. Though I am not aware of any systematic test of such a notion, it is difficult to imagine how it could be true.

The theoretical notions expressed in the above *Su Wen* extract produce untrue predictions about the relative strengths of the limbs and senses on the left and right sides, therefore the theory cannot be correct. Also, the notion that left is *yang* simply because when we face South, the East is on our left, and the sun rises in the East, which is the beginning of the day's *yang* period—this is arbitrary. And when the five phase correspondences were applied in the abdominal diagnosis example (p.270), this contradicted the above and confirmed that left is *yin*, since the theory predicted that the liver is on the left, and the lungs on the right. However, this theory also proved to be wrong (since the liver is on the right), which casts doubt on the validity of the directional correspondences (East, West, etc.) in five phase theory.

For all these reasons, this book follows the practical observations and also the experimental data mentioned on pages 282-283 above, disregards the above *Nei Jing* theories, and adopts the convention that left is *yin* and right is *yang*.

Needling techniques

Monthly meridian prohibitions

Chapter 41 of the *Ling Shu* expresses the theory that each of the twelve "meridians" are associated with a particular month, and that each month "dominates" its particular "meridian"—due to the rotation of the twelve "earth branches" through the year. Therefore it is advised that the acupoints on certain "meridians" should not be used during certain months.

Extract from *Ling Shu*, Chapter 41

During the first, second and third month the [influences] of man are on the left, and it is not appropriate to pierce the *yang* [meridians] of the left foot. During the fourth, fifth and sixth months the [influences...] are on the right, and it is not appropriate to pierce the *yang* [meridians] of the right foot. In the seventh, eighth and ninth month the [influences...] are on the right, and it is not appropriate to pierce the *yin* [meridians] of the right foot. In the tenth, eleventh and twelfth month the [influences...] are on the left, and it is not appropriate to pierce the *yin* [meridians] of the left foot.[42]

There is certainly nothing in my own clinical experience that could support this theory. And there is nothing in the theoretical aspects of this book (on how acupuncture works) that could support it either. No substance that resembles the "influences" flows in the "meridians" anyway (pp.42-47); and according to this book's intelligent tissue hypothesis, there could not possibly be any monthly variation in the effectiveness of acupoints on either the left or right meridians. The *Nei Jing* theory appears, to me, to be untrue. However, if practitioners chose to adhere to the theory, there would be no significant adverse consequences—in most situations. The only downside would be that practitioners would need to be constantly aware of the date, which would then dictate whether they used the left or right meridian—rather than both, as is the common practice today.

Elsewhere, I have written on the issue of whether to needle an acupoint on both limb meridians (left and right) or simply on one, and expressed the opinion that, in my clinical experience, it is generally not necessary to needle on both sides.[43] Therefore, one interpretation of the above *Ling Shu* passage is that perhaps this was also the practice at the time of the *Nei Jing*, and the passage merely offers advice on which side to choose, left or right (even if the theory itself appears to have no basis).

Needling according to season and moon phase

The following passage offers advice on when to needle and not to needle, depending on the season, climate, and phase of the moon.

Extract from *Su Wen*, Chapter 26

When heaven is warm and when the sun is bright, then the blood in man is rich in fluid, and the [defensive influence (*wei chi*)] is at the surface. When heaven is cold and when the sun is hidden, then the blood in man congeals so that its flow is impeded, and the [defensive influence] is in the depth. At the time of beginning crescent moon, blood and [influence] originate as essence, and the [defensive influence] begins to move.

When the disk of the moon is full, blood and [influence] are replete; the muscles and the flesh are firm. When the disk of the moon is empty, the muscles and the flesh wane, the [meridians and collaterals] are depleted and the [defensive influence] leaves. The physical appearance exists all by itself. It is therefore that one follows the [four seasons] in regulating blood and [influences].

It is therefore that: when heaven is cold, do not pierce, when heaven is warm, do not hesitate. At crescent moon, do not drain. At full moon, do not supplement. When the disk of the moon is empty, do not treat. This is the so-called regulation at the right time.[44]

Is the above literally true? Overall, most of the content seems to be derived from theory, rather than from practical observation, and since the theories are untrue (as described below), the content is misguided. However, the first two sentences may well be based on practical observation.

In contemporary physiology, when the environmental temperature is low, or when our internal heat production is low (such as with lack of exercise), then *vasoconstriction* is stimulated by sympathetic nerves. This decreases the blood flow near the body's surface to conserve heat.[45]

This correlates with the first two sentences in the above *Su Wen* extract. At that time, bloodletting was commonly used (along with needling and moxibustion). And it is possible that practitioners noticed that it was harder to let blood during Winter. Of course, the blood was not let from the "meridians"; it was let from the veins, but the *Nei Jing* authors believed that the veins were the superficial part of the "meridian" network (p.29). From this, they may have theorized that both the blood and influences retreat to the deeper portion of the "meridian" network during cold seasons. That is, rather than flowing in the veins (collaterals) both these substances then flowed mainly in the "meridians", which were thought to be the deepest part of the network. Apart from the misconceptions about the existence of the various influences, this deduction had an element of truth—in that the blood *was* less near to the surface (which would have perhaps made bleeding the patient more difficult).

As to the third sentence of the extract: "At the time of beginning crescent moon, blood and [influence] originate as essence, and the [defensive influence] begins to move," this appears to be a theoretical deduction. The "meridians" do not carry influences, or defensive influence anyway (at least, not if these *Nei Jing* terms are interpreted literally), so that the sentence could only be theoretical—and also untrue. I have said that "defensive influence" could be regarded as being analogous to the active elements of the immune system (p.46), and the notion that the effectiveness of the immune system waxes and wanes in accord with the phases of the moon is not credible, so that even in analogy, the sentence could not be interpreted as true. This sentence, and the following paragraph, also seems to suggest that the production of blood (in men as well as in women) varies through a monthly cycle, which again is not credible. Therefore, it also seems that the entire second paragraph of the extract (on the "meridians" being full and empty of blood at certain times of the month), could only be an incorrect theoretical deduction.

The advice of the third paragraph, not to needle when the climate is cold or when the disk of the moon is empty, seems to be misguided; that is, rather than being based on practical observation, it seems to be based on incorrect theories. At least, in my own clinical experience I can recall no practical observation of my own that might coincide with this *Nei Jing* theory.

As to the advice to not "drain" or "supplement" during certain phases of the moon, this, too, seems to be based on the same incorrect theories.

It could be argued that the reference to "do not pierce" referred to letting blood, which might then lend the passage more credibility. But the extract refers to defensive influences as much as to blood, and it also sates "At full moon, do not supplement," which also seems to relate to the treatment of influences rather than blood. Therefore "do not pierce" may refer to both acupuncture *or* bloodletting, depending on the context.

Needling techniques to "drain" and "supplement"

The following extract offers advice on how to drain ("reduce") a repletion (an "excess"); and how to supplement ("reinforce") a depletion (a "deficiency").

> **Extract from *Ling Shu*, Chapter 1**
> To drain, that is to say: One must hold the needle firmly when inserting it; then it is let loose and removed again. This way it is possible to reach the *yang* realm with a needle, and to drain the [harmful influence]. If one were to exert pressure when withdrawing the needle, then this would be termed an "internal accumulation". The blood would not be able to disperse, and the [influence] would not be able to come out.
> To supplement, that is to say: Follow them; follow them! With an intention as if one were to deceive them. As if there was something moving and exerting pressure, like a mosquito that stands still. Like staying, like turning around; leaving as if a string had ruptured. One sees to it that what is on the left is associated with what is on the right. These [influences] will stop as a result. The outer gate is firmly closed. The [influences] inside are replete. No blood should be permitted to remain. It must be quickly removed and done away with.
> The WAY to hold the needle, a firm grip is most valuable. A correct posture of the fingers goes along with a straight insertion; there must not be a needle movement to the left or to the right. The spirit is concentrated on the minutest detail.[46]

Today, each practitioner uses their own approach. Clearly, the author of the above extract invested a great deal of thought and practice into forming his own intricate needling techniques. Much of this technique appears to be based on the theoretical notions that the needle is inserted into "holes" or "openings" in the "meridians", through which various types of vapour (some of which are pathogenic, such as "wind influence" or "cold influence") and blood flow; and that the objective is to release harmful, or replete, influences or blood through these holes in the "meridians"; or to "close the gate" to prevent their escape. As regards these theoretical notions, they are all untrue. No such influences flow in the "meridians", nothing is released through an acupoint (p.308), and the effect that acupuncture has on the organ functions is probably produced by a simpler mechanism that is unrelated to any of these factors (according to this book's intelligent tissue hypothesis—p.372).

However, none of the techniques described above would detract from acupuncture's effects on the organs. That effect is produced when the acupoint is stimulated, and anything beyond this is a personal choice of the practitioner (and, in effect, is for their benefit only). This, at least, is the conclusion I have reached from my own clinical practice.

In today's Chinese medicine, students are often taught to use different needling techniques to either "reduce an excess" or "reinforce a deficiency".[47] As a student, I was never entirely convinced of the need for such techniques, though, of course, I tried them out once I started my own practice. However, I soon found that inserting the needle, obtaining a sensation, then simply leaving the needle alone, produced the desired effect on the related organ—even in "excess" situations. In other words, that there was no need to actively "reduce" an excess, since the organ automatically made whatever adjustments to its function were needed.

In such "excess" situations, the intensity of the needle sensation is usually proportional to the amount of excess, and this is without manipulating the needle in any special way. To intensify the sensation even further would certainly have the effect of inducing nervous movement and vocalization in the patient (often of an unrepeatable nature), but in general would seem to not enhance the treatment. However, all practitioners develop their own particular approach, and once we have convinced ourselves that a particular technique is required, we will continue to use that technique, even though it may not add anything to the treatment.

I suspect that this is the explanation for this particular *Nei Jing* author's intricate specifications about his frame of mind, the pressure and position of his fingers, and the tendency for his spirit to be "concentrated on the minutest detail". When reading such passages, it might be beneficial for students to consider whether the description seems to be an over-elaboration, rather than a necessary part of basic technique.

The nine different needles

The following extract describes the uses of nine different needle types.

Extract from *Ling Shu*, Chapter 1

The spade needle: It has a big head and a pointed end. It serves to remove and drain *yang* [influence]. The rounded needle: This needle is shaped like an egg. It is used to rub in partings of the [muscles]. It does not harm muscles and flesh; it serves to drain [influence] from the partings of the [muscles]. The arrow-point needle. Its end is pointed like the tip of a millet grain. It serves to exert pressure on the vessels without having them cave in, so that their [influence] can be reached. The sharp point needle: Its pointed end is triangular to make chronic illness dissipate. The lancet needle: Its end is shaped like the pointed end of a sword. It serves to remove massive amounts of pus. The rounded and sharp needle: It has the size of a hair. It is both rounded and sharp. In its central part it is slightly widened. It serves to remove violent [influence]. The fine needle: It is pointed like the beak of a mosquito. It is moved forward calmly and slowly. Being so small it may remain in place for a long time and provide nourishment. It serves to remove painful blockage-illnesses. The long needle: It has a sharp point and a thin body. It enables one to remove remote blockage-illnesses. The big needle: Its pointed end resembles a club. Its sharp point is slightly rounded. It serves to drain water from the joints. This is all there is to the nine needles.[48]

Two of these needles clearly had non-acupuncture uses. The "lancet needle" was used to remove pus (and interestingly, the term to "lance a boil" is still used today), and the "big needle" was used to drain "water" from the joints. Apart from these, it seems that all the other needles were used for acupuncture, in situations where we would use a single, standard needle today. This suggests that the *Nei Jing* habit of using all these different types of needle was an over-elaboration. For example, the suggestion that a special needle type was required to "make chronic illness dissipate" is untrue, since today's single, standard needle does this. And the same could be said for any other of the uses mentioned in the extract.

The practitioners of that time may well have obtained good results using all these separate needles in different situations, but that does not mean it is necessary to use all those types of needle to obtain the same effects.

On the other hand, this chapter of the *Ling Shu* may be the result of the over-elaborated technique of a single author, and other *Nei Jing* authors could well have used only a single needle type for acupuncture. It is clear that there was great variety amongst practitioners, since some *Nei Jing* authors rank the abilities of other practitioners depending on their choice of technique—both in needling and also in diagnostic technique.[49] Indeed, the author of the above extract does just this, several paragraphs before the extract. He states "Unrefined practitioners guard the physical appearance. Outstanding practitioners guard the spirit.... As long as an illness is not carefully observed, how can its origin be known? The subtle secret of [needling] lies in varying speed. The unrefined practitioners guard the trigger. Outstanding practitioners guard the inner mechanism."[50]

Note that Unschuld suggests that these last two sentences are allegory, probably comparing the art of needling to the use of a crossbow, since the following lines in the text clearly refer to Warring States military tactics; and military metaphor was often used in the *Nei Jing*.[51]

Choose acupoints and needling depth according to season

The following extract features the *Nei Jing* notions that influences may be released through acupoints; that influences tend to gather at certain acupoints in certain seasons; that diseases take the form of harmful influences lodged within the "meridian" network; and that these harmful influences (and presumably also the "meridians") adopt different depths beneath the skin in different seasons.

> **Extract from *Ling Shu*, Chapter 2**
>
> In Spring one selects for treatment the [collaterals], all the [*ying*-spring acupoints], where the flesh parts. In serious cases one penetrates deeply and removes the [influences]. In less serious cases one pierces only superficially to remove the [influences].
>
> In Summer one selects for treatment all the [*shu*-stream acupoints], the tertiary network vessels* are to be pierced from the skin above the muscle flesh.
>
> In Autumn one selects for treatment all the [*he*-sea acupoints]. In addition the same measures apply as in Spring.
>
> In Winter one selects for treatment the section covering all the [*jing*-well acupoints] and all the [*shu*-stream acupoints]. One should pierce into the depth and have the needle remain there.

* The "tertiary network vessels" 孫絡 are the small vessels that branch off from the collaterals. In other words, tiny superficial veins, which flow into the collaterals (other superficial veins), which were thought to then flow into the "meridians" (p.29).

> This is to outline the sequence of the four seasons, with the locations of the [influence], the places where diseases settle, and what befits the [appropriate applications of the needles].[52]

Is it factual that in different seasons, different classes of acupoints are more effective?

As a general rule (when considering this book's "intelligent tissue" explanation of how acupuncture works), this could only be true if in each season, only illnesses occurred which were of a type that produced tenderness at the prescribed acupoints. For example, in Spring, people would need to only suffer illnesses that produced the most significant tenderness (amongst all the acupoints that happened to be tender on that occasion) at the *ying*-spring acupoints. These are Lung-10 (*Yuji*), Pancreas-2[*] (*Dadu*), Heart-8 (*Shaofu*), Kidney-2 (*Rangu*), Pericardium-8 (*Laogong*), Liver-2 (*Xingjian*), Large-intestine-2 (*Erjian*), Stomach-44 (*Neiting*), Small-intestine-2 (*Qiansu*), Bladder-66 (*Zutonggu*), Lymphatic-system-2[†] (*Yemen*), and Gallbladder-43 (*Xiaxi*).[53]

These acupoints cater for the treatment of every organ. Therefore the extract is not relying on the fact that one of the *yin* organs tends to dominate during each season (p.244) and that therefore that organ is generally the most likely to become stressed during that season. This is *one* seasonal pattern. Beyond that, the extract is suggesting another pattern, one where any of the organs may become ill during any season (which is quite plausible), but that the organs always suffer from a condition of a particular type. In Spring (judging from the actions of the *ying*-spring acupoints), this condition might be generally described (in Chinese medicine terms) as one featuring excess *heat*, such as "Stomach heat" (p.457), "Heart fire" (p.454), or "Liver fire" (p.455).

In my clinical experience, there are no practical observations that could support such a suggestion. Such illnesses may, of course, occur during Spring, but there would also be a great variety of other conditions, far higher in number than these *heat*-related conditions. And these same *heat*-related conditions, in most people, would be just as likely to occur in other seasons.

Such statements (as this one in the first paragraph of the quoted extract) seem to me to be theoretically constructed, rather than being based on practical observation, and hence are not usually literally true.

The quoted extract also relies on other *Nei Jing* theories, which themselves are not literally true—such as the notion that diseases take the form of harmful influences lodged within the "meridian" network (see pages 44 and 277 above); and that influences flow within the veins and "meridians" and hence can exist at different depths.

It is true that a needling sensation can be obtained at different depths of needling on the same acupoint, which may give the impression that "influences" can exist at different depths. However, in my experience, a needling sensation can almost always be obtained from the most shallow of needling, even though it is also possible to needle deeper at the same acupoint and obtain a sensation. This seems to suggest that obtaining a sensation does not depend on the depth of the needling, and that the needling depth is not therefore an indicator of the location of

[*] Also called Spleen-2.

[†] Also called *San-jiao*-2, or Tipple-burner-2, etc.

the "meridian", nor of any (imaginary) influences.

When practising acupuncture today, it is easy to gain the impression that the "influences", and hence meridians, lie at different depths; and in the same way, the *Nei Jing* authors may have gained this impression. This may be the thinking behind the statement that in Winter, one should needle more deeply.

As a practitioner, there is no harm in embracing such thoughts. The therapy will work just as well now as it always has done, whatever theoretical notions the practitioner has. But if contemporary science is ever going to stand a chance of understanding Chinese acupuncture, it is important for its practitioners to be aware that such notions may not be literally true—however convincing they seem.

As to the statement that "In serious cases one penetrates deeply and removes the [influences]. In less serious cases one pierces only superficially to remove the [influences]," this was probably inspired by the *Nei Jing* notion of how pathogens enter the body and then gradually travel the "meridians", until, if they have not been removed, they lodge in the *yin* organs, when serious illness results (p.277).

There are lots of inherent contradictions here, such as, if the pathogen is lodged in the organ, how can needling a distal acupoint, even needling it deeply, "vent" the pathogen from the organ? But such contradictions only become an issue (or apparent at all) when all *Nei Jing* passages are interpreted literally, or assumed to be true. In my experience, shallow needling is just as effective at correcting a serious illness, as deep needling may be.

Harming tissue, causes serious disease in the related organ

The following is a long extract (almost the entire *Su Wen* chapter), but it is worth quoting in full since the passage's structure and content clearly suggest that it was not derived from practical observation but was theoretically constructed—hence it demonstrates this principle well.

Extract from *Su Wen*, Chapter 50

The diseases include those at the surface and others in the depth; piercing includes shallow piercing and deep piercing. Always go to the respective structures; never go too far on this way. If one goes too far on this way, then this results in internal harm; if one does not reach it, then this generates external congestion. Once there is a congestion, then [harm] will follow there.

When the proper measure of shallow or deep piercing is not achieved, contrary to one's intentions this will cause severe injury and excites the five [*yin* organs (*zang*)]. This will generate a serious disease subsequently.

When piercing the finest body hair and the interstice structures, do not harm the skin. When the skin is harmed, then internally this excites the lung. When the lung is excited, then that person will suffer from warmth-malaria in Autumn. He shivers from cold in a *su*-manner.

When piercing the skin, do not harm the flesh. When the flesh is harmed, then this excites the [pancreas] internally. When the [pancreas] is excited, then that person will suffer from abdominal distension, vexation, and a lack of appetite for 72 days[, during the last 18 days of each season].

When piercing the flesh, do not harm the vessels. When the vessels are harmed, then

> internally this excites the heart. When the heart is excited, then that person will suffer from heartache in Summer.
>
> When piercing the vessels, do not harm the sinews. When the sinews are harmed, then internally this excites the liver. When the liver is excited, then that person will suffer from heat and slackened sinews in Spring.
>
> When piercing the sinews, do not harm the bones. When the bones are harmed, then internally this excites the kidneys. When the kidneys are excited, then that person will suffer from distension and lower back pain in Winter.
>
> When piercing the bones, do not harm the marrow. When the marrow is harmed, then it melts away and the shins turn sore. The body turns *jie-yi*-like and one cannot go away.[54]

This entire passage seems to provide a clear example of content that was entirely constructed from theory, rather than being based on practical observation, and as a result is untrue. The general notion is that diseases exist at different depths, and that if you do not needle to the correct depth, this will cause a serious problem in the local tissue; and if you should damage that tissue, this will cause a serious disease to develop later in the related *yin* organ.

In my own clinical experience, this whole notion is simply untrue. The notion that if the skin is harmed at an acupoint, this will later cause the lungs to develop a serious illness (such as "warmth-malaria"), this is simply nonsense; or that if the muscle is harmed, this will cause poor pancreas function during the last part of every season for the following year; or that if the "meridians" (being imaginary artery-like tubes) are inadvertently harmed, this will produce "palpitations" during the Summer; and so on. These notions are all clearly theoretically constructed, based on the five phase associations, and, unsurprisingly, are completely untrue. Unsurprising, because there was no practical observation that guided the theory. It seems to be theory for theory's sake. In such writing, it is as though the passage was constructed by an intellectual with no practical knowledge of acupuncture, who extrapolated his essay from the five phase associations alone, which is suggested by the choice of words.

He starts "When piercing the finest body hair." This, if nothing else, gives the game away immediately. No-one ever acupunctures a hair, which would not even be possible—and it is clear from the passage's construction that he means the "hair" and not a hair follicle.

It is true that the "skin and body hair" are associated the "lungs" and "Autumn" in the five phase correspondences (p.265), and this alone seems to have convinced the author that if the "skin" were harmed, this would cause a "lung" disease in the "Autumn". And using the same logic, he goes on, stating that if the "flesh" were harmed, this would cause a "pancreas" disease in the "[last 18 days of each season]"; and that if the "vessels" were harmed, this would cause a "heart" disease in "Summer"; and if the "sinews" were harmed, this would cause a "liver" disease in "Spring"; and if the "bones" were harmed, this could cause a "kidney" disease in "Winter". And he even ends with a caution not to harm the "marrow". In practice, it is difficult to imagine how bones might be harmed during acupuncture, let alone the marrow. It seems clear that all the above are lifted directly from the five phase correspondences, and have no bearing on reality.

Another element of the passage's construction is that he progresses through the body tissue, as listed in the five phase correspondences. So, starting at the most superficial level, he imagines that the practitioner's objective might be to "pierce the finest body hair and the interstice structures", but that if the practitioner were not careful, this might result in damage to the skin. Next, when the objective were to "pierce the skin", damage might be caused to the "flesh". Then, when "piercing the flesh", damage might be caused to the "vessels" (i.e. the "meridians"). Then, when "piercing the vessels", damage might be caused to the "sinews". And he continues this down to "When piercing the sinews, do not harm the bones," and, finally, "When piercing the bones, do not harm the marrow". It appears to have not occurred to the author to ask a practitioner if they would ever have the objective of acupuncturing the sinews or the bones. To an intellectual, with no practical knowledge of acupuncture, who derived his knowledge entirely from the five phase correspondences, such statements might seem sensible. But in the real world, the resultant passage is complete nonsense—and should certainly not be interpreted literally today.

However, I would add one caveat. It is possible to find an element of truth in the passage. On page 221, I said that the organs appear to be capable of "remembering" incidental symptoms. This means symptoms that occur at any location along an organ's related meridian. This means that if a trauma occurs to the tissue along that meridian, particularly at the acupoints, and the effects of that trauma are not cleared, then it is possible that this *could* affect the function of the related organ. But this is meridian specific, rather than being tissue specific—so is an entirely different concept to the one the author of *Su Wen*, Chapter 50, had in mind. His idea was that the *type of tissue* damaged, caused damage to the organ which corresponded to that tissue type in five phase theory, not to the organ whose related meridian the damage occurred along. And also, his idea was that the organ damage would result only when the season (in five phase correspondences) associated with that organ and tissue, finally came along. This means that if the local trauma occurred in Spring and it was the "bones" that were damaged, then the related organ (the kidneys) would not feel the harm until Winter arrived. It would be difficult to fit these circumstances into the notion of the organs "remembering" incidental symptoms—no matter what intellectual gymnastics are attempted. And anyway, this notion of "remembered" symptoms probably relates most to the *Nei Jing* notions of "blockage-illness", "obstruction-illness" or "impediment-illness" (p.219), which seem to be far removed from whatever thoughts may have been in this author's mind.

Frame of mind while needling

The following passage recommends the frame of mind that the practitioner should adopt while needling.

> **Extract from *Ling Shu*, Chapter 3**
>
> "When causing a repletion or a depletion, this is to act as if something were gained, and as if something were lost" is to say: supplementing is to be done such that one is happy, as if he had gained something. When draining, this is to be done such that one is irritated as if he had lost something.[55]

In my own clinical practice I have never routinely adopted a particular frame of mind when needling, and the treatments have always been effective. It is true that I have sometimes (even often) felt happy while working, but this state of mind would have applied to all acupoints needled at that time. And I can not recall a single occasion when I felt irritated while needling. Instead, what I have consciously noticed is that the treatment seems to work best when the minds of both the practitioner and patient are unoccupied.

This has been graphically demonstrated to me countless times in the following situation. I find that when needling, the sensation the patient feels usually occurs either immediately, or within a second or two of the needle being inserted. But there is a certain class of patient where a curious scenario frequently arises. Without fail, these are patients who have poor pancreas function; in other words, patients who are used to constantly thinking. With such patients, I have noticed that sometimes the needle sensation does not occur as normal, and several seconds might elapse after I have inserted the needle (perhaps around four or five seconds), and still the patient has not felt a sensation. The curious aspect of this is that, almost without fail, when I then ask the patient if they can feel anything, at the moment I start to speak, the needle sensation occurs. This scenario has happened so routinely that when I needle a patient with poor pancreas function, whom I know usually has this particular trait, I will often make a comment or ask them something just before I needle, so that their mind is distracted; and I find that the needle sensation usually then occurs instantly, as with most other patients.

I have said that I believe the needle sensation is caused when the related organ begins to change its function, which then causes the local tissue at the acupoint to reflect that change (p.223).

My understanding of the above scenario is that when the patient's conscious mind is heavily using the organ functions (particularly the pancreas, but also the other organ functions), then perhaps this blocks those organs from being open to change—hence the organs do not respond to the stimulation at the acupoint. But as soon as the person's conscious mind is distracted, this then frees the organs to respond.[56]

These experiences suggest that it is important for the practitioner (and patient) to remain calm and to have an open, clear mind during treatments. And that the above extract is probably therefore a theoretical construction. Or alternatively, that the author *was* in the habit of using that mental technique (which he probably deduced theoretically), but that it amounts to an over-elaboration, since it certainly is not a necessary technique.

The outcomes of blood letting

The following passage theorizes about the circumstances that can sometimes arise when blood is let. Here, the term "pierced" means using a specialized "needle" (see p.289 above) to incise the collaterals (i.e. the superficial veins—p.29) to let blood. The outcomes described are fact based (the patient does fall to ground, turn green, etc.) but the theories offered to explain these outcomes are all untrue, for the reasons given following the extract.

Extract from *Ling Shu*, Chapter 39

When the vessels abound with [influence], while the blood is depleted, if the patient is pierced in such a condition then he will lose [influence]. When he loses [influence], then he falls to the ground....

When one has just ingested a beverage, the liquid seeps into the [collaterals]. If they are pierced before the liquid of the beverage has merged with the blood, the blood will appear, but a juicy liquid will come out separately. If the patient has not just ingested a beverage and if there is water in his body, after an extended period of time this will generate a swelling.

The *yin* [influence] collect in the *yang* realm. The [influence] follow the [collaterals]. Hence, when piercing them, the [influence] will move first before the blood appears. Hence a swelling results.

When *yin* and *yang* [influence] have just begun to interact, but have not merged yet, and if in such a situation they are drained, then both the *yin* and the *yang* [influence] are lost. The exterior and the interior regions are separated from each other. Hence the patient loses his complexion and assumes a greenish colour.[57]

The reasoning in the first paragraph relies on the theory that influences flow through the "meridians" and superficial veins (collaterals), which form different branches of the same network. But no influences flow in this "meridian" network at all (pp.41-47), so this supposed vaporous substance cannot be affected by the piercing of a superficial vein. This is a fundamental mistake of *Nei Jing* metabolism and physiology, so any further theory that relies on this mistake can only itself be untrue. It is more likely that that patient simply fainted because they do not like the sight of their own blood being let.

The extract's second paragraph is based on a fundamental misunderstanding about how beverages are incorporated into the body by the digestion, and also about how blood is formed. The *Nei Jing* theory is that beverages taken in by the stomach, somehow directly "seep into" the veins, and are then gradually merged with the blood that is already in the veins. It is true that about 55% of blood is plasma, which itself is around 90% water (p.42). The water is absorbed into the blood via the small intestine.[58] In the various *Nei Jing* theories of metabolism, the small intestine plays no part in absorbing nutrients, including water, and its only role is in managing waste (p.203). Even though the *Nei Jing* notions of metabolism are largely untrue, it is true that, in some sense, "beverages" do "seep into" the veins from the digestive process—even if the *Nei Jing* is unaware of the true roles each organ plays. However, there is no time needed for this water to "merge" with the existing blood, since the moment the water is transferred to the blood by the small intestine, it is already an integral part of blood plasma. Therefore this imagined delay for an ingested beverage to merge with the blood could not be the explanation for the "juicy liquid" that was sometimes seen to "come out separately" from the blood. This liquid is more likely to be fluid from the surrounding tissue—assuming that the incising needle were not so fine that *only* the vein was pierced, rather than piercing the surrounding tissue as well.

The third paragraph's explanation for the resultant swelling is also fundamentally flawed. Influences do not flow in the superficial veins (the collaterals) at all (nor flow in the "meridians" either), so they can play no part in the formation of any swelling that results after a superficial vein is pierced. Such swelling would most likely be due to the build up of either body fluid or blood, released from inadvertently pierced nearby veins or capillaries.

The final paragraph's explanation for the patient turning green is also flawed for similar reasons. The "*yin* and *yang* influences" refers to the blood and influences that were theorized to simultaneously flow through the superficial veins (collaterals) and "meridians". The offered explanation involves the not-yet-complete merging of these two substances, in the veins. But the substances do not merge at all, anywhere in the body, and the influences do not flow in the veins anyway, so this imagined "merging" never takes place. Therefore its disruption cannot be responsible for the patient turning green. I have no doubt that some patients would turn green while watching their own blood being let, but, again, the reason for this would most likely be rooted in their aversion to having their blood let.

Conclusion

The extracts quoted throughout this chapter, and throughout this book, are certainly not exhaustive examples of the incorrect theories, over-elaborations, or untrue statements in the *Nei Jing*.

There is a great deal of valuable information in the *Nei Jing*. In fact, the insights described in the *Nei Jing* still form the core of Chinese acupuncture today. But these are the fact-based observations.

In this book I have sometimes provided my own suggestions as to how the *Nei Jing* authors may have formed the theories they did—such as five phase theory, its misapplication in medicine, and the general misguided ideas on metabolism. And in other passages I have demonstrated how to differentiate between the *Nei Jing's* fact-based content and its unreliable content. It is up to each student, when reading good quality translations of either the *Nei Jing* or *Nan Jing*, to decide for themselves which content is probably fact based and provides genuine clinical insights, and which is probably theoretical and does not apply in reality—in other words, is simply untrue.

To put this in perspective, over recent decades several academics (who do not practise Chinese acupuncture) have produced hypotheses on how acupuncture works, which have transpired to be misguided and untrue (pp.373-374 and 401-407). Hence the untrue theories in many of the *Nei Jing* chapters may be compared to today's scientific papers on acupuncture—and on many other topics. The fact that academics and intellectuals produce untrue theories, has doubtless always happened, certainly happens today, and probably always will in the future. There is nothing unusual in this.

Chapter 15. Pulse diagnosis

In Chinese medicine the practitioner can diagnose problems with the organs by taking the organ "pulses".

At the time the *Nei Jing* was written, it was the practice to monitor the "movement" in every one of the twelve meridians, so as to determine various states in the health of each organ.

> **Extract from *Su Wen*, Chapter 17**
> Squeeze the vessels to determine whether their movement is excited or quiet, and observe the [patient's "spirit" in their eyes]. Investigate the five complexions. Observe whether the five [*yin* organs (*zang*)] have a surplus or an insufficiency, whether the six [*yang* organs (*fu*)] are strong or weak, and whether the physical appearance is marked by abundance or decays. All this is brought together to reach a conclusion concerning [the prognosis of the illness]. Now, the [meridians], they [indicate whether the blood is present in large or small amounts*]. The movement in the [meridians], if it is extended, then the [influence] is in order. If it is short, then the [influence] has a disease. If it is frequent, then the heart is vexed. If it is big, then a disease is advanced. If it is abundant above, then the [influence] is situated high in the body. If it is abundant below, then this is a distension because of [influence]. If it is intermittent, then the [influence] is decreased. If it is fine, then the [influence] is diminished. If it is rough, then the heart aches.[1]

The "movement of the influences" in a particular "meridian" was determined by pressing the "meridian" at one of its key acupoints. However, it is clear that different practitioners used different acupoints.

Section 1 of the *Nan Jing* begins "All the twelve [meridians] have sections where the movement in these vessels can be felt."[2] Commenting on this, in 1361, Hua Shou listed the acupoints that he used on each "meridian" (listing several choices of acupoint on some), as follows:

- lungs: LU-1 (*Zhongfu*), LU-2 (*Yunmen*), LU-3 (*Tianfu*), LU-4 (*Xiabai*);
- large intestine: LI-4 (*Hegu*), LI-5 (*Yangxi*);
- heart: HE-1 (*Jiquan*);
- small intestine: SI-16 (*Tianchuang*);

* The "meridians" were thought to consist of artery-like tubes that lay deep to the *pathways on the skin* (which pathways are what we today regard as the meridians); and that both blood and influences flowed in these "meridians" (p.29).

- pericardium: P-8 (*Laogong*);
- lymphatic system: LS-22* (*Erheliao*);
- pancreas: PAN-11† (*Jimen*), PAN-12 (*Chongmen*);
- stomach: ST-5 (*Dajing*), ST-9 (*Renying*), ST-30 (*Qichong*), ST-42 (*Chongyang*);
- kidneys: KID-3 (*Taixi*), KID-10 (*Yingu*);
- liver: LIV-3 (*Taichong*), LIV-10 (*Zuwuli*), LIV-11 (*Yinlian*);
- gallbladder: GB-2 (*Tinghui*), GB-33 (*Xiyangguan*).[3]

Some other commentators listed different acupoints, which were favoured by them.[4]

It should be noted that the only circulatory system then known was the "meridian" network. This included the superficial veins, which were called "collaterals" and "tertiary network vessels" and were thought to branch off from the "meridians", which were thought to be deep artery-like tubes (p.29). Hence, whenever a "pulse" was felt in a vein or literal artery, it was believed that this "movement" represented the movement of the blood and influences through the "meridian" network. This implies that all the above mentioned acupoints were located where it was possible to feel the pulse in a nearby vein or literal artery. And perhaps this varied from patient to patient, or with the sensitivity of the practitioner, which could explain why more than one acupoint was often specified for a particular "meridian"—so as to provide alternative locations for the organ's "pulse" to be felt.

This was the practice in the *Nei Jing*, but in the *Nan Jing* the innovation was introduced of feeling all the pulses only at the wrists. This was controversial and was argued over by commentators for almost two thousand years, with some conservative practitioners insisting that the *Nei Jing* should be strictly adhered to.

> **Liao P'ing (in 1913) commented**
> The ancient scriptures issued severe prohibitions against a diagnosis solely relying on the inch-opening. In the treatise "Cheng ssu-shih lun" of the *Su Wen* it is stated: "If someone grasps only the inch-opening, what illness can he perceive? He will give foolish names to the patient's condition, and he is bound to remain in the realm of dilettantism." The same treatise states further: "If someone sits down and grasps the inch-opening for diagnosis, he will not find out the origins of the hundred illnesses in the five vessels." ... Thus, if we talk about diagnosis in accordance with the ancient methods, it is essential to examine the locations where the movement in the vessels of all the twelve [meridians] can be felt.[5]

However, today all the organ pulses are usually taken only at the wrists. The pulse positions are shown in Figure 2 below. At the patient's left wrist, the practitioner places the first three fingers of their right hand along the radial artery (which, at the wrist, coincides with the path of the lung meridian), and under their first finger they feel the pulse of the heart; under their second, the pulse of the liver; and under their third, the pulse of the kidneys. And they use their left hand to take the other pulses at the patient's right wrist—the lungs, pancreas and *kidney yang*.

* Also called *San-jiao*-22, Triple-burner-22, Triple-heater-22, etc.

† Also called Spleen-11 and Spleen-12.

In each position, the quality of the pulse varies to indicate different states in the function of that organ. The qualities may include the pulse's width, strength, depth, the nature of each beat's rise and fall, and so on. And these qualities will often be different at two adjacent positions on the same artery, even though the positions are only about two centimetres apart.

Early in my training, I began wondering how this might be possible. It was the same blood flowing through the artery, yet by the time it flowed only two centimetres along the artery, the pulse adopted a different quality. This seemed counter-intuitive. And also, how did the flow of the blood adopt a quality that reflected the functioning of the organs (other than the heart)? The following observations and experiments shed light on these questions.

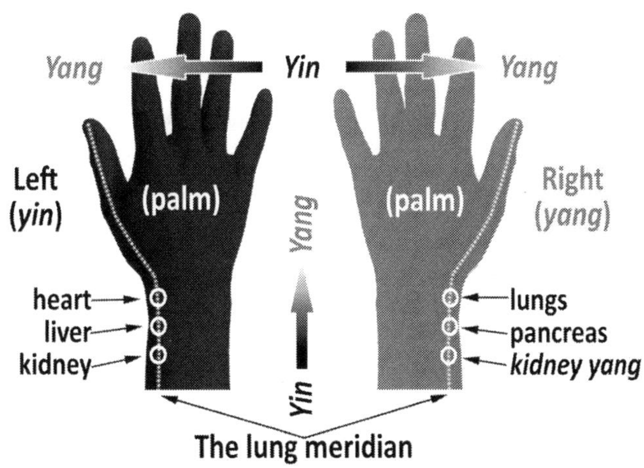

Figure 2. The organ pulse positions at each wrist

The particular finger used determines which pulse is felt

As an experienced practitioner, when I took a patient's pulses and there were notably different qualities on adjacent positions (say, the first and second positions on the left wrist—which reflect the function of the heart and liver respectively), I tried changing the finger I used to feel the pulse, and the quality of that pulse would change. For example, the first finger of my right hand would usually feel the patient's heart pulse (at the first position on their left wrist), and my second finger would feel their liver pulse (at the second position). But when I used my first finger to feel the pulse at the *second* position, the pulse would be similar to the pulse I felt at the *first* position. That is, the patient's heart pulse had now moved to where their liver pulse would normally be. I would then move my fingers back to the usual positions, and the pulses would change back.

This experiment suggests that the particular pulse felt at any position is dependent on which finger the practitioner uses. In other words, it is the practitioner's action of reading the pulse that *creates* the pulse, rather than the particular organ pulse being an intrinsic quality of that location on their radial artery.

The yin-yang hierarchy of the pulse positions

On Figure 2 above, the left hand is *yin* while the right is *yang*;[*] and each location along the hand progresses from *yin* (at the body end) towards *yang* (at the fingertips). This is reflected in the position of the organ pulses. The pulses on the left wrist are more *yin* than those on the right; and the pulses on both sides progress from *yin* to *yang*. For example, the kidneys are the most *yin*, the liver comes next and then the heart, which is the most *yang* of the organs whose pulses are on the left (see Table 6 on p.348). On the right, the same progression is from *kidney yang*[†] (the most *yin* of the organs reflected on the right), to the pancreas, then the lungs, which is the most *yang* of the organs on the right.

When the pulses are taken, the practitioner uses their first finger (the most *yang*—see Figure 2 on page 301), to take the pulse at the position nearest to the patient's thumb—where the most *yang* of the three organ pulses appears. This means that the *yin-yang* hierarchy of the three fingers corresponds exactly with the *yin-yang* hierarchy of the three organ pulses. And since it appears that it is the particular finger used by the practitioner that determines the pulse they feel, this suggests that it may be the *yin-yang* hierarchy of the practitioner's fingers that determines the pulse felt at each position.

The geometry of the patient determines which wrist a pulse appears on

The *yin* pulses are felt at the patient's left wrist, and the *yang* at their right. I wondered whether this was determined by the particular hand the practitioner used to take each pulse, or by the geometry of the patient, since this had implications concerning the mechanism that produced the pulses. And this was clarified by the following observation.

Ordinarily, when taking the pulses at the patient's left wrist (the *yin* pulses), the practitioner uses their right hand, and vice versa for the pulses at the right wrist. However, when the patient lies face-down on the treatment couch and their pulses are taken during the treatment, their wrist is rotated, so that the practitioner now uses their left hand to take pulses at the patient's left wrist, and vice versa. However, the *yin* pulses still appear at the patient's left wrist, and the *yang* at their right. This suggests that the choice of wrist that the *yin* or *yang* pulses appear at is not determined by which hand the practitioner uses but by the geometry of the patient.

How the pulse shape is produced

In each position, the quality of the pulse indicates different states in the function of that organ, which, as said above, is counter-intuitive and needs to be accounted for. And equally strange are the peculiar sensations that some patients, particularly the more sensitive ones, experience when their pulses are being taken. They may feel tenderness under the

[*] See page 275 for an explanation of why left is *yin*.

[†] See page 305 for an explanation of the pulse term *kidney yang*.

practitioner's finger when the organ associated with that particular pulse is stressed; or the action of a particular pulse being taken may cause the patient to feel a sensation at a remote acupoint related to that organ, or to have a general feeling of discomfort—but again, only when the related organ is stressed in some way.

What might explain these phenomena?

The effects are produced when the practitioner takes the pulses, so there must be some interaction between the practitioner and information from the patient's organs. But how might this interaction take place?

A meridian ends at the tip of each finger. And the practitioner's fingers are placed on the patient's lung meridian, which, at the wrist, runs directly over the radial artery (Figure 2, p.301 above). One possibility is that the phenomenon may be produced by the interaction between the electromagnetic field of the current at the practitioner's fingertips and the field around the patient's radial artery or in the tissue that constitutes the lung meridian (p.355), and/or the lung-related primo vessel. The electrical wave in the sheath of the lung-related primo vessel only reflects information from the lungs themselves, so this must be ruled out as the source of the information about the patient's organs—since it could only provide information about the lungs. However, the radial artery contains much connective tissue (described below), and it is assumed that the general connective tissue of the body has a direct current flowing through it whose electrical wave contains the combined information from all the organs (p.367).

It therefore seems most likely that this is the source of the organ information used to produce the pulses (but see page 304 below).

Connective tissue in the radial artery

As depicted in Figure 3 below, the outermost layer of an artery (*tunica externa*) is composed of connective tissue. Inside this layer is the *tunica media*, which is formed by a layer of smooth muscle and variable amounts of connective tissue; and then a second layer of elastic fibres is located beneath the smooth muscle.[6]

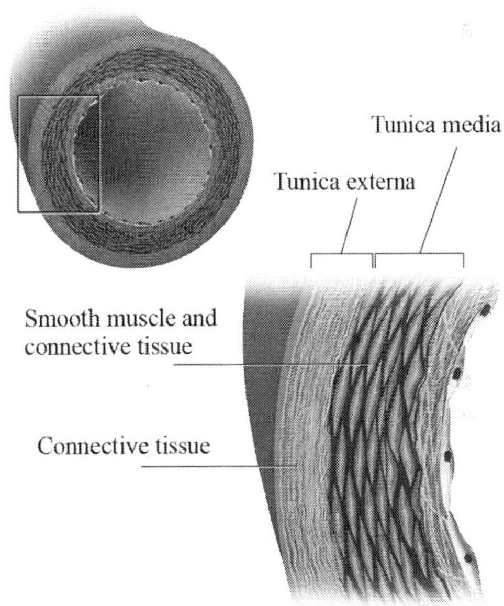

Figure 3. Structure of an artery's wall[7]

Separating an organ's information

On page 299, it was demonstrated that when moving the same finger to a different pulse position, this changed the organ pulse the practitioner felt at that position. This indicates that the organ information reflected in the pulse is not an inherent quality of any particular pulse position, and that some aspect of the process of taking the pulses must therefore *produce* that organ information (and hence the particular pulse shape).

The electrical wave in the artery's connective tissue would contain the combined information from *all* the patient's organs, therefore the information to produce the required organ's pulse must be separated out (filtered) from this combined wave.

The mechanism of "resonance filtering" is defined on page 356, which may have been responsible for determining the layout of the meridians on the body as the body evolved. The filtering was based on the symmetry between the geometry of the limbs and the hierarchy of the organs. Since this same symmetry also exists between the hierarchy of the organs and the combined geometry of the practitioner's hand and the patient's body, it may be that this same mechanism performs the filtering of the patient's organ information based on which finger the practitioner uses. However, rather than this being a slow, evolutionary process, the filtering is performed live—just as it also is when we feel the influence of another person's energy and our body adopts some of their organ-related symptoms (p.363).

How the pulse shape may be produced

Figure 3 above, shows that the connective tissue is also intertwined with the smooth muscle wall that acts to contract the artery when needed. It has been demonstrated that bodily tissue is able to interpret organ information conveyed on an electromagnetic wave (p.333). The process of the practitioner placing a particular finger over the radial artery, appears to filter the organ information already present, so as to emphasize the information from a particular one of the patient's organs, and when this happens it may be that the smooth muscle wall of the artery interprets this new organ information, causing it to adopt a shape that represents that information. And as soon as the practitioner lifts their finger, the influence clears and the artery muscle returns to its previous state.

An alternative connective tissue location

Still using all the above principles, it is possible that the source of the electrical wave representing the combined activity of all the organs is not the connective tissue of the artery wall, but the connective tissue of the thin muscle layer between the artery and the skin. I suggest that this would be just as capable (or perhaps even more so) of producing the effects described above. Normally this muscle would move involuntarily to reflect the shape of the pulse in the nearby artery, but when the electrical wave in the muscle's connective tissue is changed under the influence of the practitioner's finger and the muscle then interprets this new information, this may modify the muscle's involuntary movements so that they now reflect the function of the organ whose pulse was being taken. It seems probable that the effects would be the same. It may only be possible to determine which is the true source with careful testing. But since the principles and effects would probably be the same in both scenarios, the question is perhaps only of academic interest.

These same principles would apply at any bodily location

As stated on page 299 above—at the time of the *Nei Jing*, each organ's pulse was felt at locations along its related meridian. If the above explanation of the mechanism that produces the pulse is true, then the same mechanism would also be capable of producing an organ's pulse at any location along its meridian as it passes near to a vein or artery. In this case, the connective tissue of the muscle along the path of the meridian (or in the sheath of the organ-related primo vessel) would contain an electrical wave that represents the function of that organ *only*, rather than a combined wave representing *every* organ's function. Therefore, it may have been easier for the practitioner to feel such organ pulses, since the electrical wave would not need to be filtered at all—in the way that it needs to be when taking pulses at the wrist only.

The taking of pulses is not a passive activity

The following experiences indicate that the taking of pulses is not a passive activity, which supports the notion that the practitioner's hand creates the pulse shape they feel in the patient's artery.

The taking of pulses is a skill that can take years to learn

Different practitioners have different abilities, and the reading of pulses is a skill that is usually only acquired after much practise. Ordinarily, a total novice would not be expected to be able to read pulses at all. Anyone may place their fingers in the correct positions on the patient's wrist, but the pulse a novice feels would most likely be the same in all positions and would only enable them to gauge the pulse rate. The *qualities* of that pulse would not therefore represent the functioning of the organs. After practising this technique as a part of studying any form of energy-based medicine (such as Chinese acupuncture), most practitioners find that the skill develops in them over the span of a few years. Gradually, the pulses become distinctive and adopt qualities that do represent the function of each organ.

The patient feels the interaction with their organs

Patients sometimes tell me they can sense when I take their pulses. Some say that as soon as I place my hand on their wrist, their head starts to feel "woozy", or that it makes them feel strange in some other way. With one patient, when I first met her (which was while doing some sampler acupuncture sessions at an event), as soon as I placed my hand on her wrist to take her pulses, she said her head started to spin. She took her hand away and went to drink some water; it was when she came back that she told me the effect it had had. If the taking of pulses was passive and had no effect on the patient, such phenomena would not occur.

What does the *kidney yang* pulse position relate to?

The *kidney yang* pulse position is controversial. Amongst contemporary practitioners, there is disagreement about what this pulse relates to. Some say it reflects the function of the kidneys (just as the same position on the left wrist does); others say it reflects the *yang* aspect of the kidney function while the corresponding position on the left reflects the *yin* aspect.

Commenting on Section 1 of the *Nan Jing*, Ting Te-yung (in 1062) wrote "The foot-section [i.e. third position] at the right hand is where the movement of the vessels of the [pericardium] and of the [*san jiao* (i.e. lymphatic system)] appear." And (in 1269), the commentary of Li Chiung confirmed this.[8]

Though the above statements seem to differ, in essence they are all saying the same. The lymphatic system (*san jiao*) plays a key role in the immune system (p.212) and therefore could be regarded as reflecting the hormonal activity of the "kidneys" (which regulate and enable the immunity and hence the function of part of the lymphatic system—p.154). In other words, this pulse reflects the *yang* aspect of the kidneys. Hence, all the above descriptions of this third pulse position are very similar and are consistent with the *yin-yang* progression of the pulses described in this chapter.

In most patients, I find that the *kidney yang* pulse tends to be very low, or even undetectable—except when the patient is particularly excited about something in their life, in which case the pulse is strong. And sometimes this pulse can also be strong when the patient is taking steroidal (or similar) pharmaceuticals. In both these instances, the patient is in an unusually stimulated state, which would usually correspond with "kidney" hormonal activity; that is, being in an adrenalized state (p.154). This would correlate with the *kidney yang* description, since hormones represent one of the *yang* aspects of the kidney function (p.177). And since such an overexcited state would be harmful to the patient's heart, their body would respond protectively, either with increased activity of the pericardium or the lymphatic system, which would correlate with the other classic description for this pulse.

Some clinical experiences of my own suggest the pulse (or its superficial aspect) relates to the lymphatic system. On one patient, who had a low *kidney yang* pulse (as was usual for him), I needled the acupoint Ren-5 (*Shimen*) and immediately, his *kidney yang* pulse became high. Ren-5 is the *front mu* point of the lymphatic system. This seems to confirm that the *kidney yang* pulse reflects this immune-system aspect of the "kidney" function (since the "kidneys" regulate the immunity, and the lymphatic system is a key part of the immunity).

It should be noted that at each pulse position, two pulses can sometimes be felt, one at the superficial level, and the other located more deeply. The superficial pulse relates to the *yang* organ, and the deeper pulse to the *yin* organ in the *yin-yang* pair of organs reflected at that position. In my own experience, I only notice the superficial pulse when the *yang* organ is stressed, and perhaps stressed in a way that is different to the way the *yin* organ is stressed. Otherwise, I would only normally notice a single pulse in each position.

The uncertainty about exactly what this pulse reflects is perhaps only of academic interest, since the pulse appears to have little clinical significance. Pharmaceuticals aside, the pulse could be seen as merely an indicator that the patient is currently in an excited state, or that an aspect of their immunity is (or has been) particularly active. However, I say the pulse has little clinical significance because whenever I feel such a pulse at the start of a treatment, once the patient's main organ functions have been normalized by the treatment, the *kidney yang* pulse always returns to its usual low state.

Chapter 16. Acupuncture treatment of viral and bacterial infections

To be able to explain how acupuncture successfully treats viral and bacterial infections it is necessary to first understand how the Chinese medicine concepts of *wind* and *heat* relate to contemporary physiology.

The term "heat"

In Chinese medicine the term *heat* is used to describe all bodily phenomena that produce signs or symptoms of unusual warmth, redness, dryness, or itching.

Here and elsewhere, Chinese medicine focuses on the *appearance* of signs, rather than on how those signs are generated at the cellular level. Such concepts, as we know them today, did not exist over two thousand years ago.

The term "wind"

In Chinese medicine, the term *wind* is most often used to describe the literal wind outside. This was considered to be a pathogen that was capable of penetrating the body and thus causing a "wind invasion", which is the Chinese medicine term for a common cold or influenza.

However, the term is also sometimes used to refer to the movement of the "influences" from a particular organ, as in "liver *wind*", "heart *wind*", and so on.[1] And in today's Chinese medicine, the term *wind* is also used to describe any phenomena in the body that is characterized by sudden movement. These include the internal signs produced by a *wind* invasion, such as sneezing and shivering, but also such phenomena as trembling and facial tics. All these are considered to be produced by *wind*. In the case of trembling and facial tics, the *wind* is considered to be produced within the body, usually within the liver (as in "liver *wind*"), rather than having invaded us from outside.

When comparing these ideas with the concepts of contemporary physiology, this begs the questions

- What do these Chinese medicine concepts of *wind* and *heat* correspond to in contemporary physiology?
- If all these terms are simply describing pathogens, are the Chinese medicine terms of *wind* and *heat* equivalent to

the contemporary terms of virus and bacteria?

Are the ancient and contemporary terms for pathogens equivalent?

A pathogen is any substance that is harmful to us; i.e. is capable of causing *pathology* (which term is derived from the Greek word *pathos*, meaning suffering). In Chinese medicine the main pathogens are *wind*, *heat*, *cold*, *dampness* and *phlegm*; and in contemporary physiology, the main pathogens are viruses and bacteria. Is there any correlation between these?

Heat is the presence of unusual warmth, redness, dryness or itching. Sometimes its production is in response to an invading pathogen and sometimes not. For example, when a person's muscles are worked hard, this will produce signs of *heat*; or when a person becomes angry, this will also produce signs of *heat* (such as a red face) but also possibly signs of *wind*, such as facial tics and trembling. Even though the person is displaying signs of *heat* and *wind*, there is no bacteria or virus involved and in this case the *heat* and *wind* are, in effect, generated by the person's liver. Whatever the physiology may be, the emotion of anger and the accompanying signs are the result of the person's liver attempting to remove what it perceives as an obstruction (p.109).

In other situations, there may be signs of *heat* and *wind* produced when there *is* a virus present, such as when a person suffers a common cold or influenza. In this situation, Chinese medicine considers the pathogen to be *wind* while in contemporary physiology it is considered to be a virus. This does not mean that the term "virus" is equivalent to the Chinese medicine term *wind*—or that the term *bacteria* could be used as a translation of the term *heat*. This cannot be the case, since the signs of *heat* and *wind* are often present in the body when no invading virus or bacteria are prevalent.

These ancient and contemporary terms for pathogens should not be considered as directly equivalent, or even translatable into one another. Instead the different terms reflect the different approaches of the two systems. Chinese medicine takes an overview and (when viewed from the perspective of contemporary physiology) its notion of pathogens is more a description of how the body *responds* to the pathogens (such as viruses and bacteria), rather than trying to describe the pathogens at the microscopic level. The body responds with signs of heat, redness, swelling and itching—all of which Chinese medicine simply calls *heat*, and it often views this *response* as the pathogen itself.[2] And to tackle the problem, it strives to restore normal organ function which then enables the body's defences to clear the pathogens (whether these are *heat*, viruses, bacteria, or any other pathogens).

Does acupuncture vent pathogens from the body?

The above raises the following question. When acupuncture successfully treats conditions where viruses and bacteria are involved, has the acupuncture somehow addressed those pathogens? There are many clinical situations where acupuncture treatment *appears* to vent such pathogens from the body, and also where the body *appears* to utilize acupoints to vent pathogens. But is this really what is happening?

The common cold

When a person is in the early stages of developing a common cold (or influenza), they will start sneezing, may feel cold or have hot and cold flushes, and may feel unwell. In Chinese medicine, this condition can be clearly felt in the patient's lung pulse, which would have a "floating" quality. If a patient is treated at this early stage, this usually prevents the cold from developing.

I have also observed this in myself many times. When I have the above symptoms, I usually treat this by needling my own left Large-intestine-4 (*Hegu*) and left Lung-7 (*Lieque*), which are the same acupoints generally used on patients. And after about fifteen minutes of the treatment, I usually feel "cleaner" inside, as though an irritant had been cleared from within me. And I feel completely well from that moment and the cold does not develop.

These experiences give the impression that acupuncture clears the pathogen from the body. But it seems more likely that the following is happening.

The acupuncture immediately returns the function of the organs to normal, including that of the lungs and "kidneys", which provide the immunity (and it is clear that this corrected function happens within around one second of an acupoint being stimulated, since the effect can be detected in the patient's organ pulses). Once this is done, the body's normal defences are then able to clear the invading pathogen and the cold does not develop.

This is exactly what happens (without acupuncture treatment) in a strong and healthy person who is exposed to the same pathogen. Because their immune system is working normally, it fights off the pathogen and they do not get a cold. But in a person who is perhaps stressed and has become run down, the function of their organs would certainly not be normal, and it is such people who succumb to the cold.

The fact that the patient usually feels noticeably better at the end of the twenty minute acupuncture session could be attributed to the fact that their organ functions have returned to normal. However, on the other hand, the sudden disappearance of the person's general symptoms could also be attributed to those *symptoms* having been cleared by the acupuncture (rather than being "vented"). The situation is clarified in the following example.

Hay fever

When a patient suffers the acute symptoms of hay fever (such as sneezing; red, itchy, watering and/or puffy eyes; itching at the back of the throat) an acupuncture treatment usually clears a significant amount of these symptoms within about one minute of the needles being inserted (patient's often comment on this, since they are so surprised at the sudden relief). In the long run it is clear that acupuncture treats hay fever by normalizing the patient's "kidney" function, which then enables the patient's normal immunity to fight off any pathogens—as happens with people who do not normally suffer from hay fever. But the dramatic improvement in the acute symptoms during an acupuncture session appears to suggest that the acupuncture vents the pathogens (or, at least, the body's *response* to the pathogens—the soreness, itchiness, redness).

A key acupoint I use in this situation is Lymphatic-system-6* (*Zhigou*), which is located on the outside of the patient's arm, and its meridian ends at the side of the eye. It is said that this acupoint is able to clear *heat* from anywhere in the body, and particularly from the eyes.[3] Here, *heat* would be the signs and symptoms of redness, itching or swelling of the eyes, and itching of the throat. The relief of such signs and symptoms often starts within a few seconds of this needle being inserted. This effect seems too quick for it to be attributed to the patient's immune function returning to normal, so what might account for it?

Page 221 provides an account of how an organ seems to "remember" the distal symptoms that occur along its meridian (which may be incorporated into the fine detail of the organ's function—or malfunction). And once the organ is treated with acupuncture, so that its functions return to normal, this appears to also clear such distal signs and symptoms, by normalizing the function of the local tissue anywhere along the organ's meridian (which is the same mechanism that immediately clears tenderness at key acupoints when the related organ is treated with acupuncture, even where the acupoint that was tender was not needled—p.369). In the hay fever example above, this mechanism would be enough to explain the rapid clearing of the acute signs and symptoms, since the lymphatic system was treated, and its meridian ends beside the eye—the site of the local signs and symptoms. In other words, the tissue in this location is returned to normal function, which then clears the itchiness and redness that was previously being produced by that tissue.

* Also called *San-jiao*-6, Triple-burner-6, Triple-heater-6, etc.

Local swelling and redness

Another common situation where acupuncture *appears* to vent an infection is where there is local swelling and redness, often with associated pain. In these situations acupuncture usually reduces the swelling and redness and clears the pain—and with many patients these effects occur before the end of a twenty-minute treatment. On first appearance, it would seem as though the inserting of fine acupuncture needles had cleared a "bacterial infection". But instead, this could also be accounted for by the above explanation. When the local signs and symptoms occur on a meridian, stimulating an acupoint on that meridian would tend to normalize the related organ's function, which, in turn, would tend to normalize the function of any local tissue along that meridian. This alone would usually have the effect of rapidly calming any swelling, redness, and easing any pain. But added to this, the general effect of the acupuncture treatment would be to restore the normal function of all the patient's organs and systems, which would then enable the patient's normal defences to clear any invading pathogens that *may* be present, and to also rapidly repair any local damage.

Does the body utilize acupoints to vent pathogens?

Practitioners of Chinese acupuncture are aware of the paths of the meridians and which organs they are associated with. When pimples, boils or eruptions of pus appear in certain locations, knowledge of the meridians often enables us to associate these signs with the malfunction of a certain organ.

For example, the meridian associated with the stomach begins below the eye, descends to the side of the mouth, follows the line of the jaw, rises to the top of the head, then descends again, down the side of the neck, down the front of the body, to end at the feet. When the stomach suffers the condition known in Chinese medicine as "Stomach heat" (p.457), red spots (usually with pus) may appear along this stomach meridian, often near its beginning—on the front of the face, around the jaw line, down the sides of the neck, or even as far as the chest. "Stomach heat" might occur as a result of food poisoning, of eating too much spicy or greasy food, or as a result of the stomach being "invaded" by the liver during a woman's premenstrual phase (p.253). In all these situations, the patient's stomach is "overheating"; its tissue is literally warmer than it should be, which is a pathogenic situation—that is, is harmful to the stomach if it continues for any length of time. As a result, the red spots appear along the stomach meridian (often on the face and neck), which are a direct reflection of the *heat* in the stomach.

When recognising the connection between these spots and the "Stomach heat", it is tempting to imagine that the stomach has utilized the meridians to vent this pathogen from itself. Indeed, this *seems* to be common sense, and is an observation frequently made by patients and physicians. They imagine that the body is expelling something through the skin and that the situation, though cosmetically undesirable and even distressing, is beneficial to our health. The pathogen is "better out than in".

Some other common examples of this phenomenon are red patches appearing around heart acupoints, particularly Heart-7 (*Shenmen*) or Heart-8 (*Shaofu*), when the heart is suffering "Heart fire" (p.454); or redness and even eruptions of pus at lung acupoints, such as Lung-11 (*Shaoshang*), following a serious lung problem; or small white pus-spots on large intestine acupoints (often beside the nose, which is where the large intestine meridian ends) when there has been excessive intake of unhealthy foods.

The above phenomena are common, and it is a common observation that they *appear* to be the result of the body venting pathogens, but the following seems a more likely explanation.

When any of the organs are stressed, this stress is reflected at specific acupoints on the meridian associated with that organ. It is considered (in this book) that this disrupts some aspect of the local tissue at those locations, and this alone would be able to account for all the local signs—the redness, swelling, pus or other discharge.

When the organs are stressed and (for example) "Stomach heat" (p.457) or "Heart fire" (p.454) or any condition affecting any of the organs, results in red spots, pus, or other eruptions on the skin—I believe the phenomenon is simply an indication that those organs are stressed. The appearance of the red spots and so on, does nothing to *relieve* the stress of the organ—and for this reason this phenomenon cannot be viewed as the venting of the organ's stress through the skin.

In time, the red spots or blisters clear, due to the body's normal repair mechanisms. But these would *continue* to appear if the organ remained stressed—which confirms that the spots did not vent the stress.

In a similar way, certain acupoints become tender when the associated organ is stressed, but the presence of this tenderness appears to have no function. It does not in any way relieve the stress of the organ; it so happens that by utilizing the same resonance that created the tenderness, acupuncture is able to persuade the organ to cancel out the malfunction in itself that caused the location to become tender. But if that location were not stimulated, this healing would not take place, therefore the tenderness does not, in itself, appear to perform any healing or venting action. And in the same way, the appearance of red spots or even pus at specific acupoints when the organs are stressed, also seems inadvertent. It appears to have no function and certainly does not represent the venting of the stress of those organs, nor of any related pathogens. Such eruptions from the skin are an indicator that healing is required, rather than being a *part* of the healing process.

But further, this phenomenon usually appears at precise acupoints, and for it to be considered that this process *were* due to the organs utilizing the meridians to vent pathogens such as pus from the associated organ, it would be necessary for the pathogen (in this case, pus) to be somehow encoded into an electrical wave which would be propagated along the meridian on an electrical current, then decoded back into pus at the acupoint, so that it could then be released through the skin. This is the only way that such a pathogen could be transmitted along the meridian. But the encoding of such things into an electrical wave seems too unlikely for this scenario to be tenable.

But even if such encoding *did* take place, it would not *embody* the pathogen anyway—such that the substance itself were transported *from* the organ *to* the distal location. A good analogy of this is when an electrical wave (representing sound) travels along a metal wire, such as happens in any electronic amplification system. In this case, the electrical signal in the wire was not formed by *extracting* the physical sound from the air around the microphone. That is, the electrical recording of that sound did not in any way *diminish* the original sound. That sound still existed around the microphone and would have continued on past it until it hit other physical objects. And in the same way, the pathogen in an organ would still exist in the organ, despite its presence being *represented* at a distal acupoint (that is, supposing pus, etc., *were* transmitted along a meridian, *from* an organ).

Other similar phenomena

The above analysis suggests that the meridians and the acupoints along them are not used by the body to vent pathogens. However, apart from the above examples, acupuncturists commonly encounter other phenomena that *do* suggest acupoints vent pathogens. The following are three of the commonest examples.

1. Energy released from acupoints

When acupoints are needled and you place your hand over the needle, it is sometimes possible to feel a funnel of energy rising from the acupoint, as though something were being released, or vented. This is most noticeable on the *back shu* acupoints when the treatment is correcting a significant, long-term malfunction in the related organ.

2. Energy released during treatment

During many acupuncture sessions, the area around the patient often seems to fill up with "bad energy". That is, energy that seems to be emanating from the patient, which the practitioner can feel and which induces an unpleasant feeling in the practitioner. All sensitive practitioners feel this, and this is why it is common for the acupuncturist to leave the room after the needles are inserted. The impression is that this "bad energy" is being vented from the patient due to the acupuncture.

3. Trauma released from organs

When the organs are treated with acupuncture, sometimes this appears to release trauma from an organ which the patient then feels in their muscles or joints along the meridian associated with that organ. For example, this commonly occurs when a patient's lungs are weakened due to them suffering a bereavement (it is the lungs that feel loss—p.136), and after their lungs are treated with acupuncture and the patient starts recovering from their loss, some weeks later they may develop a muscular weakness, often accompanied by pain, somewhere along the lung meridian, typically at the wrist. This weakness and pain remains lodged in that location until the patient's lungs recover further, when the symptom resumes its journey along the meridian till it reaches the tip of their thumb, when it ceases. This common phenomenon gives the impression that the organ is using the meridian to vent "emotional pathogens" from itself (see the patient example on page 254).

However convincing these experiences seem, there is a simpler explanation for what is happening.

Explanation for example 1

The phenomenon of "bad energy" being released from acupoints is most noticeable with the *back shu* acupoints. When an organ has malfunctioned for a long time, this would have also impeded the function of some aspect of the tissue at its associated acupoints for all that time. With the *back shu* acupoints, this effect would be more pronounced, since the functional pattern of the whole organ is focused on that single acupoint (rather than being spread along an entire meridian, which happens with the limb acupoints—p.359). And when one of these acupoints is needled, and the organ function begins transforming, this would also tend to clear any longstanding impediment to the function of the local tissue. And it is possible that it may be some aspect of this process that causes the local tissue to emit the funnel of energy (or extra warmth) that can sometimes be felt. The effect may be due to either the *return to normal function* in the local tissue (which then emits an unusual warmth for a while), or due to the tissue reflecting this transformational process in the organ. This alone would be enough to account for the extra energy that sometimes radiates from acupoints during treatment, and there is no reason to think that pathogens are being vented.

Explanation for example 2

During an acupuncture treatment, there *seems* to be released from the patient "bad energy" which fills the room and can be felt by sensitive practitioners, but the following seems a more likely explanation.

The functioning of the patient's organs is transformed during the session, and their general energy also increases due to this. Electromagnetic waves continuously radiate from us, representing the organ functions (p.367). This energy would be picked up by any sensitive practitioner, but in this case something unusual is happening in the patient's organ functions. Any "bad" functioning would be much more evident than usual, since it is being highlighted by the treatment—the organs are being persuaded to normalize their functions, which inevitably highlights any malfunctions, as they start to change. And I believe this is the explanation for what sensitive practitioners feel during a patient's treatment. It is not that "bad energy" is vented through the acupoint into the room. Instead, the energy from *all* the patient's organs is radiated into the room (as usually happens), only now, one or more of those organs is transforming from malfunction into normal function, and this process is what a sensitive practitioner feels.

Explanation for example 3

When a patient is treated following an emotional trauma, it appears that the "trauma" is released from the organ concerned and slowly travels along its associated meridian until it reaches the tip of a limb and is finally released from the patient's body. But the more likely explanation for what is happening is very similar to that in the previous example.

Initially, the organ's function was affected by the emotional trauma. Following treatment, the organ's function begins to gradually return to normal. In the case of such a deep trauma, the function would not return to normal immediately, but the process may take some time—several days, weeks, months, or even longer, depending on the patient. During this process, the remaining poor organ function would be communicated to certain acupoints along the organ's associated meridian. When poor organ function is reflected at an acupoint, this would usually disrupt the function of some aspect of the local tissue (which is what causes acupoints to become tender). In the type of transformation that takes place following the treatment of an emotional trauma, it appears that the disruption of local tissue is such that it causes muscular or joint pain or weakness, or both. As the weeks go by, and the organ function becomes more normal, the location of the weakness moves along the meridian towards the tip of the limb (the more *yang* part), which reflects the fact that the disruption in the organ's function is becoming less deeply ingrained (less *yin*). Hence it is reflected to a more *yang* acupoint on the meridian (one nearer to the tip of the limb). And the rate of this movement indicates the strength of the particular organ and its ability to recover. If it is strong, it can recover quickly and the progress along the limb would be quick. The pain appears to be simply a barometer of what is happening in the organ. In other words (again), it is an indicator that healing is either still required or is taking place, rather than being a *part* of the healing process.

Chapter 17. Scientific investigation of the meridians

Research into the underlying structures

For over two thousand years it was thought in China that a network of "meridians" existed beneath the skin and were associated with the internal organs.

The Nei Jing notion of a "meridian" was that they consisted of artery-like tubes, through which the blood and influences flowed (p.29). It is now known that this notion was wrong, and today it is the *pathways on the skin* that are considered to be the meridians (p.29). However, until recently, contemporary science had failed to find any anatomical structures that might correspond with these meridians—causing some to doubt they existed.

In the 1950's a German medical doctor, Reinhard Voll (1909-1989), pioneered the scientific detection of acupoints. He found that at an acupoint, the electrical resistance of the skin dropped significantly.[1] This has since become a well-known phenomenon, though some scientists remain sceptical,[2] despite the prevalence of inexpensive machines that can electronically detect and stimulate acupoints. Hence this phenomenon provided evidence that suggested acupoints exist and that one feature of them is a change in the electrical properties of the skin, but so far no anatomical structure under the skin had been found that might correspond to the meridians, or to the acupoints.

In 1962, Bong-Han Kim (born 1916), a North Korean medical surgeon at Pyongyang Medical University, published the first scientific evidence of structures that seemed to be associated with the meridians. And up until 1965, he produced four further articles detailing his extensive research into these structures. His findings were detailed most thoroughly in his last two reports, of 1963[3] and 1965[4], which were both translated into English.

However, his reports did not describe the methods necessary for his experiments to be duplicated. In particular, the new anatomical vessels he identified were extremely fine, almost transparent and required the use of a specific blue dye to render them visible under a microscope.

In 1967, S. Fujiwara, a Japanese anatomy professor, was able to reproduce some of

Kim's results[5] (locating these new vessels inside blood vessels and on the surfaces of organs), but later recalled that it took him about six months of hard work to obtain these limited results.[6]

Kim's reports described a range of completely new anatomical structures, including node-like structures at the acupoints which were connected with fine vessels that extended to the internal organs. And these same vessels also existed within blood and lymph vessels and throughout the nervous system. The vessels were reported to circulate embryonic-like cells which transformed into the various cells required by the body's organs and tissues, the maturing of the cells taking place in the node-like structures. The purpose of the entire system was said to be the continuous repair and regeneration of key cells in the organs and elsewhere.

However, these astonishing claims were then neglected worldwide until the year 2000, when Kwang-Sup Soh, a physics professor at Seoul National University, set up a team to investigate Kim's finding, and they identified the new vessels

- floating within blood vessels,[7,8]
- on the surface of rabbit intestines and the bladder,[9]
- on the surface of a rabbit's liver,[10,11]
- floating inside lymph vessels, [12,13]
- in the bovine heart,[14] and
- in the brain, spinal cord and nerves of rats.[15]

It has also been confirmed that the fluid circulated within these vessels is abundant with immune cells such as macrophages and mast cells; and also contains very small embryonic cells, similar to stem cells.[16]

Kim originally named these new vessels *Bonghan ducts*, and the nodes *Bonghan corpuscles*. The embryonic cells he named *sanal* (which is a Korean word meaning "live egg"). But the following convention has now been adopted by researchers. The vessels are known as *primo vessels*, the nodes as *primo nodes*, the entire circulatory system as the *primo vascular system* (PVS), and the embryonic cells as *primo microcells* or *p-microcells*.

Characteristics of the primo vascular system

The superficial primo vessels (which are said to underlie the meridians) consist of very fine tubes which are almost transparent and have a diameter of about 30 microns (about the diameter of a human hair). Within each vessel there are several subvessels, and a semi-transparent, tacky liquid (known as *primo fluid*) is circulated within them at the rate of about 0.3 millimetres per second[17] (which equates to 18 millimetres per minute, or 1.08 metres per hour). The flow is in one direction only.

Around each subvessel is a layer of smooth muscle-like cells, which move spontaneously to circulate the fluid; and the entire vessel is encased in a sheath of fibrous connective tissue[18] (Figure 4).

These vessels usually run deeply in the dermis (the deep, inner layer of the skin), but do sometimes run beneath the skin; and they connect the superficial primo nodes.[19] But at some nodes, a further primo vessel also descends into the muscle layer, connecting these superficial primo vessels with those that run more deeply in the body.[20]

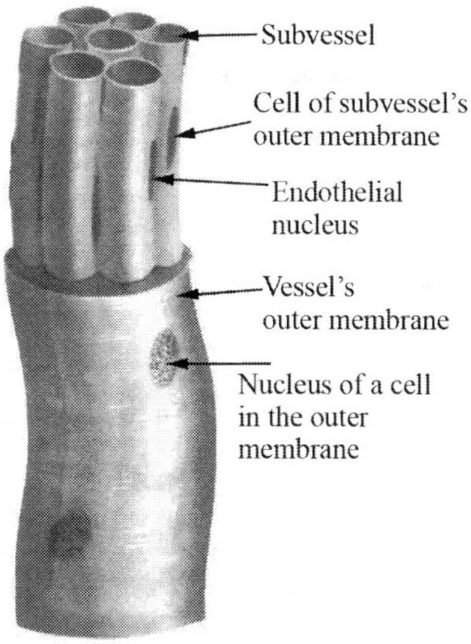

Figure 4. Depiction of a superficial primo vessel [21]

The primo vessels throughout the body

The primo vessels enter the body cavity (the ventral cavity) and join with the organs (Figure 5 and Figure 6). They form a net around each organ and send out various branches to the other organs.

In structure, these vessels are similar to the superficial primo vessels, and are also covered with connective tissue. The vessels run freely on the surface of the internal organs, rather than adhering to the surface.[22]

Primo nodes occur along these vessels at intervals, and they are similar in structure to the superficial primo nodes. They either occur as a swelling on the primo vessel, or as a junction, connecting several primo vessels,[23] and it is only at these junctions that the system tends to adhere to the surface of the organs. The primo vessels then enter deeply into the organs from these nodes.[24]

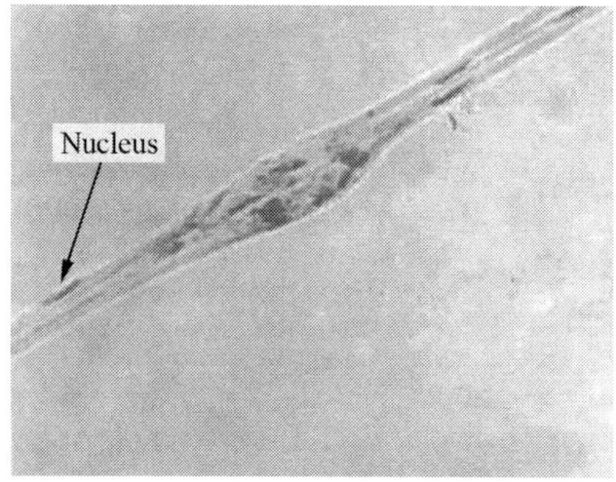

Figure 5. Primo vessel on organ surface (Feulgen reaction) (x400)[21]

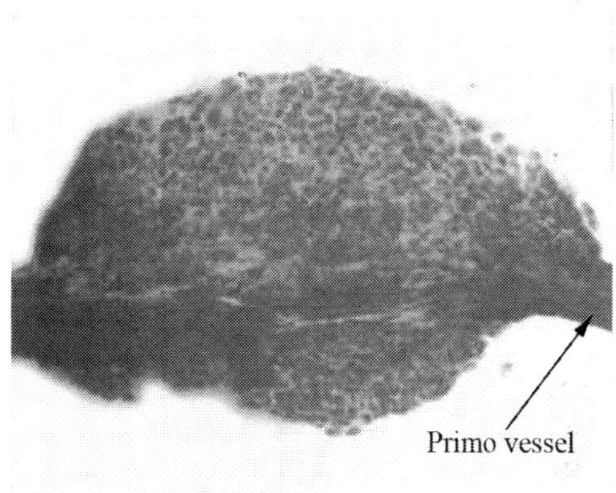

Figure 6. Primo node on organ surface (x160) [21]

The primo vessels within arteries and veins

Primo vessels and nodes also exist within the blood vessels and within the chambers of the heart—the cardiac cavity[25] (Figure 7). Interestingly, in the larger blood vessels, a primo vessel may enter and leave the blood vessel through its wall. And these primo vessels also enter deeply into the organs along with the blood supply.

Each of these *internal* primo vessels also has several subvessels within them, but the overall vessel (unlike the *external* primo vessels) is not encased in connective tissue.[26]

There may be several primo vessels within a single blood vessel; and the primo vessels float freely within the blood and are very soft and glutinous, due to the absence of surrounding connective tissue.[27]

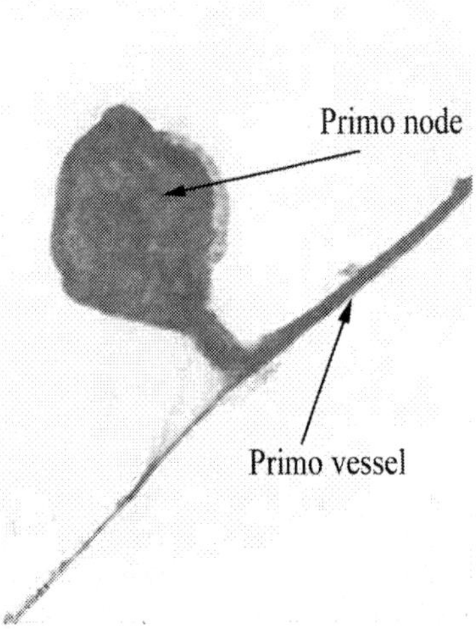

Figure 7. An internal primo node and vessel within the cardiovascular system (x63) [21]

The primo vessels within organs

Inside the organs, the primo vessels connect to minute *terminal* primo nodes (Figure 8), and fine *terminal* primo vessels then connect directly to the cell nuclei in the surrounding tissue (Figure 9).

Inside each cell, the terminal primo vessel gets thinner and enters the *cytoplasm** (penetrating the cell membrane), then penetrates into the *karyoplasm*† through the nuclear membrane. And these vessels seem to form a network in the nucleus. A fine primo vessel then comes out of the cell nucleus and again passes through a terminal primo node. Many terminal primo nodes are located in the organs, each of them only connecting to cells within a limited range.[28]

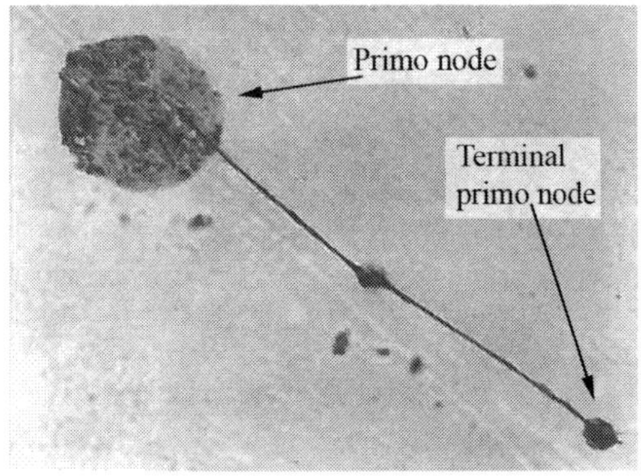

Figure 8. Terminal primo node within an organ (in the suprarenal body) (x160) [21]

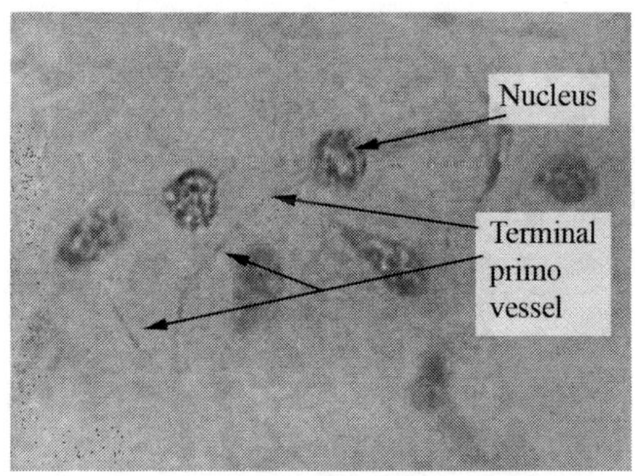

Figure 9. Primo vessel entering a cell nucleus (in the suprarenal body) (x1,000) [21]

In a similar way, the network of primo vessels extends to every part of the body and is found throughout the lymphatic and nervous systems (Figure 10); and Kim even traced

---

* The cytoplasm is the living contents of a cell, other than its nucleus.

† The karyoplasm is the nucleus part of the cell's living contents (also called the nucleoplasm).

the paths of primo vessels through many areas of the brain.[29]

Contents of the primo fluid

Kim found that the primo fluid circulated by this system contains a great deal of DNA and RNA, nitrogen, lipids, reduced sugar, much hyaluronic acid, 20 kinds of free amino acids, 16 kinds of free mononucleotides,[30] adrenalin, noradrenalin, corticosteroid, 17-ketosteroid and oestrogen.[31]

The p-microcells within the fluid were found to contain much nucleic acid, especially DNA, and a considerable amount of protein. And of particular note was the fact that the amount of DNA contained in one p-microcell was nearly equal to that contained in one chromosome.[32]

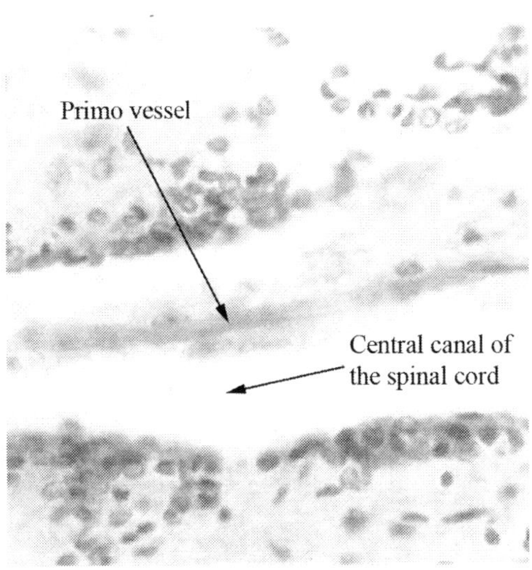

Figure 10. Primo vessel in the spinal cord (Van Gieson stain) (x400) [21]

The circulation of p-microcells through the PVS

Kim studied the behaviour of the p-microcells and their circulation route through the primo vascular system.

With the cells of liver tissue, he found that many p-microcells were formed in a single tissue cell; these then burst free from the cell, which then perished. At this stage, each p-microcell measured about one micron and they moved independently of each other. In the liver of a rabbit, about 2-4 percent of the total liver cells were in this state of metamorphosis at any one time.

Some of these p-microcells remained in the local tissue and gradually matured into new liver cells. But the remaining p-microcells entered a terminal primo vessel and circulated through the primo vascular system, to the superficial primo vessels and the primo nodes, where they matured into new liver cells. They then resumed their journey through the primo vessels, back to the liver, when the mature liver cells returned to the organ tissue through the terminal primo nodes and vessels.[33]

After a period of time, the liver cell again went through the same process, so that the cells were being constantly renewed—which also makes it clear that the origin of the p-microcells was within the cells of the target tissue themselves.

To verify these observations, Kim conducted the following experiments. A p-microcell from a rabbit liver was observed in vitro. The p-microcell grew and fused into a nucleus-like structure in 4-12 hours; and in 72-120 hours the cell membrane formed to complete the formation of a new liver cell. Then, after about 6-8 days, this new cell then produced many p-microcells and perished, completing its lifecycle.

A p-microcell from a nerve cell of a rabbit brain was also observed. It began duplicating and in 4-6 hours had become six p-microcells, and by 8-12 hours had become 12-13 p-microcells, assuming the shape of a long bunch of grapes. In 52 hours, these had fused to form a single, nucleus-like structure, having clear cytoplasm and a distinct membrane. Out of this cell body grew three projections, one of which became an axone (a nerve fibre).[34]

The primo-vessel path from the liver, following the course of the meridians and back again (via the gallbladder and liver meridians) is around four metres, so that the primo fluid would only take around 4.3 hours to make this entire journey (p.316). This would not allow enough time for a p-microcell to transform into a mature liver cell, which may explain why these cells pause in the primo nodes to complete their transformation.

Confirming the meridian-to-organ path

The path taken by p-microcells through the PVS was traced by tagging the matured cells with radioactive P32. The paths were traced from the primo vessels into the cells of the related organs.[35]

In another experiment, p-microcells were harvested from the superficial primo nodes in 79 different regions of the human body and the cells grown to maturity in culture. It was found that p-microcells taken from different regions grew into different cell types, and the cell types corresponded with the particular organ whose meridian path the p-microcell was taken from. This confirmed that each organ did, indeed, have a primo vessel associated with it which travelled to the skin, then followed the meridian route identified in the *Nei Jing*.[36]

Kim conjectured that the reason why p-microcells travel to the primo nodes in the skin to mature may be due to a beneficial photochemical influence exerted on the p-microcells, due to them being located much nearer to the surface of the body. To test this theory he harvested p-microcells from liver cells and cultivated them in both normal light and in a dark chamber. Under normal light 104 new cells were formed in 96 hours, whereas in the dark chamber only 32 were formed. And when p-microcells taken from the spleen were cultivated in the same way, 69 cells were formed in 96 hours under normal conditions, whereas in the dark chamber the multiplication of p-microcells stopped utterly in 72 hours and no more cells were formed thereafter.[37] A 2005 study also found that p-microcells react to light in the UVA range.[38]

Primo vessels maintain the body's cells

Kim found that severing an intra-organic primo vessel (one entering an organ) caused histological changes (changes in the microscopic structure) in cells within that organ.

When a primo vessel entering the liver was severed, within one day the related liver cells enlarged, their cytoplasm became turbid, and *karyolysis*[*] occurred to some cell nuclei, leading to the destruction of the cells. And three days later, serious *vacuolar*[†] degeneration of the related liver cells took place.

[*] Destruction of the nucleus.

[†] A vacuolar is a fluid filled cavity in the cytoplasm of a cell.

When the primo vessels (including those within the blood vessels) supplying the kidneys were severed, *necrosis** of the *convoluted uriniferous tubules*† and of the renal corpuscles was observed in the cortex of the kidney, and the uriniferous tubules lost their nuclei completely, while preserving their form; and the *epithelial*‡ nuclei of the uriniferous tubules in the *medullary substance*§ disappeared entirely or were destroyed partly (Figure 11).

When all the primo vessels supplying the adrenal glands were severed, initially the terminal primo nodes (connected with nuclei) in the most superficial layer of the adrenal cortex (*zona glomerulosa*) disappeared, and then the nuclei become *pyknotic*** and were destroyed or lost. And the same observations were made in the middle and inner-most zones of the adrenal cortex (*zona fasciculata* and *zona reticularis*).[39]

When a *neural* primo vessel (flowing within the sheath of a nerve) was severed, within thirty minutes the reflex time became unstable but was generally prolonged, and gradually lengthened with time. And twelve hours after the primo vessel was severed, changes in the microscopic structure of the myelin sheath and axon were observed, and the changes extended to the distal portion of the nerve, rather than being limited to the region where the primo vessel was severed.[40]

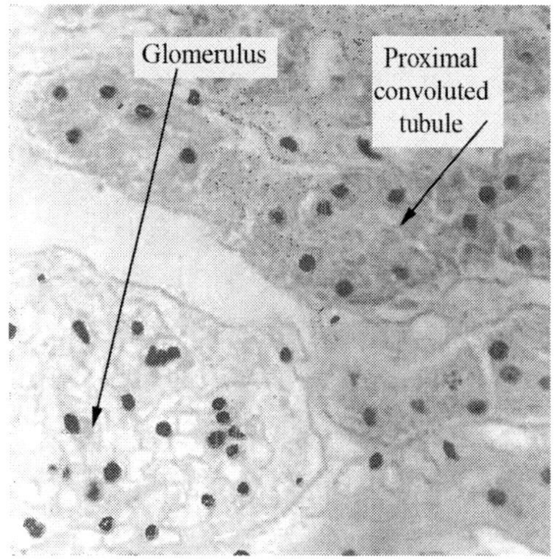

Figure 11. Changes in nuclei of kidney cells after primo vessels were cut (x400) [21]

The PVS is the first system to form in an embryo

Kim also researched the formation of the PVS in chick embryos. The formation of primo vessels had begun by five hours of incubation, and after ten hours the primitive cells of primo nodes had formed, and primitive cells of the primo vessels were differentiating rapidly. After only 10-15 hours of incubation, the entire primo vascular system was basically intact. What was remarkable was that the primitive beginnings of the organs had not yet started to form. After 20-27 hours of incubation, blood vessels had formed *around* the internal primo vessels. The primo vessels not only developed earlier but also completed differentiation and formation more rapidly than the blood vessels and nerves.[41]

The fact that the PVS forms before any other major system in the body could be taken as indicating that the presence of the PVS is a prerequisite for the health and proper function of every other system in the body.

* Death of the related cells.

† Conveying urine.

‡ Epithelial cells form thin layers (sometimes only one cell thick) covering other structures.

§ The *medulla* is the innermost part of a structure.

** A degenerative state of the cell nucleus.

The physiological purpose of the primo vascular system

Kim's team found primo vessels in mammals, in other vertebrates, in invertebrates, and even in plants; and they are assumed to exist in all multi-cellular life forms.[42]

Overall, Kim's team concluded that the purpose of the primo vascular system was to enable the continuous regeneration of the cells of the organs. It is also clear that the purpose of the superficial primo nodes is to allow time for the p-microcells to mature into the cells of their target tissue. And the same is true of the many other primo nodes within the body, which provide regions for the p-microcells to pause to allow further time for them to mature.

Does the PVS play a role in producing acupuncture's effects?

Despite the recent extensive study of this previously unknown circulatory system (p.316), no researchers had yet managed to describe the mechanism whereby stimulation of an acupoint regulates the function of the organs.[43] The physiological function of the PVS seems clear: constant regeneration of tissue cells. When Kim's work first began to be accepted around 2,000, it was assumed that the superficial primo vessels may equate to the meridians. But this now seems unlikely, and the part the PVS plays (if any) in producing acupuncture's effects is discussed in the following three chapters.

The association between acupoint impedance and organ stress

The phenomenon of low electrical impedance at acupoints has been widely studied since the 1950's (p.315). And the low impedance has also been found to decrease further in acupoints whose associated organ is diseased.

In 1978, Serisawa[44] found that in 50 patients with pulmonary tuberculosis, points of reduced impedance existed along the lung meridian on the upper arm.

In 1980, Oleson *et al*[45] found that in 40 patients, areas of reduced impedance at auricular acupoints could be used to diagnose (with 75.2% accuracy) musculoskeletal pain in the patients.

In 1981, Rosenblatt[46] found that acute physiologic changes in heart rate were reflected in acute changes in impedance at acupoints associated with the heart, while no change in impedance at another acupoint nearby and a non-acupoint occurred.

In 1985, Sullivan *et al*[47] found that in lung cancer patients, there was a change in the impedance at the acupoints Lung-10 (*Yuji*) and Lung-11 (*Shaoshang*) when compared to patients with healthy lung function.

In 1993, Saku *et al*[48] found that in patients with acute myocardial infarction, there was significantly reduced impedance at the auricular cardiac acupoint in 28 out of 30 patients (compared to only 2 out of 19 patients in the control group).

These findings suggest that when an organ's function is weak, this is reflected in reduced impedance at its related acupoints.

Investigation of the intelligent tissue hypothesis

The above findings are consistent with the intelligent tissue hypothesis (p.372). The hypothesis states that organ states (either normal function or malfunction) are reflected at an organ's related acupoints in real time. The above studies were not concerned with real-time states, and simply recorded that the general impedance at acupoints tended to be lower when the related organ functioned poorly (without measuring any real-time fluctuations in that impedance).

When there is any change in the local tissue at an acupoint (or elsewhere), this results in a change in the impedance. Therefore, monitoring the real-time impedance at acupoints enables the *pattern* of any tissue changes to be recorded, and this pattern can then be compared with the pattern of change in organ function.

The first study described below did not record the impedance changes in real time, but simply demonstrated that the impedance at an organ's related acupoints was proportional to the strength of that organ's function (in this case the stomach). And the other studies described below, monitored acupoint impedance in real time to demonstrate that an organ's states were reflected at the organ's related acupoints in fine detail and in real time. Hence, the experiments validated this aspect of the intelligent tissue hypothesis.

Increased stomach function produces increased impedance at its acupoints

Figure 12 below shows the impedance readings taken from right Stomach-36 (*Zusanli*) and Stomach-37 (*Shangjuxu*) throughout the day while the subject continued his usual daily routine.[49]

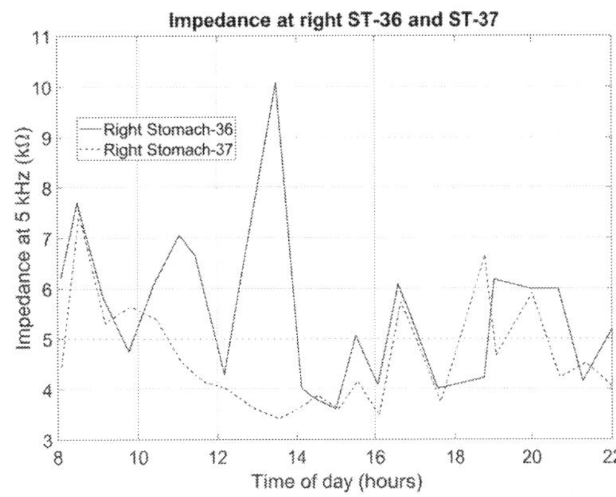

Figure 12. Impedance at right ST-36 and ST-37

Throughout the day, the peaks in the Stomach-36 plot of Figure 12 corresponded exactly with the times when the subject ate a meal, and the highest peak was produced when he ate his main meal at 13:30.

The Stomach-37 plot showed a notably different pattern between 10:00 and 15:00, and produced its highest peak at around 8:30. Even though Stomach-37 is on the stomach meridian, it is said to also heavily influence the large intestine. In other words, the large intestine function would also be reflected at this acupoint, as well as some aspects of the stomach function. At 8:22, the subject had his only bowel movement of the day, and at around this time, the Stomach-37 plot produced its highest peak.

The above results suggest that the impedance level at an organ's key acupoints is proportional to the strength of the organ's function. And the correlation of the highest peak at Stomach-37 with the time when the subject's large intestine (and rectum) was most active, was consistent with the classic indication for that acupoint. This not only confirmed the notion that the impedance at an acupoint is proportional to the strength of the related organ's function (in this case, the large intestine), but this result validated the classic indication for Stomach-37, and vice versa.

Evidence of real-time organ information reflected at acupoints

In the following study, conducted by myself in 2018,[50] the impedance at bilateral Stomach-19 (*Burong*), Stomach-21 (*Liangmen*) and Stomach-36 (*Zusanli*) was monitored in real time (taking 1,000 samples per second) while the subject drank chilled water on an empty stomach. Each acupoint was monitored at its centre and at a distance of 6 millimetres away, perpendicular to the meridian.

Figure 13 below shows the impedance at left Stomach-36. The two vertical lines to the left of the plot mark the start and end of the subject swallowing the chilled water. It takes around one second for swallowed water to reach the stomach,[51] and the inset in the plot shows that at one second after the first mark, the impedance at left Stomach-36 dropped by about 3 . This decline lasted for about one second, and then a second dip occurred, followed by a recovery.

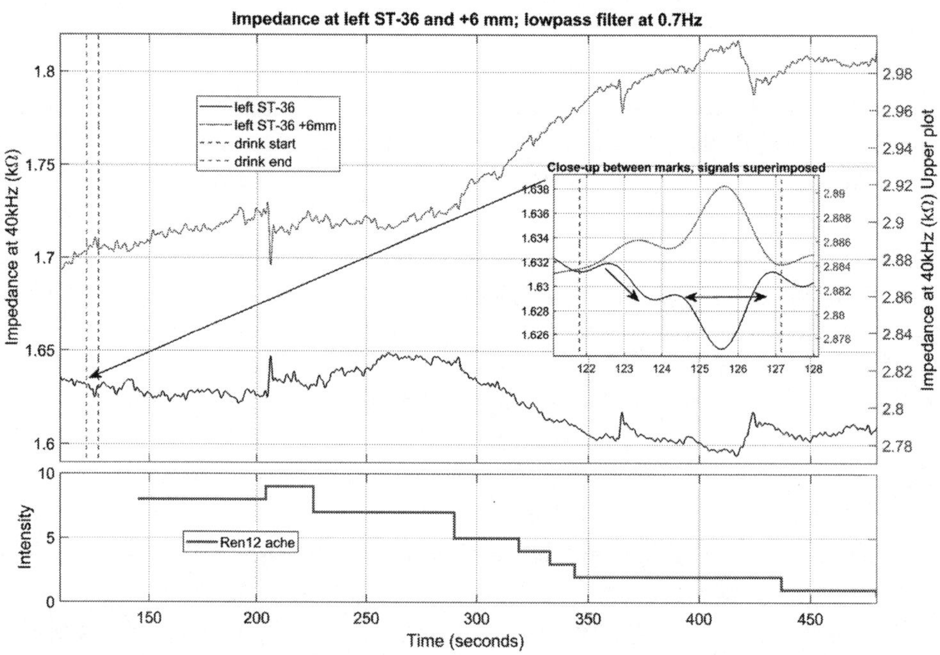

Figure 13. Impedance at left Stomach-36 after the subject drank chilled water

All the stomach-related acupoints monitored in the study registered a response to the chilled water reaching the stomach. In the case of left Stomach-36, even though the acupoint was around 74 cm below the subject's stomach, there was no discernible delay in the response (within the limitations of this particular study's design). The results demonstrated that the communication between an organ and its related acupoints certainly travelled at a rate well in excess of one metre per second.

It has been established that when the impedance pattern at an acupoint is a reflection of organ-related information, the pattern follows a "V" shape, with the impedance falling towards the centre of the acupoint.[52] This means that when dual impedance readings are taken, one from the acupoint's centre and the other at a short distance away (in this case 6 millimetres), the resultant plots tend to move in contrary motion. This can be clearly seen in the general trends of the plots in Figure 13, and also in the inset. This contrary motion pattern helps to establish that the impedance features were the result of genuine organ-related signals conveyed via an electromagnetic wave, rather than being artefact* of any kind.

When the subject drank the chilled water, this induced an ache at his Ren-12 (*Zhongwan*) acupoint, and the intensity of the ache is shown in the lower plot of Figure 13. The notable feature is that at 204 seconds, the subject reported the ache increasing in intensity, and at that same moment, a clear, contrary-motion spike appears in the impedance at left Stomach-36. This result confirmed that stomach states are reflected at Ren-12; and also, again, demonstrated that the impedance pattern at left Stomach-36 reflected a real-time change in the stomach's state (since it was that changed state that produced the increase in the intensity of the ache at Ren-12).

Remarkably, at every monitored acupoint, other features of the stomach's routine functioning were reflected. The "slow wave" contractions of the stomach and also the duodenal contractions were clearly visible. These features at right Stomach-21 are shown in Figure 14 on page 327 below.

In the figure's inset, it can be seen that the amplitude of these duodenal waves notably decreased while the subject drank the chilled water; and that the impedance at right Stomach-21 began to fall at about 125 seconds, which is about two seconds after the chilled water reached the inner surface of the stomach. This response occurred about two seconds later than the response at left Stomach-36, which responded immediately. The extra two second delay may reflect the time taken for the chilled water to reach the start of the duodenum, which is located at the exit from the stomach (but see below for an alternative explanation—p.326).

At right Stomach-21, the duodenal waves were more prominent than at the other acupoints monitored (being at least twice the amplitude). This probably reflected the fact that this acupoint is noted to be able to correct signs and symptoms related to problems with intestinal transport (i.e. the duodenal contractions). If this is the case, this would provide an explanation of how the acupoint achieves this effect. Since the real-time functioning of these duodenal contractions is strongly reflected at this acupoint, any irregularities with the contractions would also be reflected; and stimulating the acupoint would encourage these intestinal contractions to return to normal function (using the same logic that explains how acupuncture works—p.372).

* In such experiments the term "artefact" is used to describe any signal other than the signal the experiment intended to capture, such as due to electrical "noise" or from other sources in the body.

In Figure 14 below, the plots at the acupoint's centre and at its 6 millimetres radius can be seen moving in contrary motion, which confirms that these captured impedance features represented genuine organ-related information conveyed on an electromagnetic wave, rather than patterns picked up as artefact from the duodenum, either due to the physical movements of the duodenum muscles or the electrodes directly picking up the electrical potential from either the duodenal pacesetter, or from the intestinal muscles themselves (p.325).

As can be seen in the lower plot, the stomach's "slow wave" was also reflected in the impedance, with a wavelength of 10.88 ± 2.98 seconds*. This was reflected more strongly at Stomach-36, as shown in Figure 15 below, which may reflect the fact that ST-36 has a greater effect on the general stomach function than ST-21 does (which, again, would demonstrate a correlation between an acupoint's function and the impedance pattern at that acupoint). Here, the wavelength was 10.36 ± 2.65 seconds.

To mix ingested food (chyme), the stomach walls regularly contract in peristaltic waves, known as slow waves. But there is controversy over the exact wavelength. This has often been assumed to be around 20 seconds. However, in 2011, Rhee et al[58] used intracellular recordings to measure these spontaneous slow waves in the fundus muscles of the stomach, and found them to be 10.4 ± 1.7 seconds (n=12). This is consistent with the 10.88 ± 2.98 second impedance waves recorded at right Stomach-21, and the 10.36 ± 2.65 second waves at left Stomach-36. This suggests that the recorded waves reflected the slow waves in the subject's stomach.

The variable time taken for local tissue to respond to organ information

In the above study,[50] it was found that none of the "duodenal" impedance waves recorded at the six test acupoints were in phase with one another, and that at each acupoint it was rare for two consecutive waves to have the same length (in contrast to the contractions of the actual duodenum, which are relatively regular). When comparing the same wave at two separate acupoint locations on the same meridian, the phase could sometimes shift by as much as two seconds in either direction, and the leading wave could appear at either acupoint, interchangeably (so that the acupoint furthest from the organ often led the acupoint nearest to the organ, and vice versa).

The only explanation for the data appeared to be the fact that the local tissue at each acupoint took a variable amount of time to interpret the organ information in the electromagnetic waves, and to respond to it. The length of this delay could vary from as little as a tenth of a second, to as much as two seconds. And at each acupoint location the amount of delay varied from second to second, and the amount of delay at any one instant was different at different acupoints.

This variability in the response time of the local tissue makes it hard to draw any reliable conclusions about the apparent time taken for organ information to reach different acupoints. For example, when the chilled water entered the stomach, this information may have been conveyed to all acupoints simultaneously, but it may have registered two seconds later at right Stomach-21 than at left

* All such figures are given as mean ± SD.

Stomach-36 due to the local tissue at right Stomach-21 responding more slowly at that particular instant in time.

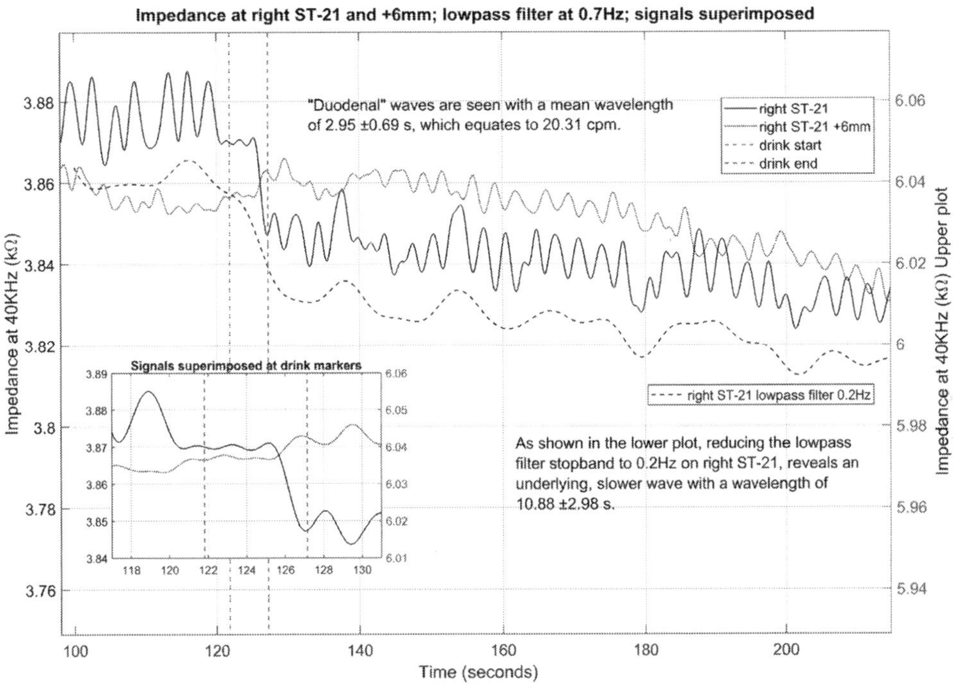

Figure 14. Impedance at right Stomach-21 after the subject drank chilled water

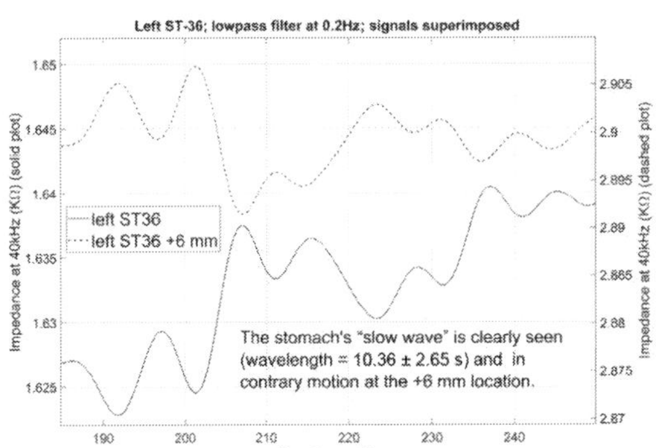

Figure 15. Impedance at left ST-36, showing the stomach's slow wave

The above results in relation to the stomach have also been confirmed in relation to the lungs. In another study from 2018,[53] the subject varied his breathing while the impedance at key lung-related acupoints was monitored in real time. He breathed deeply for 15 seconds, then rapidly for 8 seconds, then held his breath for 25 seconds. As shown in Figure 16 on page 328 below, following the 15 seconds of deep breathing, the impedance at left Lung-1 (*Zhongfu*) dropped sharply (by 38.4% over 52 seconds). The impedance at a location 6 millimetres from the acupoint's centre changed in contrary motion to this (which is the typical behaviour for dual impedance traces at an acupoint, and helps to rule out artefact of any kind—p.325); and as seen in the lower plots of Figure 16, the impedance at

29 and 35 millimetres from left Lung-1 did not feature the same sharp drop, so that the change in lung function strength was only reflected at the acupoint itself.

These results suggest that the action of taking deep, consecutive breaths for 15 seconds, fatigued the subject's lung function, and this fatigue was reflected in the reduced impedance at left Lung-1, the function gradually weakening over the following 52 seconds as the lungs recovered from the activity. Hence the changing state of the lung function was reflected at this acupoint.

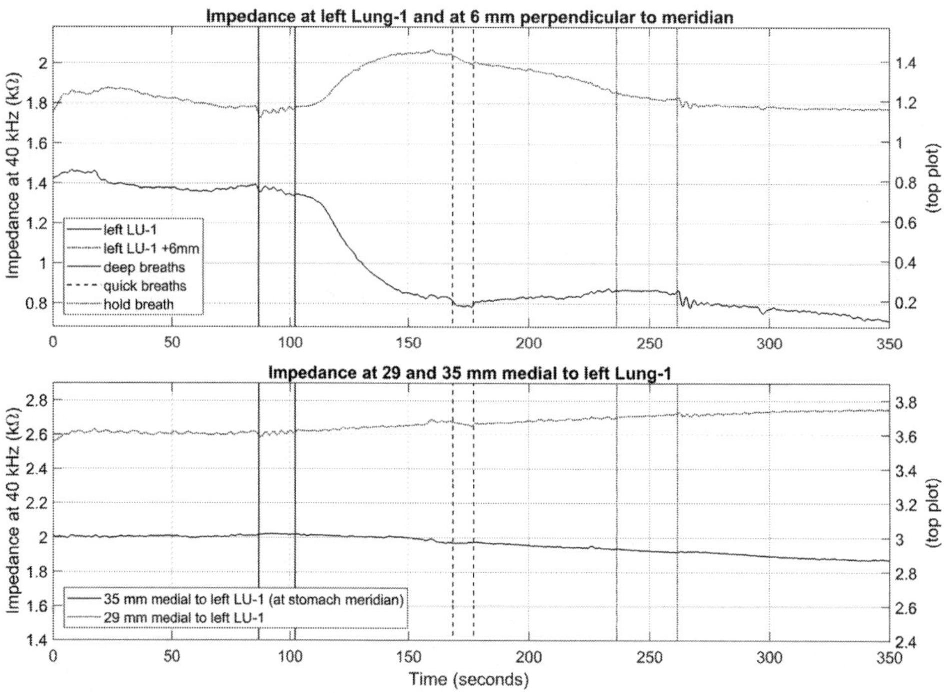

Figure 16. Impedance at left Lung-1 while the lungs were stressed

As with the impedance at stomach acupoints, which featured low-amplitude duodenal waves and stomach slow waves, the impedance at the lung-related acupoints featured low-amplitude respiration waves. And in this same study,[53] the subject's actual breathing rate was monitored and compared to the respiration waves captured in the impedance.

The study demonstrated that these impedance waves did not reflect the respiration pacesetter that is located in the brainstem (as may be expected), but instead reflected a "pace signal" that seemed to be produced by the lungs themselves. There is controversy over this topic. It is believed by many physiologists that the lungs are entirely passive in the respiratory process, which is conducted by the respiratory muscles alone (the diaphragm and intercostal muscles), which are controlled by the brainstem pacesetter. However, this study's results suggested that a separate "pace signal" plays a part in regulating the brainstem pacesetter, and this signal was probably produced by the lungs themselves.[53,54]

In Figure 17 below, the upper plot showed the actual breathing rate (and also, therefore, the rate of the brainstem pacesetter), and the lower plot showed the respiration waves captured in the impedance at left Lung-1 (the pace signal). At the start of the plot, it can be seen that these two signals had significantly different wavelengths. The pace signal had a wavelength of 3.34 ± 0.48 seconds; and that of the brainstem pacesetter was 5.58 ± 1.08 seconds.

The remarkable feature of the lower plot is that the amplitude of the pace signal increased notably in two places, which corresponded with moments when the lungs were stressed; firstly, when the subject was breathing deeply, and secondly, after the subject held his breath for 25 seconds.

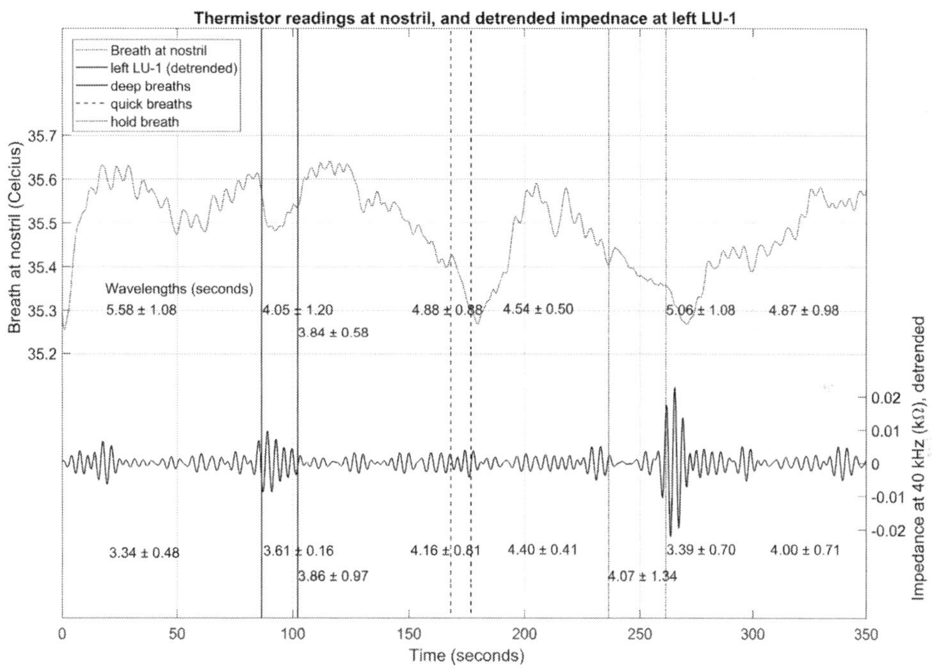

Figure 17. Thermistor readings at nostril, and detrended impedance at left Lung-1

The pace-signal waves for *all* the organs (the lungs, stomach and heart) are present body-wide. They are contained in electromagnetic waves that are superimposed on the direct current that is at every location in the body. Hence these waves would appear in the impedance taken at *any* bodily location. But their *general* amplitude varies depending on the location. When the wave relates to a particular organ, the wave is emphasized at that organ's meridian, therefore it has a higher *general* amplitude than when this same wave appears at other locations (this is further demonstrated on page 332 below).

The two *extra* instances of notably increased amplitude shown in the lower plot of Figure 17, only occurred in these waves at the left Lung-1 acupoint; and the further from the meridian, the more diminished these features were. Figure 18 below shows that by 35 millimetres from the acupoint (upper plot in Figure 18), the features were not present.

The intelligent tissue hypothesis states that all bodily tissue interprets organ information contained in electromagnetic waves, and that the bodily tissue at a particular meridian emphasizes information from that meridian's related organ. And this appears to be what was happening here. These two instances of notably increased amplitude occurred at Lung-1, because the lungs were stressed, and the stress was related to the lungs' pace signal.

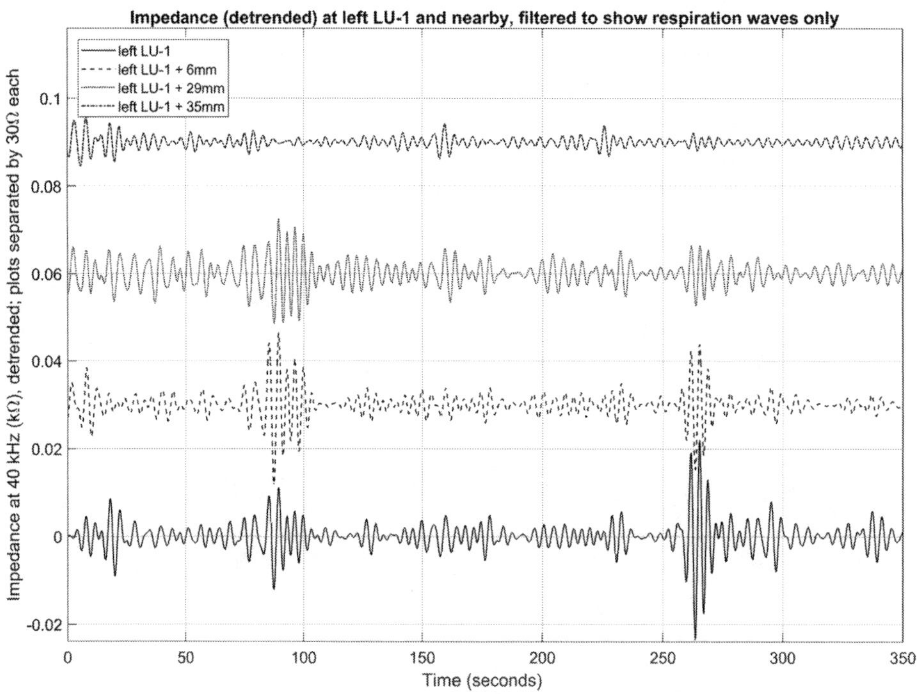

Figure 18. The notable features diminish with distance from the meridian

One possible interpretation is as follows. In the first instance, the subject's initial breathing rate was slower than this pace signal (the subject had not eaten that morning and was tired). However, during the 15 seconds of deep breathing, the amplitude of the reflected pace signal (lower plot of Figure 17) notably increased; and by the end of the deep breathing, the actual breathing (which corresponded to the rate of the brainstem pacesetter), now equalled the rate of the pace signal. The fact that the deep breathing had now adopted the rate of the pace signal, may have momentarily emphasized the pace signal—since the pace signal is (assumed to be) a part of the lungs' function and this part of the lung function was being utilized more heavily than previously at this particular moment. And after the breath was held for 25 seconds, the even larger emphasis of the pace signal wave may reflect the lungs' urgent need to resume breathing (and therefore, again impose the pace signal's rate on the brainstem pacesetter, which was currently at a standstill while the subject consciously held his breath).

In other words, since these extra increases in amplitude did not occur at other locations (locations *not* on the lung meridian), this confirmed that the amplitude of the original lung pace signal did not vary, and that these intelligent increases in its amplitude were therefore produced by the tissue at left Lung-1, which demonstrated the local tissue actively interpreting this lung-related information.

In another study,[54] which monitored the subject's breathing while he relaxed after exercise, it was clearly demonstrated that the pace signals from *all* the organs are reflected at every bodily location, so that at the lung meridian, there are not only respiration waves but also duodenal waves, stomach slow waves, and pulse waves. But because the tissue at the lung meridian (for example) emphasizes lung-related information, then the respiration waves are reflected in the tissue with a larger amplitude than, for example, the duodenal waves.

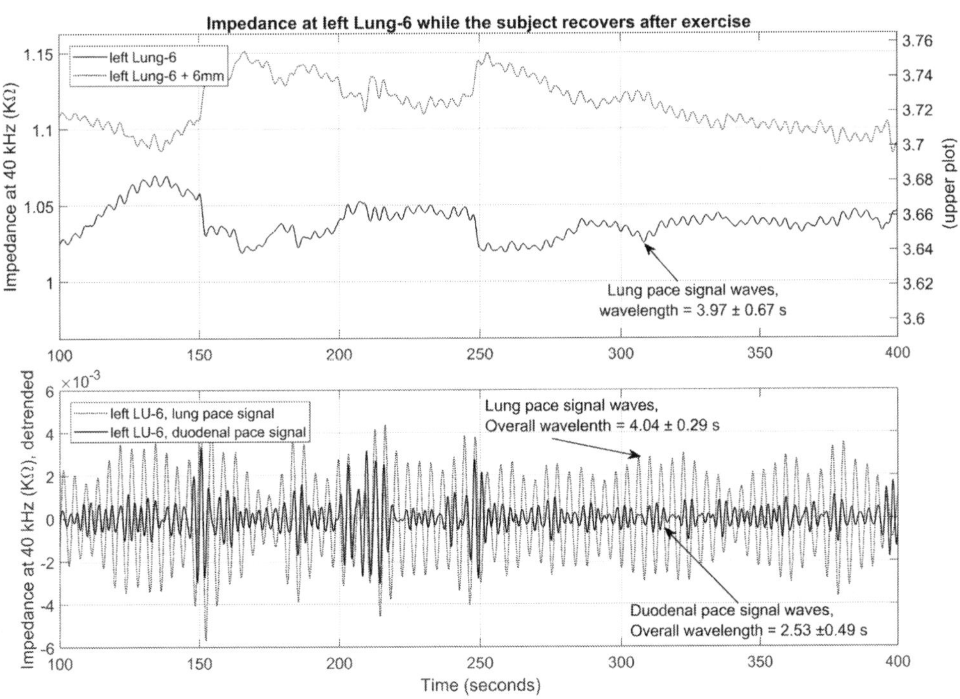

Figure 19. Impedance at left Lung-6

Figure 19 above shows the impedance at left Lung-6. The changing strength of the lung function was reflected in the general impedance level (the upper pair of plots). And superimposed on this were low-amplitude waves from all the pace setters. But since this was a lung meridian, the lung-related information was emphasized by the local tissue, which means that the lung pace signal was reflected with a greater amplitude than the (for example) duodenal pace signal, so that the waves appeared to be mainly from the lung pace signal (the small-amplitude waves visible on the upper plots).

But when the signal was filtered to separately show the lung and duodenal waves (lower plot of Figure 19), it can be seen that the duodenal waves were present, but because their amplitude (as reflected in the tissue at this acupoint) was notably lower than the lung pace signal waves, then when the waves were combined, the overall pattern consisted mainly of lung pace signal waves. In effect, the tissue at this acupoint had filtered the organ information in the electromagnetic waves, to only show the lung-related information.

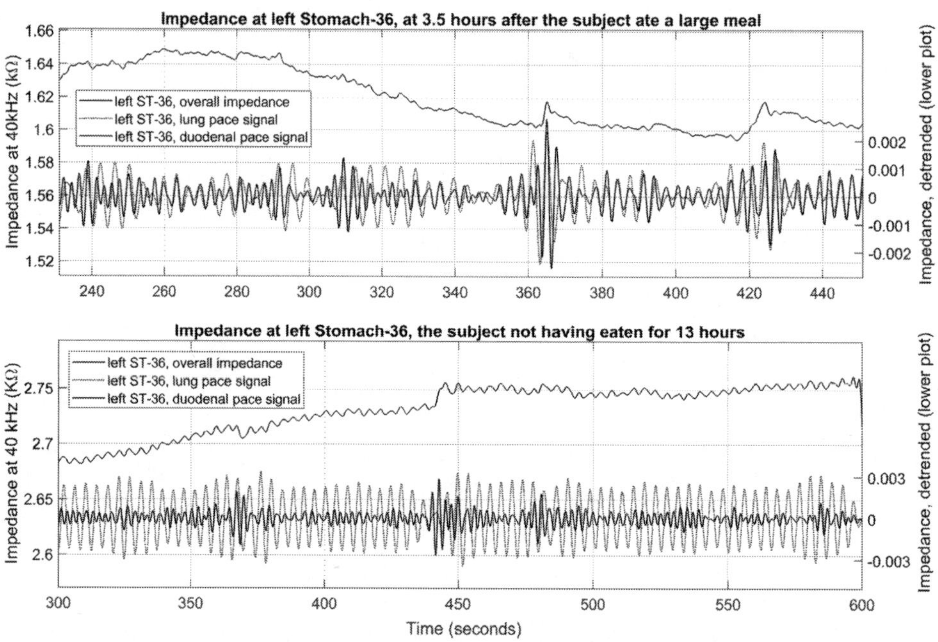

Figure 20. Impedance at left Stomach-36

However, this phenomenon also depends on the strength of the organ function. For example, the upper plot in Figure 20 above shows that when the stomach was actively digesting a meal, then at Stomach-36 the duodenal pace signal was reflected with a higher amplitude than the lung pace signal.[55] Hence, in this case, the waves superimposed on the overall impedance plot mainly consisted of duodenal waves. But when the stomach was not actively digesting a meal, then (at this same acupoint, Stomach-36) the duodenal pace signal was now reflected with a lower amplitude than the lung pace signal (lower plot in Figure 20). Hence, in this case, the waves superimposed on the overall impedance plot mainly consisted of respiration waves, even though the impedance was measured at a stomach acupoint. Also note that in the lower plot, the lung pace signal was reflected with a higher amplitude than in the upper plot. This probably reflected the fact that in the lower plot, the lungs were stressed.[54] What complicates the interpretation is that the lungs and pancreas have a "six channel" relationship (p.397), therefore it is possible that lung-related information may also be emphasized at stomach and pancreas acupoints and meridians. This phenomenon has not yet been investigated.

The above detail provides a further demonstration of the tissue at a meridian interpreting organ information contained in electromagnetic waves and emphasizing information from the meridian's related organ.

Bodily tissue interprets organ information conveyed on electromagnetic waves

Because variations in the impedance at any location would usually indicate a corresponding variation in the physical tissue (including its body fluid content), all the above results suggest that microscopic physical patterns are being constantly produced in the local tissue at every meridian location to reflect the real-time function of the related organs. The patterns reflect the pace signals related to the duodenal waves, the lungs' respiration rate, the stomach's slow wave, the pulse rate, and also the general strength of each organ's function. The speed of the response in the local tissue, and also the detail captured, suggest that the tissue is responding to organ information conveyed on electromagnetic waves (since no other known method of communication in the body could communicate organ information to *every* location at the required speed—pp.401-406). In other words, that the tissue at every bodily location is constantly interpreting organ information conveyed on electromagnetic waves.

The continuing research in this area

Since November 2017 I have been involved in a research project focussed on obtaining objective experimental data to validate all the key aspects of this book's intelligent tissue hypothesis (p.372). The results reported above were obtained in the early months of this project. The research is still ongoing and details of the latest published papers and experimental datasets can be found at:

www.curiouspages.com/research.

The following chapters discuss the electrical energy in the body, how organ information is superimposed upon this, and how the above phenomenon of the bodily tissue interpreting such organ information is central to many of the phenomena encountered in Chinese acupuncture; and also offers a lucid explanation of how acupuncture works.

Chapter 18. The electrical energy within the body

Chinese acupuncture achieves its effects by interacting with the meridians. The current chapter explains that a reservoir of electrical energy exists throughout the body's connective tissue network. And the following two chapters then describe how organ information is superimposed upon this current and that the local tissue along the paths of the meridians constantly interprets this information. It is this activity in the local tissue that *produces* the meridians and also enables the organ information to produce all the meridian phenomena familiar to Chinese medicine (including the diagnostic tenderness at acupoints, redness, heat or cold, boils, rough or dry skin, discomfort or shooting pains).

The body's use of electrical energy

It has been known for well over a hundred years that electrical energy flows within the body. Research in this area led to the development of the electro-cardiogram (ECG) by Willem Einthoven, who received a Nobel prize for his accomplishments in 1924. An ECG measures the electrical activity of the heart; and another organ monitored in this way is the brain, using an electro-encephalogram (EEG).

Electrical charges also feature in the routine functioning of many aspects of the body. As described in this chapter, they have been found to play a key role in the growth and repair of tissue and bones; are the force that enables the nervous system to function; and there is also an electrical charge within every cell of the body, without which the cells themselves could not function. But before discussing the body's use of electrical energy, it will be helpful to first cover a few basic concepts.

What is energy?

Energy is a mysterious thing. It is a force in nature which is everywhere and within everything, whether it be living organisms or any of the other substances that make up our world. Yet no-one really knows what it is. The science textbooks, rather than defining what energy is, get around this problem by stating what it does. Energy is defined as "the ability to do work" (or, in other words: "the ability to move something"). But as to *how* that ability comes about or what it really consists of, no-one knows.[1]

What is mass?

On the microscopic level, all matter in the universe (whether solid, liquid or gas) is made up of countless atoms. The centre of an atom is known as the nucleus. This contains most of the mass of the atom, is made up of neutrons and protons, and has a *positive* electrical charge. And orbiting around this are electrons which have a *negative* electrical charge. Each of these particles has a field around it, and due to the interaction of these fields, the particles either attract or repel one another. Again, no-one really knows why or how these forces come about; it is simply known that they exist. However, it is the interaction of these forces that holds the atom together. Each atom normally has the same number of protons and electrons. The electrons orbit the nucleus at specific heights, and one or more electrons may orbit at each of these heights. Each height is known as a shell (or energy level), and the outermost shell is known as the valence shell.[2]

What is electricity?

With each electron, the further out from the nucleus it orbits, the weaker is the force that keeps it in orbit. And the electrons in the valence shell have such a weak force holding them in place that they can easily become detached from the atom. When this happens, the detached electron then floats freely, not associated with any particular atom. And the atom it detached from is then left with more protons (which are positive) than electrons, therefore it now has a net positive charge. The detached electron is attracted to any neighbouring atom that also has a net positive charge, and takes up orbit around that new atom. It is this flow of electrons between atoms (this movement of negative charge) that we call electricity.[3]

An electrical current occurs when this flow of electrons happens over a distance—which might be along an electrical cable in the outside world or through tissue in the body. A good analogy is the current of a river. Both are a flow of matter in a particular direction, which flow has within it a certain amount of energy—this mysterious force in nature. Hence, an electrical current is simply a way of transferring energy from one place to another.

How electricity is created within the body

One electrical current is much the same as another, whether it occurs within the body or through a light bulb, washing machine or mobile phone. However, there are several ways of creating the initial force—this release of electrons from atoms. A common way is to utilize the force of magnetism—another of nature's mysterious qualities. This is how electricity is generated in power stations, for example (p.385). And another common way is via a chemical reaction, which is the way a battery produces its energy. And all living organisms (including ourselves) also use this method.

Every cell in the body contains many smaller components which make up the entire cell, one of which is a tiny structure known as a *mitochondrion*, which has the ability to create its own energy. Within the mitochondrion, a molecule known as ATP is converted into a similar molecule known as ADP and this process releases energy which the cell can then use to perform its tasks. The mitochondrion then converts the ADP back into ATP. This conversion is done using the glucose from ingested food as a fuel source, combined with the oxygen from the air we breathe, and is achieved via a series of chemical processes. In this way, the mitochondrion repeats the whole process over and over, each time releasing energy (p.387).

Some cells may contain only a single mitochondrion, but cells that have a high need for energy contain many more (a liver cell, for example, contains between 1,000 to 2,000). Mitochondria could be thought of as the energy factories of the cells; and within those, the ATP molecules could be thought of as the essential batteries which release the energy; and the food we eat is then used to continually recharge those tiny batteries.[4]

The movement of energy around the body

Once created, energy can be used locally (within that cell), to form new chemical bonds which, for example, might be needed to create new materials for use in cell repair; or the energy could be moved to elsewhere in the body, to do similar work there.

It was once thought that a true electrical current (a flow of electrons) could not occur in animals, since normally they only flow through metals. But some non-metallic materials, known as semiconductors, are capable of conducting electricity via a flow of electrons (p.389).

In 1941 Albert Szent-Gyorgyi, who received the Nobel Prize in 1937 for his work on the synthesis of Vitamin C, suggested that proteins are semiconductors.[5] At the time, it was not thought possible that semiconduction could occur in an animal's body, and that only *ionic* currents were present (where a charged molecule moves through a liquid). Szent-Gyorgyi suggested that when a great number of atoms were arranged with regularity in close proximity, such as in a crystal lattice, then electrons could be free to move between them, which implied that mobile electrons could move freely around the human body, transferring energy from place to place.

At the time, this concept (like many new ideas) was rejected by the scientific community. And the scientists who did strive to verify the claim, failed to find any evidence that electrons could be conducted through proteins. However, the proteins they studied had been prepared by dehydrating samples taken from living tissue, powdering them and pressing them into pellets; and it was later discovered that taking water out of a protein destroyed its ability to act as a semiconductor. The proteins and the water that adheres to them form a two-part semiconducting system. Electrons can move through the proteins, and protons can move through the water layers.[6]

Over the years, support grew for the fact that most of the molecules in living systems have semiconducting properties to some degree. And in 1981, Szent-Gyorgyi demonstrated that a protein called collagen is a semiconductor.[7] Collagen is the main component of the body's connective tissue, which is the material that forms the constructive fabric of almost every element of the body, down to the microscopic level. It is widely found throughout bones, ligaments, tendons, cartilage and also the coverings of the bones and muscles, which is known as the fascia. Hence, it is now widely accepted that many tissues in the body have semiconducting properties and that true electrical currents flow within them.

The nervous system probably uses more electrical energy than any other system in the body. But in this case, the nerve impulses are not achieved via a flow of electrons. Instead, a flow of *ions* is used. An ion is a permanently charged atom (such as sodium or potassium, for example), and when these exist in liquid form, the atoms themselves are able to flow, their charge causing them to be attracted to a molecule or cell of the opposite charge (p.387). The cells of the nervous system use this property to produce an electrical impulse. To do this, a nerve cell opens up gates in its cell wall, which allows ions to flow into the cell, thus quickly increasing its overall electrical charge*, and this increased charge acts as an impulse. And when many nerve cells are placed in a long string, to produce a nerve, this impulse travels from cell to cell, along the nerve. In this case, electrical energy is not being moved around the body via a flow of electrons, but rather, a signal (the electrical impulse) is being transmitted, and no flow of electrons (or other charged particles) takes place along the nerve. Instead, each nerve cell makes changes within itself, which then triggers the next cell to do the same, and so on. The significance of this will become clear in the following section.

Other evidence of the body's use of electrical energy

It has been known for thousands of years that many plants can regenerate a whole new plant from a single part of the old one. If a part of the plant's stalk is removed and planted, a whole new plant may sprout from the segment of stalk. Many animals also have a similar ability. For example, when a claw is removed from a crayfish, lobster or crab, the animal may regenerate that claw. And salamanders (a lizard with a skeletal and organ structure similar to our own) are able to regenerate whole limbs and also such parts as their jaw or even the lenses of their eyes. It is also possible for animals to regenerate parts of their intestine, liver, spleen, and, in some animals, even large parts of their heart, such as in salamanders and newts.[8]

These are examples of true regeneration, which means the growth of complex body parts, consisting of several different kinds of cells, in a fashion resembling the original growth of that same part in the embryo.

True regeneration involves an increased electrical current

Limb regeneration in salamanders has been studied extensively, starting as far back as 1823. The process is briefly as follows. A mass of cells gathers over the end of the stump. These cells resemble the unspecialized cells that make up any early embryo. Amongst this mass of cells, the ones nearest the stump begin to specialize (transform into a cell of a specific type needed to form either bone, muscle, skin, nerve, blood vessels, and so on); and the whole limb gradually grows back in the same fashion that the original limb formed in the embryonic creature, until a complete new limb is formed.

In the 1940's to 50's, while studying this process in salamanders, Marcus Singer (of Harvard Medical School) found that if all the nerves supplying the stump were cut, the

* Page 389 describes this process in detail.

stump could not regenerate; and after a series of further experiments he found that a certain number of nerves needed to be intact for regeneration to occur, but that what they supplied was not connected with the nerve's known function of communication via electrical impulses.[9] Something else was being supplied.

The "current of injury"

When an injury occurs (such as the severing of part of a limb) and regeneration takes place, there is a dramatic change in the electrical potential at the stump. Initially this falls, then several days later it returns at three times its normal value (in salamanders, the increased potential is -30 millivolts, compared to the normal potential of -10 millivolts). This increased potential then gradually decreases while the limb is regenerating, and returns to normal by the time the limb is complete. This became known as the "current of injury".

This same current of injury also occurs in plants. A.M. Sinyukhin (Lomonosov State University, Moscow) conducted a series of experiments on tomato plants and found that when a branch was cut from a plant, a change in the electrical properties occurred at the wound while new shoots were forming. And in another experiment, extra current was added from a battery, in the same polarity as the plant's own current of injury, and the plants regrew three times faster than normal.[10] The extra current was tiny, measuring only around 0.000002 amperes, which is comparable to the size of the plant's normal electrical energy.

Extra current enables limb regeneration in some mammals

In 1967, Stephen Smith (of the University of Kentucky), managed to induce full regrowth of limbs in frogs by implanting tiny batteries in the stumps. Ordinarily, frogs are not able to regenerate lost limbs, but by applying a tiny electrical current to the stump, this enabled full, true regeneration of a lost limb to occur.

Robert Becker has extensively researched the electrical current present when healing takes place (he was an American orthopaedic surgeon working from the 1960's onwards, and was initially interested in why broken bones sometimes failed to unite). He duplicated the above experiment but on rat legs. As with frogs, rats are not normally able to regenerate a lost limb. In very young rats however, there is a partial ability, but in adult rats, there is no ability (as is the case with humans—see below). By applying a tiny electrical current to the stump, Becker was able to extend this ability into older rats.[11]

Fingertip regeneration in children

In the 1970's, Dr Cynthia Illingworth (a surgeon at Sheffield Children's Hospital, UK) documented several hundred cases where children had regrown fingertips. In all cases, the tip was severed at some point beyond the final joint (a common injury in young children); the children were all aged eleven or younger and the wound was left to heal naturally, rather than skin being sewn over the wound. When the children's fingertips had regrown they were perfect in every detail with nothing to distinguish them from an uninjured finger. In 1980, Illingworth and her co-worker Anthony Barker went on to confirm that a negative current of injury was present at the stump while the fingertips were in the process of regenerating; and the current showed a remarkable resemblance to the current present when salamander limbs regenerated.[12]

Until this phenomenon had been documented, it was assumed that mammals were not able to regenerate limbs and could only regenerate bones—to replace those fractured or broken. The thinking was that this inability was due to the small number of nerves we have in our limbs—compared to salamanders, for example. This is due to our brains requiring such a large mass of neurons that there is less of this material available for the rest of the body; and since we have less nerves in our limbs, their regeneration was not thought possible, since this appeared to be dependent on something provided by the nerves.

However, the ability of children to regenerate fingertips does, of course, contradict the notion that humans are incapable of true regeneration due to us having such developed brains. This suggests that the number of nerves may not be the significant factor. Instead, it may simply be the electrical current (the extra energy) that enables regeneration to happen. If this is the case, how would this explain why children are able to regenerate fingertips while adults cannot? The simple answer may be that children have far more energy than adults.

The possible function of this extra current

Robert Becker speculated that the current of injury may be some sort of control signal that guides the regeneration process. However, an alternative and simpler explanation may be this. The task of forming all the cells necessary to regrow a particular part of an animal's body (including the muscle, bone, skin, ligaments, nerves and so on) requires a lot of energy. Therefore the increased current may merely reflect the fact that more work is being done (whatever triggers that to happen) and hence more energy is being used.

Under everyday conditions, however, the normal resting potential of a limb is around -10 millivolts. What function might this normal current serve?

The function of the resting potential

In the 1940's, research was carried out by W.E. Burge (of the University of Illinois) and also by groups of physiologists and neurologists at Harvard Medical School. They found that whenever groups of nerve cells were actively conducing impulses, the nerves also produced a negative potential (meaning that a current of electrons was also flowing along them). However, when brain cells were injured during brain surgery, there was an absence of current which appeared to prevent those cells from functioning normally (they could not send or receive impulses). And in other situations, when the normal current was depressed, by applying an external positive potential, this depressed normal nerve function, making it harder for the nerves to produce an impulse. But when small negative voltages were applied to groups of neurons, they performed better (they became more sensitive and generated an impulse in response to a weaker stimulus). In other words, when the normal electrical current that accompanies nerves is reduced, the nerves can not function properly, and when it is increased, this enhances their normal function.[13]

A group of scientists at the University of Chicago (Ling, Gerard and Libet), working with frog brains, confirmed that a true electrical current (a flow of electrons) travels along a nerve in the same direction that the nerve impulse flows along it, and that the current is conducted by structures *outside* the nerve cells; in other words, via some structure in the sheaths that surround all nerves.[14]

In 1982, Ngok Cheng *et al.* (University of Louvain, Belgium) found that applying a tiny electrical current to rat skin, dramatically increased the ability of the skin cells to produce ATP. In other words, this enabled the cells to produce more energy within themselves, which consequently increased the ability of the cells to carry out routine repair work.[15]

In 1983, Oscar Alvarex *et al.* (of the University of Pittsburgh School of Medicine), demonstrated that applying a tiny electrical current to fresh skin wounds in domestic pigs, produced a marked increase in the healing of wounds.[16] And in 1997, Linda Baker *et al.* (of the University of Southern California) demonstrated that electrical stimulation of open skin ulcers in diabetic patients, dramatically increased the rate of healing.[17]

The current enables cells to function normally

Taken together, the evidence in this chapter suggests that a tiny electrical current needs to be present in many parts of the body to enable the cells to function normally (and that when more cellular work is being done, the current in that region increases); but that when that current is absent, the cells function less well or sometimes not at all. All cells can generate their own energy, but perhaps an extra supply is also generally required.

What is the source of this current?

In 1961, Robert Becker used the Hall effect to demonstrate that the electrical currents in a live salamander's leg were being conducted by semiconduction.[18,19] And Ling, Gerard and Libet (at the University of Chicago) found that the negative potential that existed along a nerve (in addition to the electrical impulse) was a genuine flow of electrons, rather than of charged ions.[20]

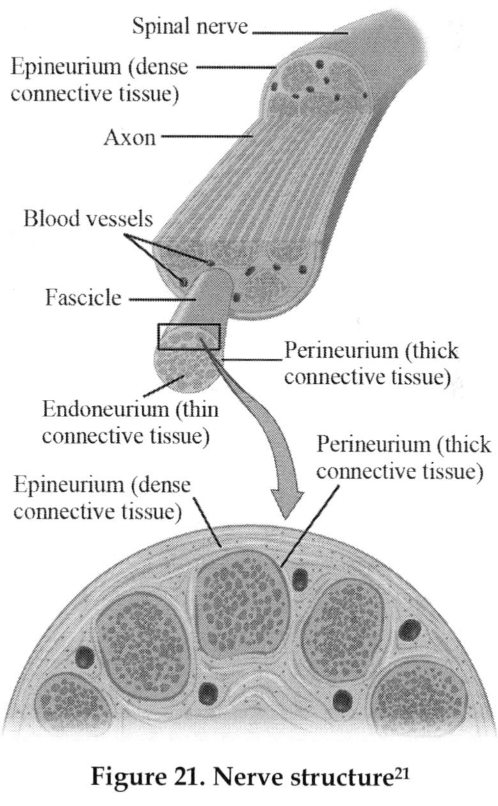

Figure 21. Nerve structure[21]

Becker also discovered that the current of injury was conducted through the perineurial sleeve of a nerve, rather than through some part of the nerve itself.[22] Peripheral nerves contain much connective tissue (which is known to be semiconducting). As shown in Figure 21 above, each nerve axon (or fibre) is surrounded by the *endoneurium*, which is a thin, protective layer of connective tissue. Several axons are then gathered together to form a *nerve fascicle,* which is enclosed by the *perineurium*, which is a thicker sheath of connective tissue formed from seven or eight concentric layers. And these may then be grouped into the larger, peripheral nerves, which are enclosed in the *epineurium*, which is the outermost layer of dense connective tissue.[23]

Primo vessels also exist within nerves

In 1965 Bong-Han Kim demonstrated that primo vessels are present in the brain, spinal cord and peripheral nerves (p.318), which was confirmed in 2010 by Byung-Cheon Lee *et al.*[24] Within nerves, the primo vessels travel through the perineurial sleeves.

However, Bong-Han Kim also found that the neural primo vessels (unlike the superficial primo vessels) are *not* encased in connective tissue (p.317). This suggests that the primo vessels themselves are not directly involved in conducting the current of injury, which instead probably flows within the connective tissue of the perineurium—as a semiconducted direct current. However, the physiological purpose of the entire primo vascular system (according to Kim) is to transport the material necessary for cell regeneration (p.322), so it is possible that this aspect of the PVS *could* play some part in the process of regenerating cells at wound sites; though the PVS also runs through blood and lymph vessels, which *are* intact in experiments where regeneration of salamander stumps did *not* take place due to the severing of nerves; and also, the PVS is thought to be primarily involved in the regeneration of organ and nerve cells, all of which casts doubt on whether the PVS is involved in the repair of the distal tissues of the body.

The meridians (and/or the superficial primo vessels) are semiconducting

The connective tissue facia is located in every part of the body, thus forming a continuous network that connects every tissue—possibly down to the individual cells. The above evidence therefore suggests that a direct current is also present throughout this extensive connective tissue network—since such a current would spread throughout an entire conductor (and the connective tissue forms a continuous body-wide network which is all theoretically capable of semiconduction). And the evidence also suggests that the current's physiological purpose may be to provide extra energy to every cell to support its normal function.

The superficial primo vessels are thought to form circuits extending from each organ pair, travelling through the skin, then returning to those same organs; and also interconnecting the organs (p.317). They are encased in connective tissue (p.316) and (as described below) it is clear that this same current is also conducted through these vessels and thus forms a direct, electrical connection between the organs and the superficial primo vessels.

In organic semiconductors the chemical doping is said to be provided by sodium-calcium (and also potassium-calcium) exchange, which happens through an *oxidation-reduction* (redox) process.[25] In other words, when there are unusually high concentrations of these ions in the connective tissue, this can be taken as an indicator that semiconduction is taking place.

In 1998, Er-Yu Chen *et al.* found that the calcium concentration on 25 acupoints of the gallbladder meridian, between Gallbladder-20 (*Fengchi*) and Gallbladder-44 (*Zuqiaoyin*), was four times more than that at non-acupoint and non-meridian areas.[26] In 2000, Er-Yu Chen *et al.* found that the calcium concentration in the area of the acupoint Gallbladder-36 (*Waiqiu*) was on average 6.80 times higher than that at non-acupoint areas elsewhere in the human body.[27] And again in 2000, Liu *et al.* found that the relative concentration of calcium at four points on the stomach meridian on the lower leg was on average 6.73 times higher than that between the points.[28]

This suggests that semiconduction is taking place either through the superficial primo vessels, or through the tissue that constitutes the meridians.

The entire skin (and also the muscles and other tissue beneath the skin) also contains connective tissue, as well as that in the superficial primo vessels; but the above experiments indicate that the degree of semiconduction is much greater along the paths of the meridians and the superficial primo vessels than in the surrounding skin. One explanation for this is that these primo vessels may require a much higher degree of current to support their function than the surrounding skin does, since the primo vascular system is engaged in the energy-hungry activity of maturing p-microcells into the various specialist cells required by the organs (p.322).

Another possible source of the above semiconduction is the tissue that constitutes the meridians. On page 355, a meridian is defined as a distal tract of tissue affected by organ function. The superficial primo vessels are separate structures from the meridians (but they may play a part in *creating* the meridians—p.355). The tissue at a meridian is constantly interpreting organ information and hence constantly making tiny physical changes in itself to reflect that organ information (p.333). It is possible that this activity may require extra energy and so may contribute to the increased semiconduction that has been detected in the vicinity of the meridians.

Replenishing the reservoir

In a 2008 article, James Oschman also wrote about this body-wide reservoir of charge, and he suggested it may be replenished by the body taking on electrons from the earth[29]. This may be one way of contributing to the charge, but there is another, more ready source of charge within the body. The liver produces an enormous amount of energy and also regulates the flow of that energy around the body (p.99), but there is evidence that it produces much more than it needs for its own functions. The activity of each organ peaks at a certain time of day; and the liver is most active between the hours of one and three a.m. (p.379). At this time, there is normally no digestive processing to be performed (which takes up a large part of the liver's activity during the day), no physical activity, no large amounts of blood to filter, and so on. Therefore, most of the tasks the liver is responsible for (in contemporary physiology) do not need to be performed at this time of day—so why should the liver be operating at its peak?

This output of pure energy is clearly required for some purpose, and this may be to assist in the repair and maintenance of the body's cells; in other words, to replenish this direct current reservoir of charge that exists everywhere in the body.

The purpose of sleep

This would also explain why the brain and nervous system are largely shut down at night. These have a massive requirement for energy (the neurons constantly generate electrical impulses, which is an energy-hungry activity). It makes sense that these should be switched off at night, so as to allow as much energy as possible for the even more energy-hungry activity of repairing worn out cells. Hence, the body goes to sleep; the brain and nervous system is switched off and we stop digesting food and make no physical movements. But even with all these systems shut down, the task of performing the body's daily cell-maintenance requires so much energy that the liver (the body's powerhouse) goes into overdrive.

The above scenario may provide an explanation for the purpose of sleep, which is to enable the body to do its daily cell maintenance work. We all know that a good night's sleep is reparative; we feel like a new person afterwards (which, in some small way, we are); and when we miss just one night's sleep, we feel drained, under par, worn out (which, again, in some small way, we *are*—our worn out cells have not been repaired or replaced).

This electrical energy does not equate to the 1970's notion of *chi*

The electrical energy discussed in this chapter does not play a direct part in producing acupuncture's effects. And it should not be associated with the 1970's notion of *chi* (p.51). Instead, this electrical energy merely provides a medium upon which organ information is able to be conveyed (p.365), and it is this organ information that produces all the meridian phenomena associated with Chinese acupuncture, and also enables acupuncture to correct organ malfunction (p.372).

Chapter 19. The relationship between organ hierarchy and the meridian locations

Chinese acupuncture relies on the association between the organs and specific bodily locations. Each organ is associated with a particular meridian, and the various aspects of that organ's function are associated with specific locations along that meridian. But what mechanism in the body was responsible for creating these associations?

This chapter examines how the arrangement of the meridians may have evolved; and the following chapter uses this information to explain how organ information may be filtered by (in effect) the geometry of the body, which then plays a part in enabling acupuncture to achieve its effects.

The remarkable layout of the meridians

According to this book's hypothesis, the meridians are merely tracts of distal tissue affected by organ function (p.355). On each limb, there are six meridians, three on the inner side of the limb (the *yin* surface), and three on the outer side (the *yang* surface; these surfaces are defined below). The remarkable feature of this system is as follows. The relationship between each meridian's location and the locations of the other meridians, follows a clear rule, and even the choice of whether a meridian exists on the arms or legs is determined by the same rule. And these same relationships also exist between the organs.

All these relationships obey a natural balancing rule in nature, which the *Nei Jing* authors referred to using the concepts of *yin* and *yang*.

The following sections describe

- the meaning of *yin* and *yang*;
- how these concepts can be used to define the relationships between the surfaces of the body, and also, in the same way, define the relationships between the organs; and
- how all these factors seem to have been used to determine the locations of the meridians on the limbs.

The meaning of *yin* and *yang*

The *yin-yang* rule is a universal rule in nature which was first described in ancient China around the 4th century BC (p.14). It was then applied to medicine, and in Chapters 4 and 5 of the *Su Wen*, many examples were given of states of *yin* and *yang* within the body.[1]

Yin-yang is a rule that describes the relationship between two interconnected qualities, and how one of those qualities changes to balance a change in the other. For example, the quality of being active would be *yang* when compared to the quality of being at rest, which would be *yin*; and as a person moves from being at rest to being more active, the *yin* states within them decrease while the *yang* states increase. In this relationship between two qualities, *yang* describes the more energetic, active, aggressive, loud, outward-looking qualities, while, in comparison, *yin* describes the more depleted, restful, passive, quiet, inward-looking qualities.

As well as activity, all other qualities can be categorized in *yin-yang* pairs, such as in the following examples:

Table 5. *Yin-yang* examples

	left	right*	
	inside	outside	
	down	up	
Yin	legs	arms	*Yang*
	land	sky	
	solid	hollow	
	backwards	forwards	

"Yin" and "yang" are states of relativity

No quality has an absolute state of *yin* or *yang*; it can only adopt those states in relation to some other quality. For example, the left hand is *yin* when compared to the right, which is *yang*. But if the left hand were compared to the left foot, it would now be *yang*, and the foot *yin*. Hence the left hand could be either *yin* or *yang*, depending on the comparison being made.

Regarding the limbs and torso, the closer a location is to the centre of the body, the more *yin* it becomes, since "inside" is *yin* and "outside" is *yang*. In this way, when considering the left hand again, its skin would be *yang* when compared to its muscles, which would be *yin*; but if the muscles were compared to the bones, the muscles would now be *yang* and the bones *yin*—so that the muscles could be either *yin* or *yang*, depending on the comparison being made.

Yin-yang classification of the body

To visualize the *yin-yang* classification of any part of the body, it is best to imagine ourselves when we still stood on four legs, since at that stage the body's shape more closely resembled the shape when the *yin-yang* surfaces were defined in early evolution.

For example, as shown in Figure 22 below, the outer surface of each leg is *yang* and the inner surface *yin*, since the outer surface faces the outside world while the inner surface is relatively more internal to ourselves. And if we were to stand with our palms resting against our legs, this would correspond to the orientation in Figure 22 (our arms corresponding to the forelegs of a four-legged animal). In this orientation, the outer surface of each of our arms (the knuckle side) would be *yang* and the inner surface (the palm side) *yin*; and the front edge would be *yang* and the back edge *yin* (page 397 explains why the head is the most *yang* part of the body, and hence why the progression is from *yin* to *yang*, along the body). When comparing the front

* This assignment of *yin* to left, and *yang* to right is controversial. See page 282 for a full discussion.

and back of the torso, the front is *yin* and the back *yang*. Again, to understand why, it is best to imagine the body when we still stood on four legs. At that stage, the back was *yang* and the belly *yin*, which reflected the fact that the belly was nearer to the land, and the back to the sky; or, in other terms, the back faced the outside world and the belly was relatively more internal to us—was the soft underbelly.

> **Extract from *Su Wen*, Chapter 4**
>
> Speaking of the *yin* and *yang* of man, then the outside is *yang*, the inside is *yin*. Speaking of the *yin* and *yang* of the human body, then the back is *yang*, the abdomen is *yin*. Speaking of the *yin* and *yang* among the [*zang* and *fu* organs] of the human body, then the [*zang*] are *yin* and the [*fu*] are *yang*. The liver, the heart, the [pancreas], the lung, and the kidneys, all these five [*zang*] are *yin*. The gallbladder, the stomach, the large intestine, the small intestine, the urinary bladder, and the [lymphatic system], all these six [*fu*] are *yang*.[2]

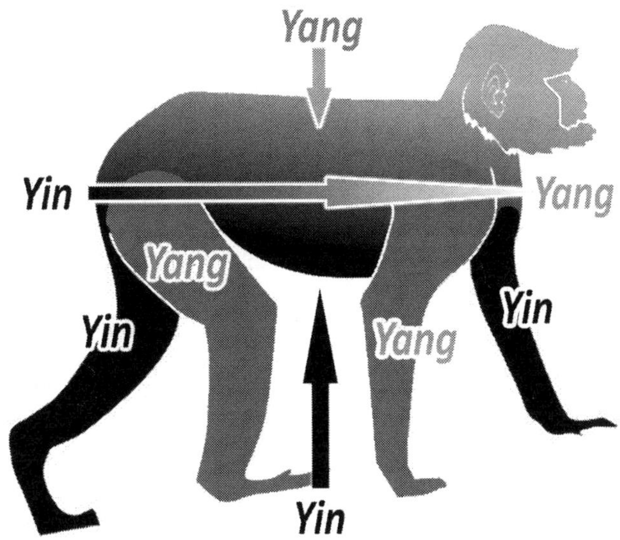

Figure 22. *Yin-yang* classification of the body

Yin-yang classification of the organs

Any surface of the body has a *yin-yang* relationship with any other surface of the body, and when considering the internal organs, their relationships with one another can also be described in this same way. Firstly, each organ is either *yin* or *yang*. As listed in the above extract from Chapter 4 of the *Su Wen*, the deeper, more important organs are *yin*, while the less important, more "superficial" organs are *yang*; and in Table 6 below, the *yin* organs are listed on the left, and the *yang* on the right. There are several other ways to differentiate between the organs, in *yin-yang* terms. These are

A. the functional pairings of organs (where each *yin* organ is paired with a *yang* organ, due to their functional relationship);

B. their position in the abdomen;
C. the features of their physical structure;
D. their depth within the body (how directly or indirectly they communicate with the outside world);
E. the nature of the substances they process; and
F. the nature of their processing.

In Table 6, all these factors have been used to determine the *yin-yang* hierarchy of the abdominal organs. In the table the organs are listed according to their progression from *yin* to *yang*. Those listed on the right are more *yang* than those on the left; and (on both sides) those higher up in the list are more *yang* than those below them. For example, in the left column, when comparing the liver with the kidneys, the liver is *yang* and the kidneys *yin*; but when comparing the liver with the gallbladder (in the right column), the liver is now *yin* and the gallbladder *yang*. And if the liver were compared with the pancreas (above it in the left column), the liver would again be *yin* and the pancreas *yang*. For details of how the *yin-yang* hierarchy of the organs in Table 6 was determined, see page 391.

Note that the liver and pancreas are bracketed in Table 6 because their *yin-yang* relationship is variable. Which is the more *yin* or *yang* organ is different depending on which criterion is used to categorize them. And for this reason these two meridians cross one another several times at different locations on the body (see page 391).

Table 6. The *yin-yang* hierarchy of the organs

	***Yin* (inner)** →	***Yang* (outer)**	
***Yang* (upper)** ↑	lungs	large intestine[*]	**Arms**
	pericardium	lymphatic system[†]	**Arms**
	heart	small intestine	**Arms**
	(pancreas[‡])	stomach	**Legs**
	(liver)	gallbladder	**Legs**
***Yin* (lower)**	"kidneys"[§]	bladder	**Legs**

[*] Page 137 describes the functional relationship between the lungs and large intestine; page 208, the heart and small intestine; and page 213, the pericardium and lymphatic system.

[†] Also called the *san jiao* or "triple burner" in Chinese medicine (p.211).

[‡] Also called the spleen in Chinese medicine (p.61).

[§] In Chinese medicine, this refers to the kidneys, adrenal glands and gonads collectively (p.153).

The locations of the meridians

This section compares the locations of the meridians on the limbs with the *yin-yang* hierarchy of the organs described above.

The meridians on the arms

Figure 23 on page 349 below shows the inner and outer surfaces of the left arm, and the meridian locations on them. Considering the darker arm first (the inner surface, which is *yin*), there are three meridians positioned on it. The arrows on the left of the diagram indicate the progression from *yin* to *yang* across the two surfaces of each arm, which progresses from the back edge (the most *yin* part) to the front edge (the most *yang* part). Therefore, of the three meridians shown on the darker arm, the lower is placed on the most *yin* part of the arm's surface, and the upper on the most *yang* part. The lower is associated with the heart; the next with the pericardium; and the upper with the lungs.

Comparing the order of these associations with the order of the organs as shown in Table 6 (p.348 above), it can be seen that the *yin-yang* hierarchy is identical in both. In other words, of these three organs, the meridian associated with the most *yin* organ (the heart) has been positioned on the inner surface of the arm in the most *yin* location, while the meridian associated with the next organ (the pericardium, which is more *yang* than the heart) has been placed in a more *yang* location on this surface. And the meridian associated with the final organ (the lung, which is the most *yang* of the three) has been placed in the most *yang* location on this inner surface of the arm.

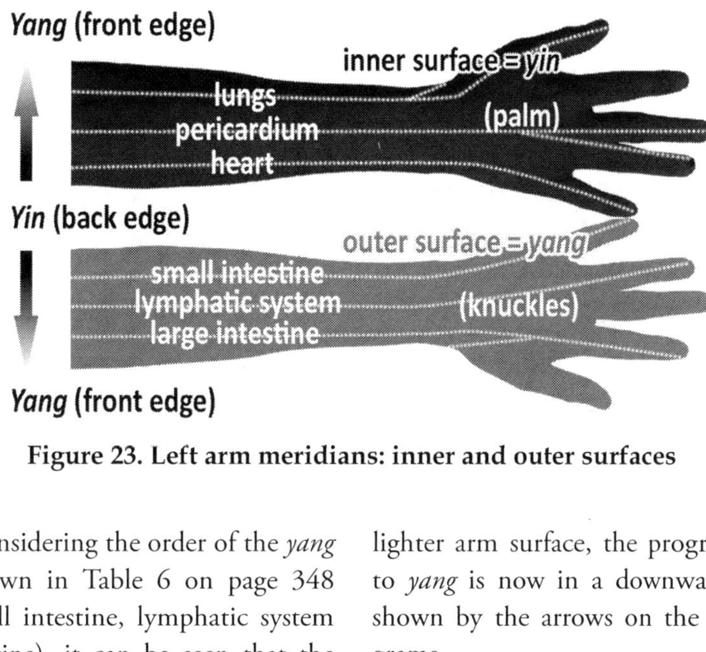

Figure 23. Left arm meridians: inner and outer surfaces

Similarly, considering the order of the *yang* organs (*fu*) shown in Table 6 on page 348 above (the small intestine, lymphatic system and large intestine), it can be seen that the meridians associated with these organs occupy locations across the *outer* surface of the arm (the lighter arm in Figure 23 above) so that the *yin-yang* hierarchy of the organs exactly matches the progression from *yin* to *yang* across the arm's surface. Note that on the lighter arm surface, the progression from *yin* to *yang* is now in a downward direction, as shown by the arrows on the left of the diagrams.

The meridians on the legs

Figure 24 on page 350 below shows the inner and outer surfaces of the left leg, along with the meridians on each surface. And in the same way as with the arms, if the order of these meridians is compared with the *yin-yang* hierarchy of the organs, as listed in Table 6 (p.348 above), it can be seen that the meridians occupy locations on the legs in locations that correspond exactly with the *yin-yang* hierarchy of the associated organs. Note that the liver and pancreas meridians cross one another at the lower leg, which reflects the variability of their *yin-yang* relationship—page 391 explains this.

Not only this, but even the choice between whether an organ's associated meridian appears on the arms or legs also obeys this same hierarchy, with the three most *yin* pairs of organs being associated with meridians on the legs (which are the most *yin* of the limbs) and the three most *yang* pairs being associated with meridians on the arms (the most *yang* of the limbs). What is the explanation for all these exact correlations?

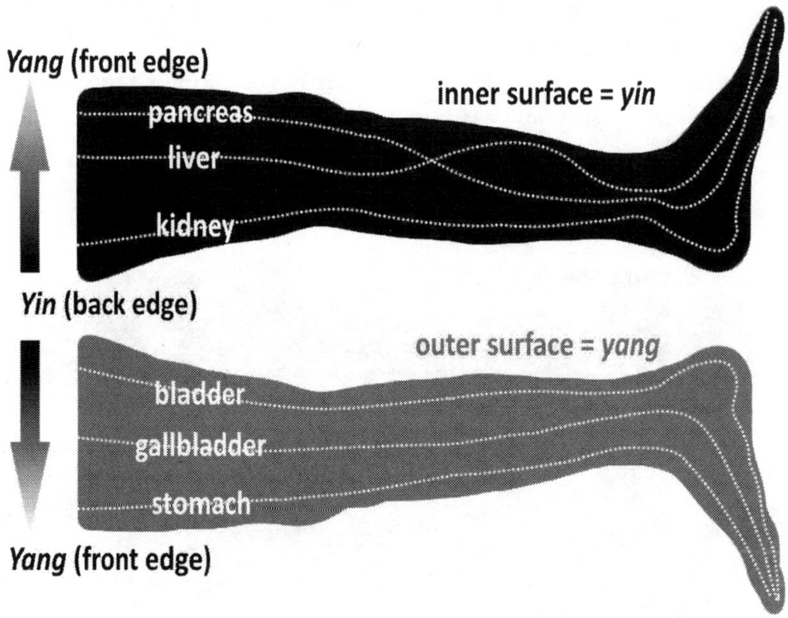

Figure 24. Left leg meridians: inner and outer surfaces

The nature of each organ determined its meridian location

Such precise correlations between the geometry of the meridian locations and the relationships between the organs could not have resulted randomly. The inference is that when the locations of the meridians were initially determined, some mechanism took account of the similarity between the hierarchy of the organ network and the geometry of that limb (and also the geometry of the body in general) and used this relationship to determine where on that limb each meridian would be located. In other words, the character and nature of the organ that was associated with a particular meridian—and also that organ's relationships with the other organs—determined which limb the meridian would exist on (hind limb or forelimb) and also the exact position the meridian would take on that limb in relation to the other meridians on that limb.

Other anatomical features reflecting this same influence

The path of the stomach meridian

The path of the stomach meridian reflects the function of the stomach. The stomach's key role is to take in food and begin the process of digestion; and its associated meridian begins at the eye, descends to the side of the mouth, follows the line of the jaw, rises up into the brain, then descends, following the line of the gullet to the stomach itself, and then down the front of the torso to the outer surface of the leg. The first half of this path follows the exact route that food takes, before and after it enters the stomach. It begins at the eye (merely looking at food is the start of the process, since this induces salivation, etc.); it descends to the mouth and follows the line of the jaw (chewing the food is the next stage); it then follows the path of the gullet, down into the stomach itself, reflecting the exact route that the swallowed food takes into the body.

There does not seem to be any anatomical reason why the path of this meridian should take this course—which suggests that the function of the stomach somehow influenced the path its related meridian adopted on the body. In other words, that some mechanism took account of the stomach's function when positioning this meridian on the head and torso.

The path of the gallbladder meridian

The gallbladder meridian also provides a graphic example of this same influence. It begins at the eye, zigzags over the side of the head several times, then down the neck, then zigzags down the side of the torso and finally down the outside of the leg. What is unusual is that this is the only meridian that zigzags. From Chapter 5 onwards I describe in detail the mental and emotional functions of the main organs. It has been observed from ancient times, and is still observable in clinic today, that the gallbladder is responsible for our ability to make decisions (that is, shall I choose this option, or that); and the path of its meridian appears to reflect this function (first going this way, then that way). It cannot be a coincidence that the gallbladder is recognised as providing us with our ability to make decisions and that *its* meridian is the only one that zigzags. And another notable feature of its path is that the most intense zigzagging takes place over the side of the head, which is the location of the thoughts which the decisions are made in connection with. (Or in another interpretation, it could be said that the most intense zigzagging happens on the head simply because this is the most *yang* part of the body.)

The head only contains yang meridians

As shown in Figure 22 (p.347 above), the head is the most *yang* part of the body (page 397 explains why this is the case). And what is notable is that every one of the six *yang* meridians extend to the head (that is, the meridians associated with the six *yang* organs—or *fu*), while not a single one of the *yin* meridians do. As with the placing of the *yin* and *yang* meridians on the limbs, the choice of the meridians that extend to the head *also* seems to reflect the *yin-yang* hierarchy of the organs—since only the *yang* meridians extend to the most *yang* part of the body. Again, it seems this cannot be a coincidence.

The positioning of acupoints

On the limbs, the positioning of acupoints along each meridian also follows similar rules and so also demonstrates the influence of this organizing mechanism. The acupoints are located to reflect particular aspects of the associated organ's health and function. As shown in Figure 25 below, each limb is *yin* at the torso end and *yang* at its tip. And the acupoints seem to be placed according to this *yin-yang* polarity, as follows.

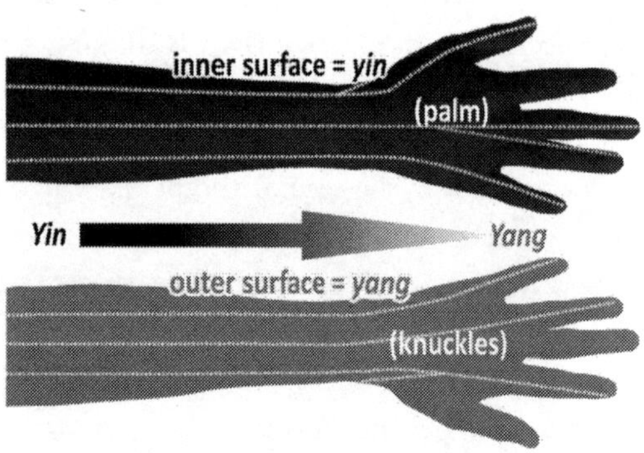

Figure 25. The *yin-yang* progression along the arm

When the various ways that an organ can malfunction are compared with one another, there is a *yin-yang* hierarchy between the malfunctions. The various factors include how long the malfunction has been present (or how deeply ingrained into the organ's functioning it is); for example, a malfunction that only recently started would be superficial and hence more *yang*, whereas a malfunction that was present for a long time would be more deeply ingrained and hence more *yin*. And if a malfunction affected the tissue of the organ, this would make it *yin* when compared to one that only affected the function (which would be more *yang*).

The *yin-yang* hierarchy of each malfunction appears to determine the position of the acupoint that is associated with that malfunction. The more *yin* the malfunction, the more towards the torso-end of the limb the acupoint is located; and the more *yang*, the more towards the tip of the limb.

Therefore, when a person's heart experiences "Heart fire",* this is a *yang* state and so would cause an acupoint towards the tip of their arm, on the heart meridian, to become tender; and the degree of the *heat* would determine how near the tip that acupoint was. But at the same time, other factors would also play a part, such as how long the malfunction was in place—the older the malfunction, the more it would be associated with acupoints towards the torso-end of the limb. This also makes sense from another point of view. The longer a malfunction was in place, the more likely it would be to affect the tissue of the organ, therefore making it a more *yin* condition and causing it to be associated with an acupoint more towards the torso-end of the limb—or, indeed, at an acupoint on the meridian where it crosses the torso itself. As an example of this, the lung *yin* (its fabric) is easily damaged, therefore when a lung malfunction is present, an acupoint on the chest, Lung-1 (*Zhongfu*), is quick to become tender.

All these factors appear to combine to determine at which location along an organ's

* The term *heart fire* is used to describe a condition that causes the heart to display signs of *heat*, which are *yang* qualities. The condition can result from emotional upsets but can also be caused by physical factors (p.454).

meridian each acupoint appears. And sometimes a condition may cause several acupoints along the limb to become tender, each to a different degree, which indicates the condition has affected the organ in various ways. For example, an acute sore throat (which is considered a lung condition in Chinese medicine) would usually cause an acupoint near the thumb, Lung-10 (*Yuji*), to become tender; but since this would be likely to affect the lungs themselves (their *yin*) the acupoint Lung-1 (*Zhongfu*) may also be tender.

But acupoints still exist even when all the organs are functioning normally. In this case, it is the hierarchy of these *normal* functions that appears to determine the acupoint locations. A good illustration of this principle is the heart meridian. The normal function of the heart is probably more *yang* than the function of any other organ, since its four chambers constantly pulse in a powerful way. And the arrangement of the acupoints on the heart meridian has a notable and unique feature. There are four acupoints clustered close together at the wrist, which is near to the most *yang* part of that meridian: Heart-4 (*Lingdao*) to Heart-7 (*Shenmen*). No other limb meridian has a similar feature, and there seems to be no anatomical reason for this cluster of acupoints, which suggests they were positioned to reflect the exceptionally *yang* nature of the heart's normal function. And the fact that there are four successive acupoints in this cluster, and also four chambers in the heart which pulse in sequence, is probably not a coincidence.

What mechanism was responsible for this organization?

As described throughout this chapter, the geographical relationship between any two surfaces of an animal's body correlates exactly with the hierarchical relationship between the two organs whose meridians occupy those surfaces. What might explain this organization?

The following chapter describes how it is possible for information related to an organ's function to be conveyed in an electromagnetic wave (p.365). And Chapter 17 described evidence that demonstrated that bodily tissue constantly interprets organ information conveyed on electromagnetic waves (pp.323-333). These two facts suggest how this organization may have come about.

In early evolution, when the primitive organs began to evolve, information about their functioning would have been present bodywide in the creature, conveyed on electromagnetic waves (p.365). Some (or perhaps all) of its bodily tissue may have been capable of interpreting this organ information. And over an extended period of time, this may have caused that bodily tissue to modify its form or even its own function, in response to the organ information. In time, this may have been the guiding force that influenced the evolution of the creature's general body shape, its limbs, and possibly even its sense organs (today, each of the sense organs are still associated with one of the five main organs—p.88). Eventually, such a process could have created the general body shape that most creatures now have, where the tracts of tissue that constitute the meridians are aligned geographically to reflect the organ functions and the hierarchal relationships between the organs.

If evolution did proceed along these lines, then every creature with similar organs would be expected to have a similar skeletal and general bodily structure, which is the pattern in nature. Whereas animals with different organ systems, such as jellyfish, have a distinctly different body form.

How was the organ information filtered?

If the above evolutionary mechanism did exist, how might the appropriate organ information have been directed to the appropriate bodily surface that it needed to influence?

Assuming that an electrical current is present throughout the connective tissue network of the entire body, when organ information is adopted by this current, the information from all the organs would be combined into a single wave (p.365). But for the above mechanism to exist, this organ information would need to be filtered so that a certain aspect of it (the information from a particular organ) only affected a certain surface of the body (the surface where that organ's associated meridian would eventually exist).

There are two possible ways that this filtering may be performed—either by the meridians themselves, or by the superficial primo vessels (since each of these is also associated with a particular organ, and is said to exist along the path of that organ's meridian). But what is the difference between a meridian and a superficial primo vessel?

The key traits of a superficial primo vessel

It is said that the superficial primo vessels now follow the paths of the meridians (p.320). As identified by Kim, the purpose of the PVS is to enable replacement organ cells to mature (p.322). New cells start as p-microcells within each organ; they then leave the organ through a primo vessel, which travels to the skin. At a primo node, the p-microcell pauses while it matures. The matured cell then progresses further along the primo vessel, which returns to the same organ, and the matured cell takes its place within the organ.

No part of this process is thought to affect the local tissue along the path of a superficial primo vessel (i.e. the local tissue along the path of a meridian).

The key traits of a meridian

Meridians have certain key traits that distinguish them from primo vessels. When an organ is stressed, tenderness occurs at one or more of its key acupoints, which are usually situated along the organ's meridian. Such tenderness feels akin to the sensation felt when bruised tissue is pressed. Other anomalies also occur on meridians, such as the skin becoming reddened, or feeling cold to the touch. Boils or pimples also occur, and sometimes aching or even shooting pains. All these anomalies occur as a result of the related organ being stressed in some way, and a certain type of anomaly is usually linked to a certain type of stress in the organ. For example, red skin indicates that the organ's stressed state features "heat" (in Chinese medicine terms); or cold skin indicates "deficiency" in the organ (in other words, poor function).

When an organ is treated with acupuncture, the above anomalies associated with its meridian tend to clear within seconds (p.369).

All these facts indicate that meridians and superficial primo vessels are different phenomena. This is because there is no known mechanism whereby a primo vessel could affect the tissue surrounding it, let alone do this dependent on real-time states in the related organ. And also, the flow rate of p-microcells within a primo vessel is 1.08 metres per hour (p.316), so that any changed contents in a primo vessel, originating from within the related organ, would take at least one hour to reach a distal acupoint. Therefore, when the organ's function is normalized with acupuncture, a primo vessel could not possibly communicate this changed organ state to the tissue at the organ's acupoints within a few seconds, so as to remove the above anomalies.

The definition of a meridian

The above facts suggest that a meridian may simply consist of a tract of distal bodily tissue that is affected by organ function.[3]

Note that in this definition I use the term "tract of tissue" rather than "path" or "channel", since this avoids the implication that something flows along a meridian.

The fact that meridians are separate phenomena to primo vessels is supported by research published in 2012 by Xiaoyu Wang *et al.*[4] who found that electro stimulation of Stomach-36 (*Zusanli*) had a significant effect on gastric motility at the duodenum (the tube through which food exits the stomach) but that electro stimulation of a single primo vessel on the stomach organ itself had *no* effect. It was also found that cutting this single primo vessel did not inhibit the effect on the stomach that stimulation of Stomach-36 had. The report concluded that the effects obtained on organ function by simulating acupoints did not appear to depend on the primo vascular system.

All bodily tissue may have this ability

When an organ's stress is strong, the tenderness at its key acupoints becomes correspondingly stronger, extends to a wider diameter, and may also affect the proper function of nearby joints—causing pain and stiffness in the joints. And experiments of my own (p.330) also indicate that a meridian (i.e. the tissue affected by a particular organ's function) extends on either side of a meridian's path by several centimetres, but that the effects diminish with distance.

These facts suggest that there is not a separate, specific type of tissue that is able to interpret organ information conveyed on electromagnetic waves, but that all bodily tissue may have this ability (unless the affected tissue is of a single type, whose malfunction is able to detrimentally affect all other tissue in the area).

Is it the PVS or the meridians that perform the filtering?

The above facts still do not define how the organ information is filtered—so that only a particular organ's information affects the tissue along the path of the organ's related meridian.

Even though primo vessels and meridians are separate entities, the PVS may play a part in creating a meridian. As stated above, the electrical current in the general connective tissue network throughout the body would contain information from *all* the organs, combined into a single wave. However, the sheath of a superficial primo vessel contains connective tissue, and such a primo vessel is said to extend from a single organ and travel along the path of its related meridian. Therefore, the electrical wave in the connective tissue of the primo vessel would only contain organ information from that specific organ. This simple fact provides a mechanism whereby the information from a single organ may influence the tract of tissue along that organ's meridian (and thereby, create the meridian).

But this simple mechanism cannot account for all acupoints, nor for the tissue that is similarly affected by organ function yet is not situated on a meridian. The exceptions are

- the powerful acupoints on the torso (the *back shu* and *front mu* acupoints) which are mostly located on meridians belonging to different organs, so that no superficial primo vessel is present from the organ pertaining to that acupoint;
- the ear acupoints, where acupoints exist for all organs and systems, yet there are no primo vessels, or meridians, extending from those organs to the ears;
- diagnostic tenderness on the palms and soles, where those areas are affected by organ function yet there is no meridian from some of those organs; and
- diagnostic signs on the tongue. These relate to all organs and also quickly respond to treatment, yet there are no meridians thought to be present on the tongue for most of those organs.

There are other situations where bodily tissue is clearly affected by live organ information, yet the filtering involved is not related to superficial primo vessels. These are

- Chinese medicine pulse taking, where the pulse shape is clearly affected by live organ information, and the process only takes place while the practitioner's finger is in place (p.299); and
- the many instances when we are influenced by the energy from another person, and may even feel some of their symptoms (p.363).

In the above situations, filtering of organ information is taking place but by some mechanism that does not involve primo vessels. The following description of "resonance filtering" is another possible mechanism.

Establishing the resonance between distal tissue and a particular organ

It has been demonstrated that bodily tissue interprets organ information conveyed on electromagnetic waves (p.333). Since bodily tissue has this ability now, there is no reason to think that it did not have this ability from early evolution.

If this was the case, and we again (as on page 353 above) imagine a hypothetical creature at the stage of evolution when its digestive organs first began to evolve, the creature at that stage would probably not yet have evolved limbs or a head, nor possibly even rudimentary sense organs. At this stage, information from the creature's newly-evolving organs would have been conveyed to every part of its body via electromagnetic waves (just as it is today; p.365). These waves would have contained information from *all* the organs, combined (that is, not yet filtered in any way). But the creature's bodily tissue, since it was naturally inclined to interpret such information, would have attempted to "make sense" of that information. And it is the process of the tissue "making sense" of the combined organ information that may have resulted in the tissue gradually (possibly over millions of years) organizing itself to reflect that information, and hence, forming the body's shape to reflect this information from the organs.

In such a scenario, the bodily tissue along each meridian would have evolved its form and function to reflect the information from the related organ (in other words, to now only work properly while under the influence of information pertaining to that organ's normal function). Thus, a resonance would have been created between the tissue at each meridian and the normal function of its associated organ. The effect of this resonance would be to now emphasize the organ information from that particular organ (since the tissue was now used to "listening for" that information—and had done this for millions of years). Hence, when exposed to a combined wave of information from *all* the organs, the tissue would pick out only the information from its related organ, which would have the effect of emphasising that information.

Today, when the everyday stresses of modern life cause one of the creature's organs to change its function, then the bodily tissue along that organ's associated meridian would no longer work properly in every way (since evolution designed the tissue to only work properly while under the influence of that organ's normal function), and anomalies may gradually appear at various locations along the meridian, such as tenderness, redness, coldness; or boils may appear; or eventually even stiff and painful joints, or shooting pains (with the anomalies worsening as the organ's stress gradually increases).

Can evolution take place in a person's lifetime?

These anomalies could be viewed as a precursor to a further evolutionary change in that tissue. If the same anomaly continued for an extended period, it is conceivable that the local tissue could modify itself so as to work well under this new organ information (i.e. it would have now evolved to work normally under the particular stress that the organ was under). This process may be the explanation for the bodily malformations that can be seen in some patients in clinic. It may be that with all people, as their life progresses, their body shape tends to change to reflect their particular organ functions. Hence (for example) people may develop malformations on their torso (such as a hump on their back) in the physical location of an organ that suffers "excess-type" stress. In some people, this influence is so strong that it could cause their ribs or spine to eventually change shape, so that their malformation becomes a permanent feature of their torso. On an evolutionary scale, this same process may resemble the process that initially caused our overall body shape to form.

Which came first, the primo vessel or the meridian?

Kim identified that the first system to form in a chick embryo is the PVS, which begins to form before the blood vessels and nerves, which then form around the primo vessels (p.321).

Due to the purpose of the PVS, which is to allow replacement cells to mature for all the main systems and organs in the body (p.322), it is also clear that its existence is essential to maintain the health of all the key parts of a creature's body.

This suggests that the PVS may have been one of the earliest systems to exist in the evolution of the first primitive creatures; and since the superficial primo vessels are thought to now follow the same paths as the meridians, this raises the question: regarding the formation of the limbs, did the primo vessels exist first and then help to create the meridians, or did the meridians determine the shape of a creature's body, including the formation of its limbs; and the PVS, like all other tissue, evolved to follow the shape suggested by the meridians?

At first sight, it seems to make sense that the PVS would have formed first (since its existence is necessary for all the other significant systems in the body to exist), and that it was therefore the superficial primo vessels in the limbs that created the meridians in the surrounding local tissue. But there is a problem with this scenario. It is thought that the superficial primo vessels travel to the skin because the exposure to light is necessary for the p-microcells to mature into organ cells (p.320). But this could take place in any location on the body's surface, particularly on the back of the torso. Therefore, there is no need for the primo vessels to travel along an animal's limbs at all. And more significantly, there is certainly no reason why the limb primo vessels should have organized themselves as the limb meridians are organized, which is remarkable, since it is unlike the organization of any similar system in the body, such as the nervous and blood circulatory systems. The remarkable feature of the meridian layout is that the relationship between the bodily surfaces where the meridians exist exactly matches the hierarchy between the organs associated with those meridians.

All these facts suggest that it was the meridians that came first (i.e. the tissue evolved under the influence of the associated organ). And that, like all other bodily tissue, the primo vessels in that region also followed this same influence and therefore the superficial primo vessel that extended from a particular organ, followed the same path that was established by the local tissue that was under the influence of that organ. In this scenario, resonance filtering (p.356) would have been the guiding mechanism.

This scenario would explain why the superficial primo vessels extended into a creature's limbs (even though this was not necessary to fulfil the function of the PVS) and formed along the paths of the meridians.

However, because the sheaths of the superficial primo vessels can convey organ information from a single organ, it is possible that the superficial primo vessels may also now play a part in filtering organ information in the vicinity of that organ's meridian (p.355).

Note that there is no experimental data to support the above hypotheses, which is why logic is the only tool available to explore such areas.

Some key torso acupoints follow a different pattern

On the back and front of the torso, there are acupoints that are not on an organ's meridian, yet they are key, powerful acupoints related to that organ. In Chinese medicine, these are known as the *back shu* and *front mu* acupoints. This raises the question: how is the organ information filtered to produce these acupoints?

The *back shu* acupoints have no primo vessel link to their organs

In a 2009 study by Hyun-Jung Han *et al.*[5] alcian blue dye was injected subcutaneously into both Bladder-23 (*Shenshu*) acupoints on twenty-four rats. Though these acupoints are located along the bladder meridian on the back, in Chinese medicine the acupoints are known as the *back shu* of the kidneys and have a powerful effect on regulating the kidney function.

Due to the slow flow rate of the primo vascular system (1.08 metres per hour—p.316), two hours were allowed to elapse before the subcutaneous areas of the whole back region and the abdomen were observed. Blue-stained primo vessels were identified but surprisingly these were not located on the kidneys or bladder but instead were located mainly on the surfaces of the duodenum, stomach, liver, the right abdominal wall and the large intestine. The beginning and ending positions of the staining in the primo vessels were not the same in each rat; and it was not possible to investigate the precise position in the skin where the blue dye entered the primo vascular system, nor trace the point at which the stained primo vessels emerged from the skin and entered the abdomen.

Importantly, this study did not detect any primo vessels directly connecting the Bladder-23 acupoints to the kidneys. There is a similar *back shu* acupoint for every organ, and they are all located along the bladder meridian as it passes down the back. However, despite there being no direct primo vessel connection to the related organs, these acupoints have a powerful effect on those related organs.

The *back shu* acupoints are produced by a different influence

How was the organ information filtered and directed to each location to create these acupoints? For most of these acupoints (except the bladder *back shu*), there is no meridian from the related organ, and also no superficial primo vessel. This suggests that these acupoints were produced by a different influence.

It is possible that resonance filtering (p.356) may have contributed to their creation, though this is difficult to visualize. However, these acupoints (and also all the *front mu* acupoints) are situated on the torso in the geographical location of the physical organ (see Table 9 on page 393), and this provides a possible explanation for the source of the influence.

Page 367 describes how organ information can also be conveyed on electromagnetic waves that then radiates from the organ. It is known that such information from the organs is emitted via electromagnetic radiation, since this is the only realistic way to explain how information about each organ's function (or malfunction) is transmitted between people (p.363). In this case, it is the organ's combined wave pattern that is transmitted (reflecting every aspect of the organ and its functions), rather than some filtered aspect, as with the limb acupoints (p.352). And this correlates with the nature of the *back shu* acupoints. Each single acupoint is able to treat any and every aspect of the related organ.

Just as with the diagnostic acupoints on the limb meridians, when an organ is stressed, this also causes its *back shu* acupoint to become tender. But unlike the limb acupoints, when the organ is particularly stressed, the *back shu* acupoint may ache to the point where the patient becomes aware of the aching. This may be because the entire organ's information is focused in one location, whereas with the limb meridians the information seems to be filtered to different acupoints along the length of the entire meridian (p.352). And the same explanation may also account for a situation that sometimes occurs when a practitioner takes a patient's pulses. When the pulse of a stressed organ is taken, the patient sometimes feels tenderness at the pulse location, which ceases when the practitioner lifts their finger. This probably happens because the *entire* organ information is expressed at that one location (p.302).

This suggests that the organ information that influenced the creation of the *back shu* and *front mu* acupoints may have been conveyed directly from the organ via electromagnetic radiation, so that no filtering was necessary. In other words, that these acupoints formed near to the physical location of the related organ. But the notable fact is that they all formed on an existing meridian related to a different organ, in the location where this "borrowed" meridian passed over the physical location of the target organ. It is possible that the acupoints formed on these "borrowed" meridians, rather than forming on the skin location nearest to the geographical centre of the target organ, because this "borrowed" meridian path was already predisposed to the creation of acupoints.

The phenomenon of Chinese medicine pulse taking also supports the above notions. In pulse taking, the information from a specific organ is filtered from the combined wave of all organ information merely by the practitioner placing their finger on the patient's wrist. Each of the practitioner's fingers terminates with a meridian from a particular organ, and it is the presence of that finger that enables the live filtering of a particular organ's information from the combined wave of all organ information (p.302). The fact that such filtering can be performed merely due to the presence of a meridian-organized finger, supports the notion that merely the presence of a particular organ may be able to produce an acupoint on the torso to reflect the information from that organ.

Chapter 20. The electrical current contains organ information

From Chapter 18, it is clear that an electrical current flows through some (or possibly all) areas of the body's connective tissue network; and this current chapter presents evidence that suggests information about the functioning of the organs is conveyed through this current. Indeed it will become clear that such phenomena as the creation of meridians and acupoints, the production of organ pulses, and the effects of acupuncture itself, are only possible *because* such information is carried by this current. This is because all these things require the communication of organ information. In other contexts, such communication is achieved via nerves and through the blood (with hormones, for example); but in the context of acupuncture, these methods are incapable of communicating the information required at the speed required (p.373), whereas an electrical current can readily achieve this.

Other energy forms that convey complex information

That complex information can be contained in a single wave is a familiar concept. For example, this is the mechanism that enables air to carry sound. But it is not easy to picture how information about the internal organs and their activity could be represented in an electrical wave. For example, what form might the wave take that represents the activity of the liver (or its physical condition), and how would this be different from the wave that represents those qualities in the lungs, large intestine, or any other organ? That is, how could such information be conveyed in a series of changes in the level of the wave's voltage? This is difficult to even imagine, let alone describe, so it might be helpful to first look at some other similar systems in nature.

What is a sound wave?

When sound travels through the air in a wave, the air itself often does not move. For example, on a windless day the air outside may be stationary, yet sound still travels through it at around 340 metres per second. In this situation, the air molecules themselves do not move geographically. Instead, the momentum of the original physical object is transferred from molecule to molecule within the air. The original object moves, and its momentum affects the pattern of vibration in the air molecule next to it. This then affects the vibrations of the next air molecule along, which then affects the air molecule next to that one, passing the momentum of the original object from molecule to molecule in the stationary air, until another physical object is reached (which may be your eardrum, for example), and the momentum is then passed to that object, causing it to move just as the original object had done.[1]

But the air around us is capable of containing countless pieces of similar information. There might be an orchestra playing a symphony outdoors, with over one hundred individual instruments; the sound of several players moving on their chairs; the rattle of the key mechanisms on their instruments; perhaps birds singing, the wind blowing, trees rustling, other people moving about, walking, the sound of children playing; and also perhaps a person sat beside us, annoyingly whispering in our ear whilst we were trying to listen to the music or perhaps catch the chatter of the children. All these separate sounds (patterns of vibrations in the air molecules) are merged together into a single wave (a more detailed pattern of vibrations), which passes through the air, hits our eardrum and is then decoded by our mind into all the individual sounds that made up that single detailed wave.

Conveying such information in an electrical current

Though there may be many hundreds of individual sounds making up such a sea of sound, there is no doubt that they are all encoded into a single wave, since this is how an audio system works. All those sounds may be picked up by a single microphone, which consists of a small disc which, when hit by the sound, vibrates. That vibration is then superimposed onto an electrical current and is represented by changes in the voltage level; and these changes are conducted through a wire. At the other end, the changes in voltage are amplified and transferred to a speaker, causing the speaker cone to vibrate exactly as the microphone disc had done, which then transfers the vibrations back into the air as sound waves.

Evidence of organ information in the body's electrical energy

ECG

In 1872, Alexander Muirhead invented the ECG (electro-cardiograph), which is a device that detects the electrical activity in the muscle of the heart as it beats. In a simplistic way, this can then indicate the overall rhythm of the heart and also some types of weaknesses in different parts of the heart muscle. An ECG is thus a crude demonstration that the activity of an organ can be represented in electrical energy, for this is exactly what is happening here.

The Human Energy Field

For well over a century there has been much serious scientific research into the various fields emitted by the human body. That these fields contain information about the functioning and physical state of the organs seems beyond doubt.

Between 1945-1950, Dr. Harold Burr published many papers in the Yale Journal of Biological Medicine, in which he described the electro-dynamic fields emitted by the human body. He described them as informational, since they were able to reveal physical and mental conditions in the patient.[2]

From the 1950's, Dr. Victor Inyushin at Kazakh University in Russia researched the human energy field and published four books on the subject.[3] He suggested the existence of a bioplasmic energy field composed of ions, free protons, and free electrons; and noted that a change in the health of patients or organisms resulted in a shift in the balance of the positive and negative particles within the bioplasma, which was otherwise relatively stable.

In 1962, Dr. Robert Becker, Upstate Medical School, published *The Direct Current Control System*, in which he described his work mapping an electrical field on the body which changed shape and strength with physiological and psychological changes in the patient.

Organ information radiates beyond the body

From the above, it is clear that some type of field radiates from the human body. And from my own firsthand experiences (described below), it is also clear that information about the functioning of the organs is also radiated beyond the body and can be picked up by other people.

Symptom transfer from patient to practitioner

In my acupuncture practice I routinely experience symptoms that have clearly been transferred to me from my patients. These could be muscular or joint pains, or such things as a cough or even hay fever symptoms, all of which are transferred to me when I am simply in the presence of the patient. Some of these sensations I feel fleetingly, for a few seconds, and others linger for a few days. The following are some examples.

Male, aged 50

I treated this patient for a few years, largely for stress. In this session, I inserted the needles and left the room to sit in the waiting area outside (practitioners often leave the room while the treatment takes effect). While sat outside, I felt an acupoint on the right side of my chest become tender: Liver-14 (*Qimen*). I had not needled this acupoint on the patient (I only needled points on his back), but I somehow knew the sensation came from his energy. After the session, I pointed to the acupoint on my chest and asked if he could feel anything around this area. He said that during the treatment he felt an intense aching and burning sensation at that location, which he could still feel now, and he described it as the most intense such experience he had had in all his treatments with me. It appears that the intense sensation he felt was somehow communicated to me while I sat outside the room.

Male, aged 46

I treated this patient for several years, primarily for hay fever. In this session, he came for an acute flare up of his hay fever symptoms, suffering from sneezing and itchy eyes. During the session, when I took his kidney pulse, I felt a soreness around the lower inner edge of my left eye. I pointed this out and he said this was where he got the symptoms most strongly.

I had noticed that when I took the pulse of a particular organ, it was then that I tended to feel some of the patient's symptoms related to that particular organ, and usually those sensations only lasted while I was taking that pulse, and as soon as I lifted my finger from the pulse, my sensing of the patient's related symptoms ceased. In this particular case, the underlying cause of the patient's hay fever was a weakness in his kidney function. Hence it was appropriate that as I took his kidney pulse, it was then that I felt in one of my own eyes this symptom of soreness.

When taking the patient's pulses, the process appears to involve the intermingling of the patient's and practitioner's energy, and the practitioner's body then filtering the patient's energy to obtain the required information (p.304), which I believe is what accounts for these experiences. In the other examples here, this same intermingling happens without there being any physical contact with the patient.

Female, aged 33

This patient sought treatment for low energy. She had a long history of painful periods and digestive problems. During this session, I felt a sensation on my *left* hip, at the acupoint Gallbladder-30 (*Huantiao*). I asked if she had a problem with her *right* hip and she said for the last few days she felt a numbness there. (For some years I noticed that when I sensed a woman's symptoms, I usually felt them on the opposite side on myself; whereas with a man, I felt them on the same side.)

During the session, I also felt an aching sensation on the left side of my neck, at the acupoint Gallbladder-20 (*Fengchi*). When I touched this location on herself and asked her about this, she said she experienced that on both sides of her neck and often found herself rubbing there.

Male, aged 42

I treated this patient for just over a year. At the start of one session, while standing over him, I felt a mild cramp-like sensation above the back of my right knee, on the kidney meridian. I touched this location on him and he said it had been tender for a few days and he was sometimes aware of it when walking. There was no visual clue to this in his gait.

Female, aged 31

I treated this patient for three years for various problems, related to lungs, kidneys, digestion and general stress. During this session, I sensed a weakness on my *left* hip. I pressed this same location on her *right* hip and she said it felt tender there (and there was no tenderness on her left hip). She said she had not noticed the problem recently, but did often get a feeling of tightness on her right hip.

Further examples

Appendix A (p.375), contains many more examples, which are too voluminous to include here.

An explanation for the above phenomena

Taking all the above incidents together (including those starting on page 375), they suggest that certain information about the health of the patient was being communicated to me via their energy, such that I was able to feel the same symptoms the patient felt. But how could this communication take place?

Before answering this, it will be helpful to first provide some basic details about what electrical waves are, and also describe the mechanics of how it may be possible for organ information to be encoded into such waves.

What is an electrical wave?

An electrical direct current (DC) is a steady electrical *potential*. A potential is a large mass of charged particles (such as electrons) that are present in one place. Each of the individual charges has energy, which provides it with the *potential* to do something, and the more charges present, the greater that potential is, which is measured in volts.[4]

These charges may be present within a conductor. For example, if the conductor were a single wire cable of twenty metres in length, the mass of electrons would spread evenly along the length of the entire conductor. All electrons have a field around them, and these fields interact with all other nearby fields, including those of the other electrons. All the electrons (like all particles) constantly move in random directions, until their direction changes due to the interaction of their field with that of another particle, when they shoot off in another random direction. However, this random movement is confined to a tiny area of space, so that the net movement of the electron would usually be zero. In this way, the electrons do not move along the cable, but stay in one place.

If the voltage level at one end of the cable suddenly changes, even by the tiniest amount (either rose or fell), this would affect the first electron, causing it to vibrate to a greater or lesser degree (but remaining, in effect, in the same location). In turn, this increased vibration would then transfer to the next electron, via the interaction of their fields. And this process would pass the increased (or decreased) voltage to every electron in the cable, so that none of them had, in effect, moved, yet they were all now slightly more (or less) excited. Such changes in voltage would propagate along the wire at near to the speed of light.[5]

When such a change of voltage happens repeatedly (perhaps many times a second, for example), the front edge of this change of voltage, propagating along the cable, is an electrical wave.

The amount of times a second the voltage changes is known as the frequency of the wave, measured in hertz (named after Heinrich Hertz, a German physicist); one hertz being one change a second.

How organ information is adopted by an electrical wave

The evidence in Chapter 18 suggests that a steady electrical potential is maintained in the body, which is probably conducted through the connective tissue (as well as elsewhere) via semiconduction.

When physiological activity takes place in the tissue of the body, or even in an individual cell, this may produce a change in the electrical charge of that tissue. Indeed, the bioelectrical activity of tissue is regarded as a reflection of its physiological activity. For example, Figure 26 on page 367 below, shows the bioelectrical activity in a segment of smooth muscle taken from the rectum of a rat.[6] The measurement was made *in vitro*, therefore the bioelectrical activity reflects the spontaneous activity of the muscle tissue.

As can be seen, the activity of the muscle tissue produces rapid spikes of electrical potential (a rapid rise, followed by a rapid fall, then a return to the resting potential). When a steady direct current is conducted through such tissue, these tiny changes in potential would be adopted by that current and propagated along the conductor. That is—assuming this current were conducted through the connective tissue network of an animal's body—these tiny changes in potential would be rapidly transferred to every location in the animal's body via its general connective tissue network. Within a single of the abdominal organs, for example, there are many different types of cells and tissue; and as these function, they would all emit bioelectrical activity in much the same way—but in a different pattern, depending on their individual function. And many aspects of an organ's tissue may also emit such bioelectrical activity when at rest, just as smooth muscle does. Within the organ, all these separate voltage patterns would combine to make a single overall pattern that represents the combined physiological activity of that organ. And this pattern would also vary continuously, just as an organ's functioning does.

When the electrical current from all the separate organs combines, the voltage pattern from each organ would also combine to make a single overall pattern that represents the function of all the organs collectively (much like a sound wave is the combination of all the individual sounds in that vicinity), and this combined wave may be present throughout the general connective tissue network of the entire body.

The propagation speed through connective tissue

The speed (or velocity) that an electrical wave propagates through a substance is dependent on the *relative permittivity* of that substance. And the relative permittivity varies depending on the frequency of the wave—that is, on how many times per second the voltage changes. Once these factors are known, the velocity is given by the following formula.[7]

$$\text{Velocity} = \frac{\text{Speed of light}}{\sqrt{\text{Relative permittivity}}}$$

Table 7 below gives the speed that an electrical wave would travel through human connective tissue, for a range of wave frequencies.* For example, if the voltage only changed once per second, the wave would travel at around 67,000 metres per second.

Table 7. Relative permittivity of connective tissue[8]

Hertz	Relative permittivity	Velocity (m/second)
1	20,058,555	66,938
10	19,921,176	67,168
20	19,517,869	67,859
60	16,056,295	74,817
100	11,857,141	87,062

To put this in perspective, nerve impulses travel in the body at about 100 metres per second. And sound travels through air at about 340 metres per second, which is 3.4 times faster than nerve impulses travel. But a one hertz electrical wave would travel through human connective tissue at almost 200 times the speed of sound.

Since this is significantly faster than nerve impulses travel (670 times faster), any change

* **Note:** There appears to be some confusion amongst acupuncture researchers over the issues of the propagation speed of meridian sensations, electron drift, charge mobility, and electrical signal propagation (which equates to electrical wave propagation), all of which issues are clarified on page 407.

in such voltages can be considered to be transferred to every location in the body instantly (in biological terms). As an example, suppose the pattern of the entire liver's bioelectrical activity had a wave frequency of between one and ten hertz, then any change in that voltage pattern would be transferred to every single acupoint on the gallbladder and liver meridians within 0.00003 seconds (assuming the furthest meridian location from the liver was around two metres). Hence, in biological terms this communication can be considered to be instant.

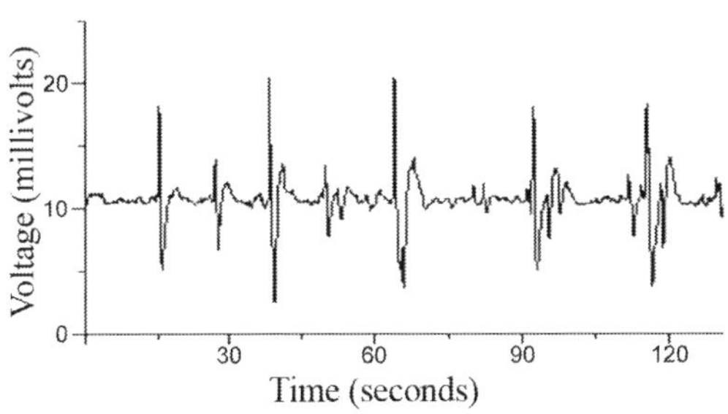

Figure 26. Smooth muscle bioelectrical activity

The transformation into electromagnetic radiation

The semiconduction of direct current through the connective tissue in the vicinity of the meridians has been confirmed (p.342), therefore it is reasonable to assume that the same current also exists throughout the body's *entire* connective tissue network—since an electrical current spreads to every location of a conductive network.

All electrical currents produce two fields around them, an electrical and a magnetic field. These are at right angles to one another, and the two fields combine to form an electromagnetic wave, which itself travels at right angles to the direction of the current flow in the conductor. These phenomena are described by *Maxwell's equations* (James Clerk Maxwell, 1831-1879), which describe how electric and magnetic fields are generated and also how they are altered by each other and by charges and currents.[9]

The body's electromagnetic radiation

Hence, whenever a direct current travels in the body, and its electrical wave represents the bioelectrical activity of the organs, this also produces an electromagnetic wave around the conductor (the particular connective tissue) which also represents that same organ information. But an electromagnetic wave can also break free from the conductor, and it then travels independently of the conductor. When this happens, the wave has become electromagnetic radiation. When this leaves the body, it travels through the air at very near the speed of light.[10]

In this way, theoretically, the body emits waves of electromagnetic radiation which contain information about the bioelectrical activity of all the organs, merged into a single wave.

How another person's energy is able to affect us

Theoretically, the organ information radiated from another person as electromagnetic radiation would be able to influence the electromagnetic fields that surround the connective tissue in our own body, which in turn would then influence the electrical current flowing through that connective tissue. In other words, the wave pattern from the other person's organs would be transferred to the electrical wave in the connective tissue network of our own body.[11] Therefore this principle is able to theoretically explain every one of the examples of symptom transfer listed on pages 363 and 375.

How the information is filtered

The information wave from another person would be added to the direct current in our own body, but it would do this indiscriminately and influence the current *everywhere* in the body—in the general connective tissue network.

But for our own body to make sense of this radiated information, the combined wave of organ information would need to be separated out into the patterns that represent the activity of each organ, such that the liver voltage pattern (for example) mainly affected the tissue along the liver meridian and also the liver organ itself. How might this be achieved?

Since the other person's voltage pattern (representing the information from all their organs, combined into a single wave) was added to the voltage pattern in our own network of connective tissue, the information from the other person's organs would be filtered in the same way that information from our own organs was. This may be achieved via resonance filtering (p.356), where the tract of tissue that constitutes a particular meridian, habitually emphasizes the organ information from that meridian's related organ. This mechanism would, in effect, filter out the information from each organ and present it to the tissue along that meridian—just as the mechanism does to the information from our *own* organs and thereby *creates* the meridians in our body in the first place (p.355).

The effects would usually be subtle

In most people, the influence from the other person's energy would usually be subtle, but it is possible that a sensitive person could be affected in all the ways described in the examples starting on pages 363 and 375 (as indeed, I am).

For example, suppose an improper function in the other person's liver produced a pain on a certain part of their body—such as on the side of their head, around or behind their eyes, on their neck or shoulder, or on the outside of their legs (which are all common areas affected when the liver is stressed—p.113). A particular pattern in their liver's bioelectrical activity would reflect this improper function, and this pattern would be present in the combined wave of all their organ functions. When this wave (now in the form of electromagnetic radiation) was combined with the wave in our own general connective tissue network and then filtered so that it influenced our own liver meridian and also the liver itself, this could then have the same physical effect on our body that a similar improper function in our own liver would have.

This may cause us to feel the same pain the other person felt—though the pain may be weaker in ourselves, since the electrical wave reflecting our *own* liver function would be more resilient than that received from the other person. The pain would perhaps feel like a ghost of the original pain (as it often does in myself when I sense a patient's symptoms) and it may only be felt fleetingly.

Feeling another person's anger

A common example of just this phenomenon is when you enter a room where an angry person is present. Most people would be able to feel the other person's anger, even before being aware of their presence. This could be accounted for by the process suggested above. Anger is often produced when the liver function stagnates (p.109), and it seems that it is this malfunction of the other person's liver that is communicated to our own body as we enter the room; we feel as though our *own* liver function were stagnated (though usually to a weaker degree) and it is this that causes the discomfort within us.

The mood of a society

The above scenario may also provide an explanation for related phenomena, such as mass hysteria or any feeling or mood that tends to pervade a society. When a large portion of the people around us feel a certain way, this would tend to produce that same feeling in ourselves. The news media tends to focus on bad news, so any person who frequently follows the news would be repeatedly given negative messages about the world they live in, which could only create feelings of fear, anxiety, mistrust and so on. And when a large proportion of society is persuaded to adopt such feelings, there would tend to be a general sense of unease, literally pervading the atmosphere, which itself would have a negative impact on *all* people within that society, particularly the more sensitive ones.

The meridian network is an ear for other people's energy

Due to the ability of our own meridian network to, in effect, interpret the organ information our body picks up from other people, the meridian network could be considered an "ear" that is able to listen for organ information from other humans (just as it does in our own body—it "listens" for organ information from our *own* organs).

The communication between organs and acupoints

Organ stress produces physiological effects at acupoints

Acupoints frequently serve a diagnostic function, in that if they are tender when pressed, this indicates the associated organ is not functioning normally and requires treatment. And these acupoints usually cease to be tender immediately the organ is treated, even if those particular acupoints were *not* used in the treatment. The following patient example is an instance of this situation that I noted in a clinical session.

> **Patient example**
> Female, aged 35. This patient usually attended for monthly maintenance treatments. During one session, I pressed the acupoint Gallbladder-41 (*Zulingqi*) on her *left* foot and she said it was extremely tender. I then pressed the acupoint Gallbladder-34 (*Yanglingquan*) below her *right* knee and she said this was also tender but not as much. I needled the acupoint Gallbladder-34 below her *right* knee, and a few seconds later I again pressed the acupoint Gallbladder-41 on her *left* foot. Even though I had not needled that acupoint, she said, "That's amazing; it doesn't feel tender at all now."

The example is typical. Since noticing this phenomenon I have tested it countless times on many patients, featuring various organs and acupoints, and found that a similar outcome occurs each time.

From the Chinese acupuncture point of view, the explanation for what was happening here is this. Both acupoints were tender because either the patient's liver or gallbladder were stressed (with this particular patient this was a typical situation, due to her lifestyle). Either acupoints *could* treat the condition—as could several other acupoints at various locations on the body. I needled the second acupoint, which quickly normalized the function of both her liver and gallbladder; and since the functions of these organs were now normal, the other acupoints around her body associated with the organs ceased to be tender, even though they had not been needled.

This demonstrates that the tenderness felt at acupoints is the result of stress in the related organ (in other words, improper function), and that this situation was communicated to the acupoint by information from the organ, since as soon as the organ stress was cleared, the organ's changed state was immediately communicated to all the related acupoints, which cleared the tenderness.

What mechanism could explain this communication, and also explain *how* the communication could produce tenderness in the local tissue at an acupoint?

Organ stress creates tissue stress at acupoints and meridians

The experimental data on pages 322-333 demonstrates that bodily tissue interprets organ information conveyed on electromagnetic waves. When an organ is stressed (is not functioning properly), this information is communicated body-wide via electromagnetic waves, and when the local tissue at the organ's acupoints interprets this information, this causes the local tissue to also cease to function properly. Apart from tenderness at an organ's key acupoints, other phenomena routinely encountered in Chinese medicine include the skin at key acupoints (or along sections of a meridian) feeling cold to the touch, appearing red, rough, or dry; or for pimples, boils, or even shooting pains to eventually occur. The dysfunction may also spread to nearby tissue, causing joints to become weak, painful, or stiff.

The exact signs or symptoms at a meridian usually mirror the type of stress in the related organ, where (for example) redness, increased skin temperature or dry skin indicate "heat" (in Chinese medicine terms—p.307); shooting pains indicate stagnation of function (typically experienced in relation to the liver—p.113); and reduced skin temperature indicates poor function.

This suggests that the local tissue adopts an anomaly that resembles the type of stress in the related organ. Therefore, when an organ is stressed, the communication is not limited to causing the distal tissue at its acupoints to also cease to function normally, but the tissue appears to intelligently duplicate the type of stress in the organ.

Yet when the organ's function is corrected with acupuncture, this new information (of now functioning normally) is also immediately communicated to the organ's related meridian and acupoints, and the local tissue in those locations also returns to normal function. Such anomalies as redness, heat, coldness, aching, or shooting pains tend to clear within seconds; but other signs, such as rough or dry skin, pimples or boils, may take several days to clear as the local tissue repairs itself.

Psoriasis lesions can occur due to this cause

In my own experience, it is common for psoriasis lesions to appear in locations where the skin recently suffered a trauma, such as an abrasion, pimple or anything similar. It seems that this trauma to the skin is then expressed as a psoriasis lesion in susceptible patients. And I have noticed in several psoriasis patients (including myself) that when a particular organ is stressed, this can cause a new psoriasis lesion centred on the very acupoint that would best treat the particular stress in that organ. The skin at that location suffered no recent trauma, and the only stimulus that prompted the lesion was the changed organ information expressed at the acupoint, now reflecting the stress in that organ. This suggests that when the local tissue at the acupoint interprets this stressed organ information, the effect this produces in the tissue is comparable to the effect that a small wound could produce. That is, it certainly causes the local tissue to cease to function normally.

Other anomalies experienced during an acupuncture treatment

During an acupuncture treatment, sensations are often felt. These could include the sensation induced at the acupoint due to the treatment. At other times, the patient may feel a tingling sensation flowing a short way along the meridian near to the needled acupoint; or they may feel warmth apparently flowing along a meridian; or sometimes a sensation akin to an electric shock is felt shooting along an entire meridian. All these sensations can also be accounted for by the bodily tissue's interpretation of organ information, and are explained on page 55.

The speed of acupuncture's effect on the organs

In recent decades, when academics have attempted to fathom how acupuncture may work, the most significant factor overlooked is the speed of its effect on the organs. In an acupuncture practice, an insight into the speed of this effect can be obtained by monitoring the patient's pulses before and after a needle is inserted. Using this technique, I have frequently noted that acupuncture corrects an organ malfunction within around one second of the acupoint being stimulated. The meridian distance from an acupoint to an organ varies, but an average of around one metre would be a fair estimate. This means that the communication from the acupoint to the organ would need to travel at around one metre per second, or faster.

However, the experimental data referred to on page 324 provides an indicator that the communication between an organ and its related acupoints travels at a much faster rate than this. Within the limitations of the experimental design, there was no discernible delay between the chilled water reaching the inner surface of the stomach, and the response at left Stomach-36 (*Zusanli*).

Theoretically, an electrical wave travels through human connective tissue at around 67,000 metres per second (p.366). However, the above experiment also established that there is a variable delay for bodily tissue to interpret organ information conveyed on an electromagnetic wave (p.326), which means that this same delay would be present when the tissue of an organ interprets the information conveyed from a stimulated acupoint. This variable delay may play a large part in determining the speed of acupuncture's effect on an organ at any one time.

Until the speed of acupuncture's effect on organ function can be accurately measured, the rate of one metre per second is a good rule of thumb for the minimum rate of communication between a stimulated acupoint and the related organ.

Acupuncture's effect is unrelated to the physiological purpose of the PVS

The liquid in a primo vessel flows at around 0.3 millimetres per second (p.316), which means it would take 56 minutes to travel one metre. But the most significant element of the liquid's content, the p-microcells, circulate much slower than this, since they mature within primo nodes. For example, liver p-microcells can take around 120 hours to fully mature into a new liver cell (p.316). This makes it clear that neither this primo fluid, nor any element of its content, could play any part in acupuncture's effect of correcting organ malfunction—since they are not capable of achieving the required speed of communication.

Another fact also supports this conclusion. The purpose of the entire primo vascular system is to enable p-microcells to mature into the specific cells required by each organ (p.322). But since acupuncture tends to correct improper organ function in around one second or less, it is clear that the improper organ function could not have been due to a cellular problem within the organ, since if it were, it could not have been corrected so quickly.

How acupuncture works

The intelligent tissue hypothesis

Organ information is communicated body-wide on electromagnetic waves (pp.361-368). Bodily tissue constantly interprets this information (p.333), which is filtered so that each organ's information is emphasized along the path of its meridian. This filtering is probably achieved via resonance filtering (p.356), which causes the tissue in a meridian location to emphasize the organ information from the meridian's related organ. The result is that each organ's states are reflected in the tissue at its related meridian and acupoints.

When an organ functions improperly (i.e. is stressed in any way), it is this mechanism that causes the local tissue at its key acupoints to also fail to function normally, producing any of various anomalies. The key acupoints may be tender when pressed; or the skin may feel cold to the touch, or feel unusually warm; the skin may appear reddened; or boils, painful joins, dry or rough skin, or even shooting pains may eventually occur along the meridian (phenomena familiar to Chinese medicine practitioners). The type of anomaly usually mirrors the type of stress within the organ, where (for example) red, dry or itchy skin indicates "heat" in the organ; or cold skin indicates poor organ function, or shooting pains indicates stagnated organ function.

By needling such key acupoints (those where the anomaly caused them to be tender when pressed), this tends to relax the local tissue (i.e. causes it to shed its borrowed stress), and thus returns it to its normal function.[12]

When the tissue at a key acupoint is caused to relax, this "return to normal function" is also communicated body-wide on the same electromagnetic waves. The wave pattern of this transformation would be specific to a particular organ (the organ that caused the anomaly at the needled acupoint), and when this pattern (of the tissue shedding the stress that was borrowed from that particular organ) reaches that organ, this appears to persuade the organ to follow this same pattern and it also returns to normal function. This may happen simply because the tissue in the organ *wants* to function normally (in the way it has habitually done for millennia), and the electrical wave pattern guides the way, since the information in the wave transforms from that particular organ's stressed state, back to its normal state (just as happens at the stimulated acupoint).

While the organ is transforming from its stressed state, back to normal function, this transformation is also conveyed body-wide on electromagnetic waves and reflected at the stimulated acupoint (and sometimes elsewhere along the same meridian), which is probably the explanation for the typical "needle sensation" (known as "de chi" in Chinese medicine); see page 55.

Alternative hypotheses

There are several other hypotheses on how acupuncture works. However they have usually been devised by researchers who are not familiar with the many common phenomena associated with acupuncture treatments, with the result that their hypotheses are usually incapable of accounting for those phenomena.

The most significant factor usually overlooked is the rapid speed of acupuncture's effect on the organs; and also that the communication takes place in *both* directions (from the organ to the acupoint, as well as from the acupoint to the organ) and at the same rapid speed (as demonstrated in the patient example on page 369).

These factors alone make most other proposed hypotheses untenable, but there are also other similar shortcomings.

The neural hypothesis

John C Longhurst champions the neural hypothesis,[13] which suggests that "the clinical influence of acupuncture is transmitted primarily through stimulation of sensory nerves that provide signals to the brain, which processes this information and then causes clinical changes associated with the treatment". But it is clear that this hypothesis is unable to account for acupuncture's effects, for many reasons.

There are sensory nerves around all acupoints that *could* indicate to the brain when that location was stimulated. But there is no direct neural input from the brain or spinal cord *to* the abdominal organs, which are largely self governing (p.88). Therefore the brain could only correct an organ's function via messages sent through the blood (such as hormones). But the flow rate of blood is around twelve centimetres per second and it takes around twenty seconds to circulate the body (p.404), which would make it impossible for this mechanism to correct an organ's function in around one second. And this proposed mechanism would not allow for communication from the organs *to* the distal acupoints at all, again making it impossible for this hypothesis to account for acupuncture's effects. These points are discussed in detail on page 401, along with other further shortcomings.

The connective tissue hypothesis

This hypothesis (proposed by Helene Langevin and Jason Yandow in 2002[14]) focuses heavily on the concept of "needle grasp", which it supposes may produce cellular changes that propagate along connective tissue planes in hypothetical channels, which are also assumed to exist but have never been identified.

This proposed mechanical signal is equated to the occasional experience that some patients sometimes feel—of a tingling sensation slowly radiating along the meridian near to the needle. But the propagation speed of this phenomena is around 18 centimetres per minute,[15] which is far too slow for this to be able to account for acupuncture's effects on the organs, which is communicated at the rate of around (at least) one metre per second. But also, the hypothesis's central concept of "needle grasp" is itself absent in many acupuncture treatments given by an experienced acupuncturist, so that it could not possibly account for acupuncture's effects—it not even being present. These points are discussed in detail on page 406.

The low hydraulic resistance hypothesis

In 2008, Zhang *et al.* proposed the low hydraulic resistance meridian theory. [16] This study found that "interstitial fluid flows freely in meridians and appears to play an important role in regulating extracellular contents". The flow rate was measured at about four millimetres per second.

This outcome is reminiscent of the studies on the primo vascular system, by both Bong-Han Kim and also more recent researchers, who found it to be a circulatory system whose fluid flowed at the rate of about 0.3 millimetres per second, which equates to 18 millimetres per minute (p.316).

In both the above cases, this flow rate is far too slow for it to be responsible for the rapid communication between an acupoint and its associated organ. This means that the "low hydraulic resistance" hypothesis, could not possibly account for acupuncture's effect on the organs.

Other related research issues are discussed on page 407.

Appendix A. Further examples of symptom transfer

Further examples of the transfer of symptoms from patient to practitioner are given here. These supplement the examples given on page 363.

Female, aged 58

I treated this patient for a few years. In this session, she sat in the treatment room and I immediately felt a sensation in my throat, at about the level of my Adam's apple; it was a tickling sensation and there was also a tightness. I pointed to this location on myself and asked if she had a cough at this location and described the sensation I felt. She said that was the exact location and type of cough she had recently. On another occasion with this same patient, when standing near to her I felt a tightness on my right hip. She had not complained of this, but when I asked her about it, pointing to the location on myself (but on my left hip—p.364), she said she had a stiff hip recently, exactly where I was pointing.

Male, aged 24

I treated this patient for migraines, hay fever and allergies. During this session, I felt a very localized itching on the inner corner of my left eye. I told him I could feel the irritation in his eye, and with the tip of my little finger, pointed to the inside edge of my left eye. He said that was exactly where he had felt it. It is important to note that there was no visual clue to this, such as any redness or swelling of his eye; and also that (until I felt it on myself) I would not have expected the *inside* edge of his eye to be affected but would rather have expected the outside edge to be affected. Hence, the itching I felt on the inside edge of my eye was unexpected.

Female, aged 56

This patient sought treatment for a shoulder pain. During the session, I felt a sudden, fleeting dizziness, which lasted for about a second. The sensation was unusual and one I had not felt before. I asked her if she ever felt dizzy, and she said recently she felt dizzy a few times a day, lasting for a few seconds at a time.

A nearby male, aged around 40

I was sat in a corridor at the clinic, taking a break, when a man walked in and started talking to the clinic manager, who was sat in the adjoining room, about six metres from me. As the man leant over the manager's desk, talking to him, I felt a tickling sensation in my throat—at the acupoint Ren-22 (*Tiantu*)—and started coughing. I had no cough at any time near that day and did not routinely cough. When the man left the shop, the sensation cleared from my throat. I mentioned to the manager that I thought the man had a cough and he said the man seemed like a heavy smoker since he could smell the tobacco whilst he was talking to him. It was notable that I could sense the man's symptom from the adjoining room at a distance of about six metres, when the man was not even addressing me and I was paying him no attention. Of course, I could not verify with the man that he had a cough, but together with all my similar experiences (which I *could* verify with patients), I have no doubt that the sensation in my throat was one of the man's symptoms which my body sensed.

Male, aged 41

This patient initially sought treatment for panic attacks, which cleared with treatment; he also suffered hay fever since childhood. On this occasion, as I stood over him during the treatment, I felt a burning in my eyes; he was suffering hay fever at that time. As I then took his kidney pulse, I felt a twinge in my lower back. I asked if he felt any twinges there and he said he was feeling one right then (such back pains are often due to poor kidney function). At the end of the treatment I felt an ache behind my right eye. I asked him about this and he said he often gets that.

This is another phenomenon I frequently notice. I not only sometimes feel a symptom my patient is currently suffering, but I can also feel the symptoms the patient is *prone* to get, or has had recently.

Male, aged 38

I treated this patient for several years, for various problems. In this session, he had recently had laser eye surgery and his eyes were still adjusting. He suffered intense pain and itching in the days following surgery. Apart from other acupoints, I needled two points near his ankle to address these issues: Gallbladder-37 (*Guangming*) and Gallbladder-44 (*Zuqiaoyin*). I then took his liver pulse, and as I did so I felt a tingling sensation on my own right leg, between these two acupoints. This sensation is what patients often feel around an acupoint during treatment, and the sensation I felt was clearly the sensation the patient was then experiencing.

There is a close functional relationship between the gallbladder and liver (and also, both these pulses are taken at the same position on the patient's left wrist), which explains why I felt this sensation when taking his liver pulse.

Male, aged 41

I treated this patient for about six months. In this session, as I felt his lung pulse, I sensed a dry, tickly sensation in my throat, at the level of Stomach-9 (*Renying*). I mentioned this to him and he said he forgot to mention it but he could feel that right now.

Female, aged 29

I treated this patient for several years, initially for panic attacks, depression, stress, and painful periods. During this one particular session, I needled an acupoint on her back:

Bladder-23 (*Shenshu*) which treats the kidneys. As I needled this point, I felt a tingling sensation at the Kidney-3 (*Taixi*) acupoint on my own right ankle, which is on the kidney meridian. I mentioned this to the patient, touching the point on her left ankle, and she said this was exactly where she felt a tingling sensation just as I needled the acupoint on her back.

Female, aged 75

This patient sought treatment for back pains she had for many years, and also vertigo, which she suffered for about five years. For about two days after her first treatment, I felt a part of her vertigo symptoms. I felt light-headed, as if about to fall over. I had never before felt this, and have not felt it since.

Female, aged 41

I treated this patient for a few weeks, primarily for high blood pressure. At the end of this session, I felt a shooting pain at the back of my *right* shoulder, near to Small-intestine-10 (*Naoshu*). I described this to her (but referred to her *left* shoulder) and she said she had been getting a problem there.

Male, aged 43

This patient sought treatment for stiff joints in his fingers and arms. After treating him, I felt a heavy feeling along the top of both my arms on the large-intestine meridian, which lasted for two days. A few days after this, the patient phoned me and while listening to his voice, this same sensation returned on both my arms. After the call, I felt my arms and noticed that the acupoint Large-intestine-10 (*Shousanli*) was tender. About two hours later, the heavy feeling in my arms had gone and the acupoint was no longer tender.

The implications of this are that either the pattern of organ malfunction was conveyed by qualities in his voice as we spoke on the phone, or that the energy that radiates between people can travel considerable distances. Chinese medicine recognises that the tone of a person's voice can indicate their main organ malfunction (p.111).

A third possibility (which cannot be ruled out) is that when talking to him on the phone, I recalled his energy, and being a sensitive person, this was enough to reproduce his symptoms within me, including the obstruction at the acupoint Large-intestine-10, since this seemed to become tender in response to the phone call.

An unknown patient

While waiting for a patient to arrive, I was stood in another treatment room, watching the traffic through the window, when I felt an acupoint near my left elbow activate; I felt a burning sensation there. The acupoint was Heart-3 (*Shaohai*), which is an acupoint that would be tender on a patient suffering emotional distress.

I realized that a talk-therapy session had been recently conducted in that room and I was stood next to the chair where the patient would have sat. As I looked down at the chair, it seemed to me that the sensation in my arm was connected with the chair; and it seemed clear I was picking up the energy of the patient, which was somehow left behind in the chair, and that the patient was suffering emotional distress while sat in that chair—and that the acupoint Heart-3 would have been tender on the patient if I could have tested it.

Female, aged 41

I treated this patient for stress and neck tension. During this session, I felt a burning sensation around my *right* ear (on the lymphatic-system meridian*). She suffered a painful neck and shoulder on her *left* side. I traced the lymphatic-system meridian on the left side of her neck (which travels over the side of the shoulder, up onto the neck and circles the ear) and she said the pain she feels often radiates up the side of her neck to her ear, exactly where I was touching.

Male, aged 40

I treated this patient for a few years, primarily for joint stiffness. He recently fell over and hurt his left wrist, which I treated in this session. I needled some acupoints on his left wrist, using acupoints on the small-intestine meridian; and immediately after, I felt a tingling sensation on my own left wrist and arm, travelling along the small-intestine meridian, and sometimes also shooting pains around Small-intestine-9 (*Jianzhen*). These sensations lasted for a few minutes, gradually fading away.

Male, aged 32

This patient sought treatment for muscular pain and stress. In the previous treatment, I needled Pericardium-6 (*Neiguan*) and after the session this same acupoint ached on myself for about an hour. And in this current treatment, I needled the acupoint Heart-7 (*Shenmen*) on his left wrist, and again, after the session I felt a sensation like cramp in my left little finger—which is where the heart meridian flows to beyond the acupoint Heart-7.

Female, aged 33

This was her third treatment session with me. During the session, I stood over her and felt an aching sensation on the *right* side of my forehead, at Stomach-8 (*Touwei*). I asked her if she had any headaches in the last few days, on the *left* side of her head. She thought about it for a moment, then said she had but she had forgotten about it. I touched her head at Stomach-8, on the left of her forehead, and she said this was exactly where she had felt the pain.

* This meridian is also called the *San jiao*, or triple-burner meridian, etc.

Appendix B. The daily cycle of organ activity – midnight to noon, ebb and flow

Chinese medicine recognises that the activity of the abdominal organs has a daily rhythm. The strength of an organ's function rises and falls throughout a twenty-four hour cycle. It peaks in a particular two hour period, and twelve hours later reaches its weakest.

This theory is known as *zi wu liu zhu* 子午流註 ("Midnight to noon, ebb and flow"). It postdates the *Nei Jing* and *Nan Jing*, and was described in a work titled *Zi wu liu zhu zhen jing* ("Zi and wu ebb and flow needle classic"), compiled in 1153 by Yan Ming-guang.[1] The two hour peak for each organ is shown in Table 8 below.

Table 8. The "organ clock"

Time	Most active organ
1 a.m. – 3 a.m.	liver
3 a.m. – 5 a.m.	lungs
5 a.m. – 7 a.m.	large intestine
7 a.m. – 9 a.m.	stomach
9 a.m. – 11 a.m.	pancreas
11 a.m. – 1 p.m.	heart
1 p.m. – 3 p.m.	small intestine
3 p.m. – 5 p.m.	bladder
5 p.m. – 7 p.m.	"kidneys"
7 p.m. – 9 p.m.	pericardium
9 p.m. – 11 p.m.	lymphatic system
11 p.m. – 1 a.m.	gallbladder

In between the highest and lowest points, it is clear that the strength of each organ's function gradually rises and falls, rather than there being a sudden drop off after and before its peak. This is because the two hour period that marks its lowest point is felt symptomatically by many patients (p.381 below), and if the level dropped off suddenly—before and after the peak—patients would not be able to clearly feel the two hour weakest period, twelve hours after the peak; instead the weakest period would last for almost twenty-two hours.

The following figure depicts the approximate change in the strength of an organ's function throughout the day (taking the lungs as an example).

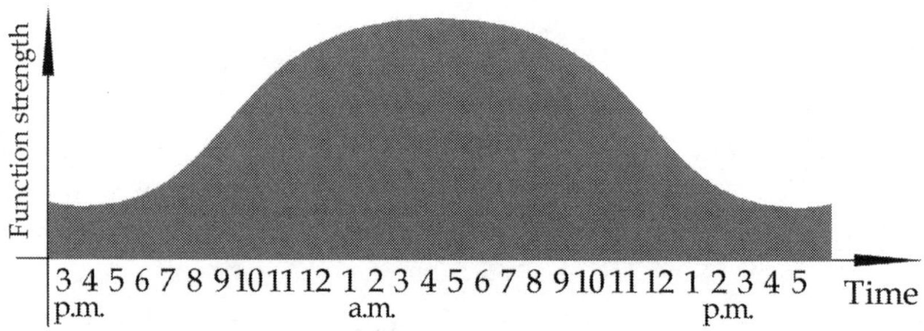

Figure 27. The daily cycle of lung resources

As shown, the lung function is at its weakest between the hours of three and five p.m. and the function strength gradually increases until it reaches its strongest between the hours of three and five a.m., when it then gradually diminishes until it reaches its weakest again at three p.m. the following day.

Why organs peak at certain times

When considering the role each organ plays, it is possible to understand why each organ's peak activity is timed to occur when it does.

The liver is probably responsible for providing the energy that drives the daily bodily repair tasks which appear to primarily take place while we sleep (p.343); hence its function is at its strongest between one and three a.m., ensuring that maximum energy is available for this essential role.

The lungs are the other organ that play an essential role in the generation of energy (in providing oxygen to enable the body's cells to produce energy—p.336), so the lung function peaks after the liver's, between three and five a.m. (for the same reason).

Generally, the *yang* organs (*fu*) tend to service their associated *yin* organs (*zang*), so in this "organ clock" the *yang* organs are always placed next to their paired *yin* organs. This places the large-intestine after the lungs, peaking between five and seven a.m. This also makes sense in terms of the daily rhythms, suggesting that throughout evolution, mammals usually had a bowel movement first thing in the morning, just prior to starting the digestive process on each new day.

The next organs to peak are the stomach and pancreas, between seven and nine a.m. and nine and eleven a.m. respectively. This places the digestive function at its strongest between these hours, so that we can most effectively digest the food necessary to provide our energy for the remainder of the day.

The heart then peaks between eleven a.m. and one p.m. This is when the highest demands would normally be placed on the blood circulation, for two reasons. This is when we might be at our most physically active, following eating (which provides us with our fuel for the day); and also the circulation would be required to assist in the digestion of food and the transportation of the fuel needed to generate the energy in our muscles. The small intestine peaks between one and three p.m., following the heart, since this is a *yin-yang* pairing. But also, the small intestine assists the heart in these circulatory functions, since the small-intestine is the interface between the pancreas and blood, allowing the nutrients to be absorbed into the blood, so that the heart can then circulate them.

The "kidney"/bladder pairing peaks next, between three and seven p.m. (the bladder first, then the kidneys). The kidneys are mainly concerned with our immediate and long-term survival. They are responsible for providing the drive for all the organs, for regulating the body's use of energy, and they also provide an emergency energy boost when needed (the adrenaline release). This is the time of day when a none-food boost may be most needed; we are still active but have already eaten and digested our main meal (which evolution clearly expected humans to eat between seven and eleven a.m., which is when the digestion peaks), so that our immediate energy supply may be running low. Our survival is clearly a top priority, and placing the kidney function peak at this time gives us the best chance of meeting whatever demands we might face in our remaining hours of activity (with an adrenaline release).

The pericardium/lymphatic system pairing peaks next, between seven and eleven p.m. These organs are concerned with our protection. This is the time of our remaining waking hours, after we have been physically active but before we sleep. Earlier in the day, when our daytime energy was higher, this afforded us some protection. But when that energy has declined, we are more vulnerable, which may be the reason why these protective organs function at their strongest during these hours.

And to complete the daily cycle, the gall-bladder peaks between eleven p.m. and one a.m., since it is paired with the liver, which peaks between one and three a.m.

The symptomatic clues to each organ's peaks and troughs

By three p.m., the lung function has diminished to its weakest, and people with poor lung function usually feel a sharp drop in their energy at this time of day. They often describe it as being like "hitting a wall", and once their poor lung function is successfully treated they no longer experience this drop in their energy.

Between five and seven a.m. the "kidney" function is at its weakest, and patients with poor kidney function will often experience their worst asthma or hay fever attacks at this time of day (and if the poor function is only slight, they may *only* experience attacks at this time of day). Poor kidney function is the usual underlying cause of asthma (of the type where it is hard to breathe in) or hay fever.

Between three and five a.m. the bladder function is at its weakest. The bladder and "kidneys" are intimately associated, and problems associated with the bladder (such as frequent and urgent urination) are usually present when patient's have poor kidney function. Patient's with this condition will often wake between these hours with an urgent need to urinate.

The stomach and pancreas function are at their strongest between seven and eleven a.m., and patient's with poor pancreas function usually find they can mentally digest facts most clearly in the morning, and as the day progresses, this ability rapidly declines (these organs provide our ability to mentally digest facts—p.71). At eleven a.m., the end of this peak, people whose organs are properly regulated also feel a strong pang of hunger, which marks the point when their digestion is at its strongest; consequently, the tradition has evolved of taking "elevenses" (the mid-morning snack) at this time. From the body's point of view this is a signal for us to eat our main meal of the day, but due to the way our lives are organized in most developed countries, the main meal is usually taken much later.

The large intestine function peaks between five and seven a.m., which is immediately prior to the time when many people feel the urge to have a bowel movement.

The liver function peaks between one and three a.m., and the liver provides us with the ability to think creatively and thus solve problems (p.107). For this reason, we often wake in the morning to find that any problems that were on our mind appear to have sorted themselves out while we were asleep. It is the liver that performed this function. The knowledge of this phenomenon has become fossilized in the language with phrases such as "sleep on it".

Appendix C. Tongue diagnosis

On page 76, I introduced the subject of tongue diagnosis in Chinese medicine and described some features present when a patient has poor pancreas function. This Appendix summarizes the common diagnostic signs on the tongue as routinely used in Chinese acupuncture.

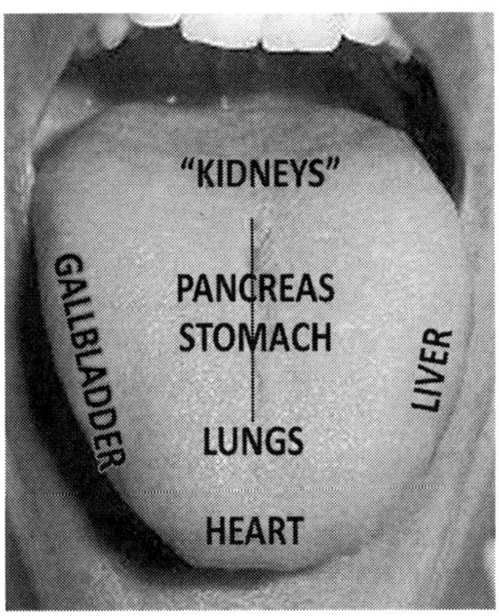

Figure 28. Diagnostic areas of the tongue

The above figure shows the areas of the tongue relating to each of the main organs. For example, when a person has stagnated liver function, this would be reflected on either the left side of their tongue, or frequently on both sides (since the function of the liver and gallbladder are so interrelated). The sides would most often appear reddened, or they may have darker "blood spots" or sometimes some other form of discolouration.[1] With stagnated liver function, the whole body of the tongue would also tend to have "stagnation dots" scattered about it, which are about one millimetre in diameter, slightly redder than the background and without a tongue coating.

With *all* organ conditions, I have noticed that any reddened area of the tongue body usually clears during the treatment session when the corresponding organ is treated.

When a person has "Heart fire" (p.454), due to emotional problems, or poor heart function, then the tip of their tongue would usually appear reddened.

When they have poor pancreas function (which is often accompanied by poor stomach function), the central region of their tongue may have a dip, and the whole body of the tongue would appear swollen, usually with teeth indentations along both sides, which are due to the simple fact that the tongue is so swollen (the tongue shown in Figure 28 above is swollen). After eating a large meal, the central region would also often become reddened, which clears as the stomach completes its part in the digestive process. This increased stomach activity, when compared to the "rest" state, might be viewed as "Stomach heat" (p.457), which explains why the "stomach" area of the tongue develops a reddened body colour after eating.

When a person has poor stomach function, there would also be a central crack on the tongue (as shown by the line in Figure 28 above), with the depth and width of the crack reflecting the degree of the weakness—the weaker their stomach function, the deeper the crack. This is quite noticeable in clinic when poor pancreas function is treated (which also treats the stomach); as the patient improves between treatment sessions, any central crack in their tongue tends to gradually diminish, until it disappears.

When a person has poor heart function, there would also usually be a central crack, which often extends to the very tip of the tongue.

The fur coating of the tongue can also reflect various states. Generally, it indicates the strength of a person's digestion; and when poor pancreas function becomes marked, the coating would often be thin, or not present at all. A thin white coating is the normal state. But the coating can sometimes become suddenly very thick, which would usually indicate the presence of a strong pathogen (such as influenza). If there is a persistent thickened coat, this usually indicates the presence of *dampness* or *phlegm* (p.76 and 202), which are both pathogens, hence the thick white coat. And a yellow coat would indicate the presence of *heat*. This would occur when the patient has a fever; or it could be due to the presence of *damp heat* (p.181).

The "root" of the coating can also sometimes be absent in patches, which appear like patches of raw flesh. This indicates the condition of "Yin deficiency" (p.200), which this book translates as: "internal production of heat". In Chinese medicine, this sign is known as a "peeled" tongue.

The surface of the tongue can also have cracks in various regions, which tend to indicate the condition of dryness (often long-standing) affecting the organ whose region the cracks appear in. For example, these are probably most frequently seen in the lung region, where the patient has long-standing poor lung function, which has affected the *yin* of the lungs (that is, the fabric of the lungs themselves, rather than simply resulting in weak function).

The general tongue body colour can also indicate various states. A pale body colour would usually indicate poor quality blood (p.199). Whereas a pinkish colour would be normal. If the body colour were too red, this would again be an indicator of *heat* being present. When *heat is* present, the tongue would usually also appear too dry. Whereas if the tongue appeared too wet, this could indicate a "deficient" condition (p.453).

The tongue is a very reliable diagnostic tool, and together with the taking of the pulses and asking the patient questions about the symptoms they might or might not have, these three techniques constitute the cornerstone of Chinese acupuncture diagnosis.

Appendix D. More detail of the body's electrical properties

Using magnetism to create electricity

There are many ways of creating an electrical current—a flow of electrons. A common method is to utilize the force of magnetism. When a wire is passed through a magnetic field, the combination of the magnetic field and the physical movement, causes a flow of electrons to occur along the wire (no-one knows exactly *why* this happens; we only know it does). This mysterious phenomenon can thus be used to convert a physical force (the movement of the wire) into an electrical force (the flow of electrons through the wire). This is how a coil microphone works, or the turbines that produce electricity in power stations, whether the turbines are moved by wind, the power of flowing water or the steam produced when water is heated by the burning of coal or by a nuclear reaction (a nuclear power plant uses the nuclear reaction purely to generate heat, which is then used to produce steam, which turns a turbine to generate the electricity). And it so happens that this process can also be utilized in reverse, so that if an electrical current is passed through a wire that is suspended in a magnetic field, the current interacts with the magnetic field to produce a physical force acting on the wire (the direction of movement is determined by *Faraday's Law*). This is how an electric motor works, or a hi-fi speaker.

The creation of electricity within the body

An electric current may also be created using a chemical reaction, which is how the body creates electricity. But before explaining this fully, it will be helpful to first summarize some basic facts about chemistry.

Atoms, elements, compounds and molecules

There are 118 different atoms (currently known), which are combined to make up the entire contents of the universe. Each atom is made up of different numbers of neutrons, electrons and protons. Curiously, every single electron is the same, as is every single proton and neutron; but when these three identical particles are combined in different numbers, this somehow causes the resultant atom to adopt different qualities and behaviour. For example, when an atom consists of:

- a nucleus of 8 protons and 8 neutrons, with 8 electrons orbiting in two shells (2 in the inner and 6 in the valence shell*), this is an atom of oxygen;
- a nucleus of 26 protons and 30 neutrons, with 26 electrons orbiting in four shells (2 in the inner, 8 in the second, 14 in the third and only 2 in the valence shell), this is an atom of iron; and
- a nucleus of 79 protons and 118 neutrons, with 79 electrons orbiting in six shells (in the pattern of 2, 8, 18, 18, 32 and only one in the valence shell), this is an atom of gold.

All the above atoms are made up of these same three basic particles (protons, neutrons and electrons), but by mixing them together in different numbers and combinations, this determines the nature of that particular atom. This nature is most dramatically influenced by the number of protons, so that adding or subtracting just a single proton produces a considerable effect. For example, mercury has 80 protons, but if one proton were removed from a mercury atom, it would then become an atom with 79 protons, which is a gold atom.

The 118 possible atoms are known as *elements*, since they are the smallest building blocks used to make up any substance. For example, oxygen is an element, since it is made up from a single atom; and this single atom is then known as a *molecule* of oxygen. These elements can be combined together to make up any number of other substances. When two elements are combined in this way, this is known as a *compound*. For example, if one atom of oxygen is combined with two atoms of hydrogen, this then creates water (whose chemical formula is H_2O); and these three atoms are then known as a *molecule* of water.

How the body converts food into energy (the mitochondrion's story)

A *mitochondrion* is a tiny "creature", very much smaller than the cells in the body. It is known as an *organelle*, rather than an *organism*, since it is much smaller than a cell and can be used as one of the many building blocks that make up a single cell of any living organism, including ourselves.

A mitochondrion has the ability to create its own energy, and to do this much more efficiently than the cells in the body can. It is thought that at a very early stage in evolution, complex cells (of the sort that make up all animals) incorporated mitochondria within themselves, as one of the many building blocks that make up each cell, so as to use them as the cell's "energy factory". It is notable that mitochondria contain their own DNA, separate from the DNA of its host cell, and that its DNA is similar to that of bacteria.

To give an idea of scale: a single mitochondrion measures about 0.0007 millimetres in diameter. In other words, about 1,400 could be placed side by side within one millimetre. Some cells only contain a single mitochondrion but other cells have many. The liver has such a high need for energy that each liver cell contains between 1000 to 2000 mitochondria, which makes up about 20% of the cell's content. And the muscle cells of the heart contain an even higher proportion of

* The valence shell is defined on page 336.

mitochondria, making up about 40% of each cell's volume.

Within these tiny organelles a series of chemical reactions take place, which generate the energy. A molecule known as ATP resides within the mitochondrion. This molecule is made up of one molecule of *adenosine* and three *phosphate* molecules (which gives it its name, *adenosine triphosphate*, or ATP). To generate energy, one of the phosphate molecules is broken off. The parent molecule is then known as ADP (or adenosine *di*phosphate, since it now only has *two* phosphate molecules). The removed phosphate molecule *was* being held in place by a chemical bond, and when the molecule is broken off, the energy that made up this chemical bond is no longer needed and is released. This released energy is then available to be used elsewhere—and this is how the mitochondria creates energy, by the conversion of ATP into ADP.

Another clever trick the mitochondrion then performs is to convert the ADP *back* into ATP, by using the glucose in the blood as a fuel, combined with oxygen (this is done via a series of complex chemical processes, known as *glycolysis*, the *Kreb's Cycle*, and the *Cytochrome System*). In this way, the mitochondrion can repeat this process over and over again, each time releasing energy which the containing cell can then use. This energy is used to do many things, including creating large molecules such as proteins that are used in the repair or regeneration of the tissues in the body.

The glucose in the blood is an essential fuel that drives this process. It is mainly extracted from the food we eat. The stomach, pancreas and small intestine break down the food and extract glucose molecules which are then circulated in the blood. The liver can also generate its own ADP and also extra glucose, which ensures a ready supply of these fuels (as described in Chapter 5).

These clever tricks performed by the mitochondria allow very much more ATP to be produced from each glucose molecule, and it is thought it was the incorporation of mitochondria into the cells of all creatures that enabled complex creatures to evolve. Without the mitochondria, there would not have been enough energy available to enable this to happen.

ATP molecules could be thought of as the essential batteries that the cells use to perform all the vital functions that make us work, and the food we eat is then used to continually recharge those tiny batteries.

The extraction of glucose from the diet

Carbohydrates (also called *saccharides*) are substances such as starch and cellulose which have very large molecules and are known as *poly-saccharides*. For these to be digested by us, they need to be broken down, first into "smaller" substances such as sucrose, which are known as *di-saccharides*; and finally into substances that are "smaller" again, such as glucose, which are known as *mono-saccharides*.[1] These can then easily pass into the capillaries of the *villi* in the small intestine, and hence into the blood stream.

The digestive process begins in the mouth. The saliva contains the enzyme *amylase*, which breaks down some of the carbohydrates (*poly-saccharides*) into *di-saccharides*.

The stomach breaks down the food further before passing it into the duodenum, where pancreatic juices are added.[2]

The pancreatic juice contains many enzymes, including *amylase*, which breaks down the remaining digestible carbohydrates into *di-saccharides*. The food then passes through the small intestine.

The inner walls of the small intestine are made up of many *villi*, whose walls contain *enterocytes*. These contain enzymes to complete the digestion of carbohydrates (as well as proteins and fats). The enzymes *sucrase*, *maltase* and *lactase* complete the digestion of carbohydrates by converting *di-saccharides* (such as *sucrose*, *maltose* and *lactose*) into *mono-saccharides* (primarily glucose), which can then be absorbed into the capillaries of the *villi* and hence into the blood stream.[3]

The nervous system, and ionic flow of electricity

Ordinarily, most atoms have an equal number of protons and electrons, and so have a neutral electrical charge. With some atoms, one or more electrons may break free from the valence shell (making the atom temporarily positive, since it then has more protons, which are positive, than electrons—p.336), but other free electrons are then attracted to the atom, take up orbit and return it to a neutral charge. This flow of *negative* electrons is what we know as electricity. But some atoms, due to their structure, have a tendency to more permanently lose or gain a single electron. These atoms are known as *ions*.

Ions and the "Octet rule"

Some atoms are more stable than others. The most stable ones do not usually lose or gain electrons. These atoms have eight electrons orbiting in their valence shell, which is a particularly stable configuration (they are known as the "noble gasses"). The other atoms naturally strive to become stable, which they do by attempting to achieve this same configuration of eight electrons in their valance shell, and they take the easiest path they can to achieve this (the so called "Octet rule").

For example, chlorine has 17 protons and 17 electrons, with 7 of the electrons orbiting in its valance shell. For chlorine to become an ion, it does this by *gaining* one electron (which is the easiest way for it to obtain eight electrons in its valence shell). Hence a chlorine ion has an overall negative charge, since it has 18 electrons but only 17 protons.

Whereas sodium has 11 protons and 11 electrons, with only 1 of its electrons orbiting in its valence shell (its shells contain 2, 8, and 1 electrons respectively). To become an ion, it *loses* one electron, so that its *second* shell then becomes its valence shell, containing eight electrons. Hence a sodium ion has an overall positive charge, since it has 11 protons but only 10 electrons.

The flow of ions

It is this positive or negative charge of ions that enables them to flow in a similar way to the way electrons flow in an electrical current. In this case, it is not the electron that flows; it is the atom itself that flows from one location to another. This is a different type of electrical current, known as an *ionic* current. This flow can only occur when the element is in a liquid form. In the body, we have several such elements, such as sodium, potassium and chlorine, which all exist in liquid form.

They body utilizes the electrical charges on these ions to perform many vital functions. For example, without this the nervous system could not function. Every cell in the body has an outer membrane which serves as the cell's skin. This acts as a barrier, letting only certain elements pass in or out of the cell while blocking others. Each cell of the nervous system also has various "gates" in the walls of its outer membrane, which enables the cell to control when certain ions may or may not pass into or out of the cell. This enables the cell to change its electrical charge, as follows.

The normal resting charge on these cells is -70 millivolts. The cells contain many potassium ions, which have a positive charge, but they also contain many more negatively charged molecules, such as protein molecules, which means that the cell has an overall negative charge. In the liquid that immediately surrounds the cell, there are many sodium ions accumulated. These are also positively charged and so are attracted to the negatively charged cell, but the membrane does not normally allow sodium ions to pass through it. When the cell wants to change its overall charge (in effect, send out a signal to a neighbouring cell), it does this by opening up *sodium channels* in its membrane, and there is a rush of sodium ions into the cell. This causes the cell's overall charge to rapidly increase to about +30 millivolts.

A nerve consists of a long chain of such cells. This increased voltage is transferred to the next-door cell. The sodium channels in that cell are triggered when they experience a voltage of a certain level (and hence are known as *voltage gated*), and this increased voltage then causes *that* cell to open *its* sodium channels, which causes sodium ions to rush into it, which then causes *its* overall voltage to suddenly rise to +30 millivolts. This signal is transferred to the next cell along, which then repeats the process. In this way the signal is transferred along the nerve (the long chain of such cells) until it reaches the end of the nerve, where some sort of action is triggered.

After each cell has opened its sodium channels, and the inrush of sodium ions has occurred, the cell then closes its sodium channels again, and another mechanism (known as the *sodium-potassium pump*) then quickly pumps the sodium ions back out of the cell, thereby returning it to its resting potential of -70 millivolts.

These voltage-gated ion channels usually remain open for only 0.0005 seconds, which is the amount of time required for the cell's overall charge to increase to the required amount to trigger the next-door cell into firing. This might seem quite quick, but when all the components of the nervous system are put together, the speed that signals travel through it is limited by various factors. An average speed would be about 100 meters per second, which itself might seem quite fast, but it is vastly slower than the speed that electricity travels through metal wires, for example (which is a true *electron-flow* current).

The body's use of semiconduction

The nervous system is one way the body uses ionic current flow (the flow of charged elements). But ionic current flow is inefficient and limited. An ion (in liquid form) can only travel a very short distance. The distance between nerve cells is short, so ionic current flow works well in nerves. But it is not a suitable system for transferring energy around the body. For this, a true electrical current (the flow of electrons) would be more suitable. Normally, this can only happen in metals. However, there is another form of conductivity, known as semiconduction, which enables a current of electrons to flow in non-metallic materials.

A semiconductor is halfway between a conductor and an insulator—a substance that electricity cannot pass through. It can only carry a small current but can easily conduct that current over long distances. Semiconduction is only possible in substances whose molecular structure is orderly, such as in crystals. In these substances, the atoms are arranged in regular lattices, which often have spaces where other atoms are included—impurities. These impurity atoms often have more electrons than the lattice atoms, and these extra electrons are then free to move through the lattice without being bound to any particular atom. It is this movement that creates a current of electrons through the substance.

In his 1960 book, *Introduction to a Submolecular Biology*, Albert Szent-Györgyi pointed out that the molecular structure of many parts of the cells in living organisms was regular enough to support semiconduction. He suggested that protein molecules, each having a "slot" for mobile electrons, might be joined together in long chains so that electrons could flow in a semiconducting current over long distances (in a similar fashion to the process of photo-synthesis, which he had also done much work on).

Due to these ideas, semiconduction in animals started to be researched (previously many biologists thought that electrical currents in animals could only occur via ionic flow). In 1974, McGinnes *et al.* showed that melanin (the pigment found in the skin and also known to be present in the brain and inner ear) had remarkable semiconducting properties, with the current occurring via a flow of electrons, rather than a flow of ions.[4] And in 1977, Shirakawa *et al.* reported high conductivity and semiconduction properties in various polymers (the protein molecules found throughout the body), and received the 2000 Nobel prize in Chemistry for their work.[5]

This story is taken up in Chapter 18, at page 337.

Appendix E. The *yin-yang* hierarchy of the organs

In Chapter 19, it was stated that the *yin-yang* hierarchy of the organs was used to determine the locations of the meridians on the body. And page 347 gives a list of the six criteria this book used to determine this hierarchy, as follows:

A. the functional pairings of organs;
B. their position in the abdomen;
C. the features of their physical structure;
D. their depth within the body (how directly or indirectly they communicate with the outside world);
E. the nature of the substances they process; and
F. the nature of their processing.

The *yin-yang* organ pairings

The functional pairings provide the most clear-cut differentiation between the organs, and determine which organs appear on the left or right of Table 6 on page 348. In each pairing, there is a *yin* and *yang* organ. The *yin* organs (*zang*) are always the more important, in that they play a more central role in producing the substances vital to our survival, which means that, functionally, they are situated more deeply within us. They also communicate less directly with the outside world than the *yang* organs (*fu*) do, all of which makes them more *yin*.

Most of the *yang* organs (*fu*) communicate directly with the outside; the bladder and large intestine excrete waste to the outside[*]; the stomach takes in food and liquids[†]; the small intestine transfers digested food to the large intestine, so has an indirect communication with the outside, but one that is still more direct than its paired *yin* organ, the heart.

The pericardium and lymphatic system are functionally paired since they are both concerned with defence. The pericardium surrounds and protects the heart, and the lymphatic system plays a key role in the immune system, protecting the whole of the body. Of the two, the pericardium is both physically deeper within the body and also communicates less directly with the outside world,

[*] In Chinese medicine, the rectum is considered to be an extension of the large intestine.

[†] The gullet and mouth are considered to be an extension of the stomach.

making the pericardium *yin* and the lymphatic system *yang*.

Some of the functional organ pairings are obvious, such as the kidneys and bladder, the liver and gallbladder, the pancreas and stomach. With each, the less important *yang* organ (*fu*) tends to only service the *yin* organ—to act as a reservoir or extension, in some way. The two pairings that are not obvious are the lungs and large intestine, and the heart and small intestine. However, there *is* a clear functional association between these paired organs, which was explained on pages 137 and 208.

Further, the *yin* organs (*zang*) tend to be "solid" while the *yang* organs (*fu*) tend to be hollow. The solid organs are *yin* because their fabric is more dense than that of the hollow organs, which are relatively less dense and hence more *yang*.

The hierarchy of the *yin* organs

Once the *yin-yang* organ pairs are determined, it is then necessary to decide which pairs are more *yin* or *yang* than the others, so as to order the pairs according to the list in Table 6 on page 348.

Criterion "B" above (the position of the organs within the abdomen) provides the most clear-cut way to determine this. The torso has a *yin-yang* progression from bottom to top (p.397), and a left and right side; and both these can be used to determine the hierarchy of the *yin* organs (*zang*). However, when the organs are situated near to one another, it is not always clear which is the higher organ. But the location of each *yin* organ affects the creation of acupoints on the torso (p.359), so that these acupoints can be used to determine the exact hierarchy, as follows.

The torso acupoints on the bladder meridian

The bladder meridian passes down the back, on either side of the spine. At the top, each branch also splits into two, so there are two bladder meridians descending the back on either side.

Why the back bladder meridian splits into two

The following is a possible explanation for why the bladder meridian splits into two on the back.

The acupoints on the outer bladder channel on the back are associated with each organ's mental and emotional functions (Table 9, p.393 below). These mental/emotional functions are far more *yang* than each organ's physical functions, so when these mental/emotional acupoints were created (which may have been guided by the presence of the electromagnetic radiation from the associated organ—p.359), the tendency would have been for them to be located in a more *yang* location than those associated with each organ's physical functions. Hence, this may have led to the bladder meridian splitting into two on the back, so as to accommodate the two sets of acupoints—the inner, physical ones, and the outer, mental ones. It should be noted that each organ's mental functions would have been utilized by all creatures, from early evolution—since these appear to be what produces the basic instincts that drive all animals (p.92).

What may have caused the "back shu" acupoints to form

On the bladder meridian as it descends the back, there is a powerful acupoint associated with each of the organs, which can treat any aspect of those organs. In Chinese medicine terms, these are known as the *back shu* acupoints. From an evolutionary perspective, these acupoints could not have been created due to the same influence that appears to have created the acupoints on the limb meridians. Instead, as explained on page 359, they may have been created due to the influence of the physical presence of each organ—which presence was directly communicated via the electromagnetic radiation from that organ. Therefore the order of these acupoints on the bladder meridian reflects the relative positions of the associated organs in the torso, and hence their *yin-yang* hierarchy. Table 9 below lists the acupoints.

Table 9. Torso acupoints on the bladder meridian

***Yin* (inner) → *Yang* (outer)**

***Yang* (upper) ↑ *Yin* (lower)**

		Acupoints of... *yin* organs / *yang organs*			Acupoints for mental/emotional functions of...
Inner bladder meridian	13	lungs	Outer bladder meridian	42	the lungs
	14	pericardium			
	15	heart		44	the heart
	18	liver		47	the liver
	19	*gallbladder*			
	20	pancreas		49	the pancreas
	21	*stomach*			
	22	*lymphatic system*			
	23	"kidneys"		52	the "kidneys"
	25	*large intestine*			
	27	*small intestine*			
	28	*bladder*			

Bladder-13 (*Feishu*) relates to the lungs and shows that the lungs are the most *yang* of the *yin* organs (*zang*)—since this acupoint is positioned at the highest location. Next is Bladder-14 (*Jueyinshu*), the pericardium, then Bladder-15 (*Xinshu*), the heart. It is clear that the pericardium is more *yang* than the heart, since it surrounds the heart (making it more superficial and therefore more *yang*). This hierarchy is shown in the order of the organs in Table 6 on page 348.

Of the remaining three *yin* organs (*zang*), the liver, pancreas and kidneys, the position of the liver and pancreas is reversed when compared to the order in Table 6 (p.348), and the kidneys are shown to be the lowest of the *yin* organs in the abdomen, which corresponds with their ranking in Table 6 as the most *yin* of the *yin* organs.

The liver/pancreas hierarchy

The *yin-yang* hierarchy of the liver and pancreas varies depending on which criterion is used to determine it (and hence depending on which part of the body is considered). It is for this reason that these two meridians cross one another at three different locations on the body.

While considering their hierarchy at the torso, the criterion that has the most influence is the physical presence of the organs (criterion "B" on page 391), which makes the liver more *yang* than the pancreas, since it is positioned slightly higher in the torso. This is confirmed by the placing of the liver acupoint, Bladder-18 (*Ganshu*), which is higher than the pancreas acupoint, Bladder-20 (*Pishu*).

The other aspect of an organ's position in the torso is whether it is placed on the left or right. Both the liver and pancreas are single organs which are not placed centrally, so their left or right positioning could also be used to indicate their hierarchy. The liver is on the right and the pancreas on the left, which makes the liver *yang* and the pancreas *yin* (p.346), and therefore *also* confirms their *yin-yang* hierarchy. (And it is even possible that it was this very *yin-yang* hierarchy that determined which side of the torso these organs should migrate towards as the early organ system evolved.)

On the front of the torso, this same factor (the organ's position in the torso) causes the liver meridian to be placed at a more *yang* position than the pancreas meridian—when the liver meridian bends to reach the acupoint Liver-13 (*Zhangmen*) on the side of the torso. The liver meridian then bends back towards the centre and crosses the pancreas meridian again to end at the acupoint Liver-14 (*Qimen*).

At this final location, the liver meridian is then at a more *yin* location than the pancreas meridian, despite the meridians being located on the torso (where it would be expected that the *pancreas* would be at the more *yin* location). However, the acupoint Liver-14 (*Qimen*) is placed at the physical location of the liver; hence the presence of the organ was probably the factor that influenced the creation of this particular acupoint (and in Chinese medicine terms, the acupoint is therefore categorised as the *front mu* of the liver). Therefore the acupoint is located there simply because that is the physical location of the liver, which would have probably overridden any influence due to the liver's *yin-yang* relation to the pancreas.

These two meridians next cross one another at the junction between the leg and torso—the liver crosses the pancreas meridian at Pancreas-13 (*Fushe*) and Pancreas-14* (*Fujie*). Hence the pancreas meridian from here downwards adopts a more *yang* position than the liver meridian does. What is the explanation for this?

This location marks the start of the body's physical communication with the outside world; it is the start of the limbs, which are the means the body uses to physically communicate with the outside. Therefore, of the criteria listed on page 391, the one that most closely corresponds with the body's geometry at this location is criterion "D", the organ's "depth" within the body (how directly or indirectly it communicates with the outside world). The pancreas receives part-digested food from the stomach, which has taken in the food from the outside. Hence the pancreas communicates indirectly with the outside, but the liver does not communicate with the outside at all, which makes the pancreas more *yang* than the liver (when using this

* Also called Spleen-13 and Spleen-14.

"communication" criterion). For this reason, as the pancreas meridian passes from the torso to the legs, it adopts a more *yang* position than the liver meridian, which is shown in Figure 24 on page 350. This correlates with the hierarchy indicated in Table 6 on page 348.

However, as shown in Figure 24 (p.350), these two meridians then cross one another again on the lower leg, the liver then adopting the more *yang* position again. This final location is towards the most *yang* part of the limb (the tip). Therefore, of the criteria listed on page 391, the ones that most closely correspond with the body's geometry at this location are the most *yang* ones, which are the last two, criterion "E" and "F", the nature of the substances the organs process, and the nature of their processing.

The liver processes energy. It regulates the production of energy by the digestive organs, and even creates its own energy when needed, and thereby maintains the smooth flow and availability of energy in the entire body; while the pancreas only completes the digestion of food—all of which makes the liver clearly more *yang* than the pancreas. To reflect this, as these two meridians approach the end of the leg (the most *yang* part), they cross over again, so that the liver now occupies a more *yang* location than the pancreas.

This changeover of the relevant criteria for determining the *yin-yang* hierarchy of the organs may also be part of the explanation for why the *yang* meridians on the legs (the gallbladder, stomach and bladder meridians) all have a kink in them at around this changeover point.

The pancreas/stomach hierarchy

Another apparent anomaly in the meridians on the front of the torso is the fact that the stomach meridian occupies a more *yin* location than the pancreas meridian. The stomach and pancreas form a *yin-yang* pair of organs, where the pancreas is the *yin* organ (*zang*), so the pancreas would be expected to occupy the most *yin* location.

However (as with the liver and pancreas), at the junction between the torso and legs, the stomach and pancreas meridians cross one another, so that for the whole of the leg, the pancreas then *does* occupy a more *yin* location than the stomach does (as would be expected). What is the explanation for this?

On the limbs, the location of the meridians reflects the *yin-yang* hierarchy of the organs, but when the meridians cross the torso, their location (and the creation of acupoints on them) is probably most influenced by the physical location of the organs. However, there is little difference between the physical locations of the stomach and pancreas, so it appears the *location* of their activity is used instead to differentiate between them. The stomach's activity takes place on the upper part of the body, starting at the mouth, then the gullet, and ending at the stomach organ itself. And beyond this point on the torso, the pancreas takes over as the most influential digestive organ, this being the location of *all* its activity—so on *this* portion of the front of the torso, the stomach is relatively inactive and the pancreas is most active, which makes the pancreas *yang* and the stomach *yin*. And the locations of the stomach and pancreas meridians reflect this.

The "front mu" acupoints on the torso

It may have been the physical presence of each organ that caused an acupoint for that organ to be created on the bladder meridian on the back as it passes over the organ—the *back shu* acupoints (p.359). In the same way, as the various organ meridians travel over the front of the torso, acupoints are created on them by *other* organs as the meridians cross the physical locations of those organs.

For example, as the liver meridian crosses the location of the pancreas, the acupoint positioned there relates to the pancreas, even though it is on the liver meridian. The acupoint is Liver-13 (*Zhangmen*), but its largest influence is on the pancreas function, so it is known as the *front mu* of the pancreas. As the gallbladder meridian crosses the location of the kidneys, it was probably the physical presence of the kidneys that caused an acupoint to be created there: Gallbladder-24 (*Riyue*). The acupoint is on the gallbladder meridian but its main influence is on the kidneys and it is therefore known as the *front mu* of the kidneys. And as the stomach meridian passes over the top section of the large intestine, this creates Stomach-25 (*Tianshu*), which is the *front mu* of the large intestine.

The remaining criteria confirm the *yin-yang* hierarchy

Any (or all of) the criteria listed on page 391 can be applied to any pair of organs to determine their *yin-yang* hierarchy. Starting on page 392, criterion "B" (each organ's position in the body) was used to determine the hierarchy between the heart, pericardium and lungs. These three organs are situated close together, so their exact hierarchy might seem difficult to determine conclusively by considering only their position in the body. In this situation, the other criteria can be applied to confirm the hierarchy. Of these three organs, the relationship between the heart and pericardium is clear; the pericardium is the protective membrane that surrounds the heart, therefore the heart is deeper inside the body, making it *yin* and the pericardium *yang*. The pericardium's physical structure is less dense than that of the heart, also making the pericardium more *yang*. And the pericardium performs a protective role, much as all the elements of the immune system do; therefore the substance it processes is more *yang* than the blood the heart processes (in contemporary physiology), which also makes the pericardium more *yang*.

And the relationship between the heart and lungs can also be similarly clarified. The lungs communicate directly with the outside via the air we breathe, making them *yang* when compared to the heart, which is then *yin*. But further, the heart processes blood, which is a *yin* substance when compared to the air that the lungs process, which again makes the lungs *yang* when compared to the heart. And the lungs are the only *yin* organ (*zang*) that communicates with the outside world, by taking in oxygen and expelling waste gasses (in contemporary physiology), which also explains why the lungs are the most *yang* of the *yin* organs—and therefore more *yang* than the heart.

The arm meridians do not cross one another

On the legs, the liver and pancreas meridians cross one another, which reflects the fact that when applying different criteria (from the list on page 391), the *yin-yang* hierarchy of these two organs sometimes changes. But none of the meridians on the arms cross one another in this way, which reflects the fact that whichever of the criteria are applied, the *yin-yang* hierarchy between the lungs, pericardium and heart (whose meridians appear on the arms) remains the same.

Why the head is the most *yang* part of the body

Table 9 on page 393 above, shows that the upper part of the torso is more *yang* than the lower part. Several factors can be used to determine which are the *yin* and *yang* ends of the body. The *yang* end tends to be more mobile, active or agile—hence, making it more *yang*. Also the primary movement of all animals is always in the direction of this *yin-yang* progression; they move from *yin* to *yang* (*yang* being the most active), with their head leading the way.

This movement also reflects the fact that the head is the most *yang* part of the body. In all four legged animals, the head is always at the highest point, making it *yang* compared to the remainder of the body. But also, the head contains all the sense organs, which are more *yang* than the abdominal organs since they directly connect us with the outside. But also, the abdominal organs are situated more deeply within us and process substances that are relatively more *yin* than those processed by the sense organs (blood, food and water are more *yin* than light, sound and scents). For all these reasons the head is the most *yang* part of the body.

The "six channel" theory

The twelve main meridians are consecutive and when considered together, they may be considered to form one complete path; and the order of the meridians in this path reflects clear functional relationships between the organs.

Because of this order, the *yin* organs (*zang*) are linked in pairs, and the *yang* organs (*fu*) are also linked in pairs. And between the two organs in each pairing, there appears to be a functional relationship, which is often seen in clinic, and which there is no physiological explanation for.

In Chinese medicine, these functional organ pairings were clearly discovered by the ancestors of the *Nei Jing* authors, since the *Nei Jing* refers to them throughout.

Instead of the twelve separate meridians, each pair of organs was considered as being associated with a single two-meridian combination (or channel), which gives a total of six channels, as in Table 10 and Table 11 on page 398 below.

To form each channel, two meridians are considered to be joined. Each channel then travels over the arms, torso and legs—with the "joint" between the two meridians being on the torso. Each of these two meridians is named according to whether it is situated on the arm or the leg section of the channel.

For example (as shown in Table 11), the *taiyin* channel is formed by joining together the lung and pancreas meridians. The lung meridian is situated on the arm, therefore it is named the "hand *taiyin* channel", or "the *taiyin* channel of the hand". And the pancreas meridian is situated on the leg, therefore it is named the "foot *taiyin* channel", or "the *taiyin* channel of the foot".

Table 10. The three *yang* channels

Channel	Alternative translations	Paired organs	Meridian names
yangming	*yang* brilliance sunlight *yang*	large intestine stomach	hand *yangming* foot *yangming*
taiyang	great *yang* major *yang* greater *yang*	small intestine bladder	hand *taiyang* foot *taiyang*
shaoyang	minor *yang* lesser *yang*	*san jiao* gallbladder	hand *shaoyang* foot *shaoyang*

Table 11. The three *yin* channels

Channel	Alternative translations	Paired organs	Meridian names
taiyin	great *yin* major *yin* greater *yin*	lungs pancreas	hand *taiyin* foot *taiyin*
shaoyin	minor *yin* lesser *yin*	heart kidneys	hand *shaoyin* foot *shaoyin*
jueyin	ceasing *yin* absolute *yin*	pericardium liver	hand *jueyin* foot *jueyin*

In clinic, this principle can often explain unexpected phenomena. For example, pericardium acupoints, such as Pericardium-6 (*Neiguan*), can often be used to treat stagnated liver function, which effect is probably due to both organs being associated with the same channel, the *jueyin*—the pericardium meridian forming the hand *jueyin* section, and the liver meridian forming the foot *jueyin* section. And this same principle applies to the heart and kidney meridians, which form the hand and foot sections of the *shaoyin* channel; in this case, I have found that the acupoint Heart-7 (*Shenmen*) is often effective in treating the kidneys (p.175), particularly on occasions when some of the key kidney acupoints seem ineffective, such as Kidney-3 (*Taixi*) or Kidney-6 (*Zhaohai*).

These channel pairings can also sometimes explain the apparent functional relationships between the organs. For example the lung and pancreas functions often seem linked in this way, as described on page 137.

The communication appears to be via the yang organs

The lung and pancreas meridians form the two sections of the *taiyin* channel. And even though there is no direct link between these two meridians (in that none of the start and end locations of these meridians coincide), there can often appear to be a clear functional relationship between the two organs (p.137). However, the lung meridian connects with the large intestine meridian (the two being *yin-yang* paired organs[*]); the large intestine meridian connects with the stomach meridian (at the side of the nose[†]); and the stomach meridian connects with the pancreas meridian (the two being *yin-yang* paired organs[‡]). Therefore it seems that any communication between the lungs and pancreas may take place via their paired yang organs, the stomach and large intestine. And if this is the case, the same may also be true for the other two channels. For example, on the *shaoyin* channel, any such communication between the heart and kidneys may take place via the small intestine and bladder.

---

[*] A branch separates from the lung meridian at Lung-7 (*Lieque*) and links with the large intestine meridian at Large-intestine-1 (*Shangyang*); see Deadman, p.73.

[†] At large-intestine-20 (*Yingxiang*) the large intestine meridian joins with the stomach meridian; see Deadman, p.96.

[‡] On the dorsum of the foot at Stomach-42 (*Chongyang*), a branch leaves the stomach meridian and joins with Pancreas-1 (*Yinbai*), also called Spleen-1, on the medial side of the tip of the big toe; see Deadman, p.126.

Appendix F. Other research into how acupuncture works

Apart from clearly explaining the key aspects of Chinese acupuncture using contemporary anatomy and physiology, this book also introduces a new hypotheses on how acupuncture works.

Why was a new hypothesis needed?

It seems that the approach used by many researchers has been to only take into account the fact that acupuncture consists of "inserting a needle into the skin" and then considering which of the systems currently known to biology may be invoked by this, so as to bring about therapeutic effects. But this approach usually falls down because it does not consider (or is sometimes not even aware of) the many facets of an acupuncture treatment.

One important facet that appears to be uniformly overlooked is the rapid speed of acupuncture's effect on the organ functions. When taken into account, this negates most of the proposed hypotheses on how acupuncture works. And another issue is that, even though the most common effect of an acupuncture treatment is its adjustment of organ functions, many researchers overlook this and confine themselves to investigating minor side-aspects of acupuncture treatments (such as pain relief in local tissue) and then find that their resultant conjectures on how acupuncture works are incapable of explaining its most common effect—the correction of organ malfunction.

For all these reasons, no-one had yet produced a credible explanation of how acupuncture works, which is why I developed the intelligent tissue hypothesis, which is summarized on page 372.

The competing hypotheses

The following sections test the competing hypotheses by examining whether they account for key facets of an acupuncture treatment.

The neural hypothesis

John C Longhurst champions the neural hypothesis,[1] which suggests that "the clinical influence of acupuncture is transmitted primarily through stimulation of sensory nerves that provide signals to the brain, which processes this information and then causes clinical changes associated with treatment". But it is clear that this hypothesis is unable to account for acupuncture's effects, for the following reasons.

The activation of skin nerves

This hypothesis clearly relies on the stimulation of skin nerves (as a direct or indirect result of the needling). But the sensation at an acupoint experienced by patients is variable.

The usual process is to tap the needle so that it quickly enters the skin without activating the skin nerves. At this point, many patients feel no sensation. My own technique is to then gently stimulate the needle until the patient feels a sensation (known as "de chi" in Chinese medicine). This could be a sting, a gentle tingling, a feeling of heaviness (similar to a toothache feeling), or a burning feeling. These sensations would obviously involve the activation of skin nerves.

Sometimes there is no immediate sensation, but around half a minute later, the patient reports feeling a tingling sensation in the meridian distal to the stimulated acupoint, or elsewhere, which indicates that the skin nerves at the acupoint itself had *not* been activated—since there was no sensation *at* the acupoint.

At other times, the sensation may consist of the patient simply starting to feel unusual in themselves, as though "something is happening" but without feeling any sensation at the needled acupoint (this feeling could be accounted for by the adjustment in the function of one or more of their organs). And at other times, even after a few seconds of stimulation of the needle, the patient feels no sensation at all. In this situation, I would then retake the patient's pulse, and I usually find that the function of the associated organ had changed, even though the patient felt no sensation at the acupoint. Both these last two examples are instances where the acupuncture has clearly changed the function of the associated organ without there being any skin nerves activated at the acupoint.

In these situations, we can be sure that the skin nerves had not been activated, since the person felt nothing (and is used to feeling a "normal" acupuncture sensation, so is waiting for something similar to happen, but feels nothing). We can be sure of this, since this is the whole purpose of skin nerves; when one is activated, the person would feel something. Yet, the organ has changed its function as a result of the acupuncture. This fact alone contradicts the neural hypothesis, but there are further shortcomings.

Bidirectional communication

All nerves only transmit impulses in a single, fixed direction. Skin nerves transmit from the skin *to* the brain; and never from the brain *to* the skin. Yet an extremely common phenomenon that is an integral part of the acupuncture mechanism requires two-way communication between the organs and their associated acupoints.

This is demonstrated in the experiment described in the patient example on page 369. The muscle at an acupoint becomes tender in response to its associated organ becoming unusually stressed (in other words, not functioning properly). And when the organ function is changed during an acupuncture treatment, this changed function is immediately communicated back to its related acupoints, causing them to cease to be tender (usually within seconds, if not almost immediately), and this happens even when those acupoints had not been stimulated in any way. This mechanism is so common and reliable that these tender locations can be used as a diagnostic device (when tender, this indicates the associated organ is not functioning normally).

This diagnostic tenderness, and its ceasing in response to changed organ function, could not possibly be communicated *to* distal acupoints from the organs via skin nerves, since they do not transmit in that direction. And also, there is no known way that a sensory nerve in the skin could adversely affect the tissue in that same location, so as to cause the tenderness (i.e. the improper function of some aspect of the local tissue). This rules out the involvement of skin nerves in this organ-to-acupoint communication.

Could motor nerves serve this purpose?

Proponents of the neural hypothesis might argue that motor nerves (*efferents*) transmit from the brain *to* the muscles, and therefore *could* be involved in producing these effects.

For this to be the case, a motor nerve would need to adversely affect a very specific portion of the muscle tissue (which coincided with the acupoint) but without in any way affecting the remainder of the muscle, and without triggering the movement of the muscle—which is the normal function of such motor nerves.

This requirement alone casts serious doubt on the proposition. But added to this are these further requirements. This damaging effect on the local tissue (some effect that causes the tissue to be tender when pressed) should only happen to reflect improper function in a particular aspect of a particular organ. And further, since such nerves are hard-wired and cannot change their function, this proposed system would presumably require dedicated motor nerves to exist which did not have a motor function at all but rather served to negatively affect some aspect of the tissue at an acupoint so as to cause it to feel tender when pressed; and to only do this when a specific aspect of the associated abdominal organ were stressed, and to do all this with no conceivable physiological purpose. And further, that this proposed system would require the *sensory* nerve for the skin at this specific location to be separately processed by the brain to modify the same specific aspect of the same abdominal organ's function—and that this same arrangement should be repeated for over 600 similar acupoints around the body.

The proposal that motor nerves could serve this purpose is not credible. Therefore it seems that the two-way communication between an organ and its associated acupoints could not be accomplished neuronally.

The following situation provides further evidence of this same communication—which equally could not be explained by the neural hypothesis.

The association between Bladder-13 (Feishu) and Lung-9 (Taiyuan), etc.

Another common phenomenon I have noted in clinic is this. When needling the acupoint Bladder-13 (*Feishu*) on the patient's back (a powerful lung acupoint), the patient sometimes reports feeling a tingling at their wrist, near to the acupoint Lung-9 (*Taiyuan*), also a powerful lung acupoint. Or when needling Bladder-23 (*Shenshu*) on the patient's back (a powerful kidney acupoint), they report feeling a tingling at their ankle, at either Kidney-6

(*Zhaohai*) or Kidney-3 (*Taixi*), or sometimes Kidney-1 (*Yongquan*), which are all powerful kidney acupoints.

In such cases, the patient did not know which acupoint I was needling on their back, and they also did not know what the acupoints on their limbs pertained to; they merely reported feeling a tingling sensation there and when I touched the acupoint to confirm this, they said that was the exact location. Also, the sensation was clearly associated with the needle I had inserted in their back, since the tingling started immediately after, and often the patients themselves linked the tingling sensation with my inserting the needle in the back acupoint, saying that they felt the tingling as I needled the acupoint on their back (patients often point out such things, since they find them so unexpected—which adds credibility to the phenomenon).

Again, nerve stimulation could not account for this communication between each specific back acupoint and the related distal acupoints at the end of the patient's limbs (nor for communication between the organs and these distal acupoints—which may be how these distal acupoints were triggered in these instances), therefore nerve stimulation must be ruled out as a possible mechanism to account for acupuncture—since it cannot account for every facet of it, including these common phenomena.

The abdominal organs are mainly self-governing

The abdominal organs are largely self-governing (p.88). There are some minor aspects of each organ that rely on input from autonomic nerves, but the organs work independently of any direct input from the brain and spinal cord. For example, on page 88, the liver's reliance on autonomic nerves is described. But even when these are cut, the liver still regulates itself under most conditions. It is only when the patient is in a stressed state (such as during the fight-or-flight response) that this autonomic nerve input plays any role.

However, in an acupuncture session the patient is usually extremely relaxed, and acupuncture routinely adjusts a patient's liver function, which suggests acupuncture does not achieve its effects on the organ functions by somehow activating nervous input from the brain, but by some other method.

Since acupuncture's main effect is on the organ functions, and the organs are mainly self-governing, a more rational mechanism to explain acupuncture would be one that influences the viscera directly, rather than a brain-centric mechanism.

The communication rate

It might be argued that the adjustment could be achieved by the brain communicating with the organ hormonally. However, I have found that, typically, a distal acupoint being stimulated changes the associated organ's function in around one second. And most such acupoints are located around one metre from the organs, which means the communication must take place at around one metre per second. It is said that the blood takes around twenty seconds to circulate the body, and has a mean speed of around 12 centimetres per second.[2] And during a typical acupuncture treatment, the patient is both lying down and is also usually extremely relaxed, so that their blood flow rate would certainly be no higher than this, which would make it impossible for any hormones originating within the brain to reach the organs in time to account for the change in organ function.

This makes it clear that acupuncture does not achieve its effects via nervous or hormonal pathways, and that some other method is used to rapidly communicate between an acupoint and its associated organ—in both directions.

And one final fact that casts serious doubt on the plausibility of the neural hypothesis is the following.

The proposed mechanism is purposefully designed and requires outside stimulation

The neural hypothesis recognises that two-way communication with an acupoint would be necessary and conjectures that perhaps motor nerves could supply the brain-to-acupoint communication.

There are various effects at an acupoint that occur as a result of the mechanism that acupuncture utilizes. The muscle at the acupoint usually becomes tender when the associated organ is stressed, and the tender muscle is usually very localized, within a diameter of around one centimetre. On other occasions, there may be tingling, or some other sensation at the acupoint, which begins in response to the function of its associated organ being changed—either during an acupuncture session, or sometimes at other times, and without the acupoint being directly stimulated in any way. And in all these situations, there is not normally any associated movement of the muscles at the acupoint.

But the normal function of motor nerves is to cause muscles to simply move. For a motor nerve to be able to initiate any of these effects it would need to be targeted on just the small segment of tissue local to the acupoint (rather than triggering a whole muscle to contract, for example), and it would need to have a specialized function. For example, one function would be to cause this local segment of tissue (or other nearby structure) to malfunction in such a way that the acupoint was then tender when pressed. And there would need to be at least one of these specialized nerves dedicated to every acupoint on the body. And these nerves would serve no other physiological purpose.

The neural hypothesis further relies on acupuncture's effects being "transmitted primarily through stimulation of sensory nerves that provide signals to the brain, which processes this information and then causes clinical changes associated with treatment". But how is it supposed that the brain performs this processing?

Again, there would have to be specialized areas of the brain that perform this processing—that monitor the sensory nerves emanating from the skin at each acupoint, and once triggered, then somehow cause that associated organ to immediately change its function. No specific brain arrangement has been proposed that might perform these changes, but whatever ones are imagined, this overall system would need to be a dedicated system that performs no other physiological role.

Apart from the arguments that acupuncture's effects are unachievable via nervous or hormonal manipulations, the other big problem with any such hypothesis is that it describes a complex mechanism that is dedicated to achieving acupuncture's effects and has no other physiological purpose.

Acupuncture meridians are said to exist in all life forms,[3] and it is assumed they must have been present from the earliest beginnings of life (since the PVS is the first structure to form in an embryo—p.321—and there are, at least, geographical associations between primo vessels and meridians). Therefore, the neural hypothesis would have to rely on the fact that over hundreds of millions of years, evolution purposely designed the complex system suggested above (with dedicated nerves and brain hard-wiring), which had no physiological purpose other than permitting acupuncture to work, required stimulation from outside the creature's body to activate it, and that evolution did all this in anticipation of humans eventually evolving and then discovering acupuncture, so that a needle could be inserted into the skin to activate the system. The notion is in no way tenable.

Any hypothesis on how acupuncture works that relies on a dedicated mechanism having been purposely evolved, which depends on external stimulation to activate it but is otherwise inactive and has no other physiological purpose, such a proposed hypothesis could never be credible (see also page 409).

The connective tissue hypothesis

This hypothesis (proposed by Helene Langevin and Jason Yandow in 2002[4,5]) focuses heavily on the concept of "needle grasp", which is a phenomenon that sometimes happens with some acupuncturists. Often, when first inserting the needle, the patient does not experience a sensation, so the acupuncturist may slowly rotate the needle until a sensation is achieved, which can sometimes cause the muscle fibres to grasp the needle. And it is hypothesised that this may cause distortion of the collagen fibres in the connective tissue which may then set up a mechanical wave that spreads through the connective tissue, which could act as a signal. But there are problems with several aspects of this hypothesis.

In my own experience as an acupuncturist, during treatment sessions the needling sensation is often obtained on first tapping the needle into the skin, with no manipulation of the needle whatsoever, and I find that this alone usually achieves the desired change in organ function—which occurs within around one second. This negates any claims regarding the importance of "needle grasp". But further, an organ's function is frequently changed by applying only pressure or heat or electro stimulation to an acupoint, all of which could not possibly involve any "needle grasp", nor "whorl" of the subcutaneous tissue, so that the focus on these phenomena appears to be misguided.

Also, in acupuncture sessions, some patients can sometimes feel a sensation slowly propagating along a meridian after an acupoint has been stimulated. And the connective tissue hypothesis has equated this with the speed that a mechanical wave would travel through connective tissue. But in both cases, this speed is far too slow for it to be able to account for acupuncture's effects on the organs. The speed of sensation propagation along meridians is around 18 centimetres per minute,[6] whereas the communication between an acupoint and its associated organ travels at around one metre per second, or faster (p.371). The researchers are clearly unaware of how fast this communication takes place, and have wrongly assumed that the occasional phenomenon of sensation propagation along a meridian is somehow equated with acupuncture's effects (see page 55 for an explanation that accounts for most meridian sensations).

The connective tissue hypothesis speculates about the possibility that signals of some type may be transduced through connective tissue, with the possible secondary involvement of other systems including the nervous system. Apart from the problems with the very slow speed of such signals, the involvement of the nervous system has also been ruled out in the analysis of the neural hypothesis.

The requirements for an explanation of how acupuncture works

From all the above, it is clear that any valid explanation should be able to meet the following criteria:

- It should not rely on a purposefully designed mechanism that has no other physiological function.
- The proposed mechanism must be able to facilitate rapid two-way communication between the organs and their associated acupoints at a rate of at least one metre per second.
- It should be able to account for a distal acupoint becoming tender when its associated organ is stressed, and for this tenderness clearing within seconds of the organ function being corrected.
- It should be able to account for how stimulation of such an acupoint (by needling, pressure, heat, or electro) can immediately correct improper function in the associated organ.
- It would probably not depend on brain involvement but rather would somehow directly interact with the viscera themselves.
- It should be capable of explaining the other common phenomena encountered during the practise of acupuncture, such as why the meridians are laid out in the unusual way they are, why each acupoint formed where it did on its particular meridian, and also account for how the Chinese medicine organ pulses are produced.

Further acupuncture research issues

Amongst acupuncture researchers, there appears to be much confusion over the concept of the propagation speed of signals in connective tissue, and any relation this may have to the propagation speed of meridian sensations that are sometimes felt by some patients.

Propagation of meridian sensations

In the 1960's Bong-Han Kim measured the flow rate of PVS fluid in the primo vessels to be about 0.3 millimetres per second, and the propagation speed of stimulation from one acupoint to the next on the same meridian to be about ten times faster than this, at three millimetres per second. But this stimulation often only travelled to the next acupoint along, and sometimes to the following one, but (in his experiments) never any further along the meridian.[7]

This fact alone would rule out any role this phenomenon may play in acupuncture's effects on the organs, since it would never reach the organs, let alone that its flow rate is far too slow to account for acupuncture's effects on the organs. (See page 55 for an explanation that accounts for most meridian sensations.)

Charge mobility in semiconductors

There is also confusion over the concepts of charge mobility (which is similar to electron drift) and the propagation speed of an electrical wave. This last concept is unrelated to the first.

Normally electrons and charged particles have no measureable geographical movement. They shoot around in random directions, but remain in roughly the same geographical location. When a direct current is applied to a conductor, the electrons or charged particles then drift very slowly along that conductor. In the case of electrons moving along metal wires, this is known as *electron drift* and is extremely slow, in the order of millimetres per hour.[8] In a piece of connective tissue where semiconduction takes place, this drift is known as *charge mobility*, and is also very slow.

Neither of these speeds provide the propagation rate of an electrical wave along these conductors. Any change in the electrical potential is passed between each charged particle along the conductor, without those particles moving geographically (in the same way that air molecules may not move geographically, but sound still travels through them at around 340 metres per second—p.361 and 365). In metal wires, the rate of propagation is very near to the speed of light; and in connective tissue, is also extremely fast. For example, when the signal's frequency is between one and 10 hertz, the wave propagates through connective tissue at around 67,000 metres per second (p.366), which is 670 times faster than nerve impulses travel. In biological terms this means that communication via an electrical wave is, in effect, instant.

However, some researchers cite the very slow rate of charge mobility in semiconductors, wrongly assume this indicates the speed that an electrical wave would propagate through connective tissue, and when this very slow rate is in the same ballpark as the propagation rate of meridian sensations, assume that the one equates to the other, and that they have thus somehow explained acupuncture's effects.

But every element of such arguments is flawed. Not only is the understanding of the science wrong, but the lack of first-hand knowledge of acupuncture also fosters its own misunderstandings.

Acupuncture's effects are unrelated to the physiological purpose of the PVS

Acupuncture's effect of correcting an organ's function could not be related to the physiological purpose of the PVS for the following reasons.

The purpose of the PVS is to enable p-microcells to mature into the specific cells required by each organ (p.322). But since acupuncture tends to correct improper organ function in around one second, such malfunctions could not be due to a cellular problem within the organ—since if they were, they could not be corrected so quickly.

The liquid within the primo vessels flows at around one metre per hour (p.316), which means it could not possibly communicate with an organ in around one second. But the most significant element of the liquid's content, the p-microcells, circulate much slower than this, since they mature within the primo nodes. For example, liver p-microcells can take around 120 hours to fully mature into a new liver cell (p.316).

These facts make it clear that neither the primo fluid, nor any element of its content, could play any part in acupuncture's effect of correcting improper organ function.

Could acupuncture be intended as a self-healing system?

When an organ is stressed, its related acupoints are tender when pressed; and by pressing these points, this tends to correct that organ's function. Therefore, it might be supposed that the acupuncture system was purposefully created by nature to act as a self-healing system, whereby we (or any animal) stimulated these tender locations to bring about self healing. But there are several problems with this argument.

Patients are usually unaware of the tenderness—*until* an acupuncturist presses the exact acupoint for diagnostic purposes. Therefore, the opportunity for a patient to perform acupressure on themselves is not normally available; and for nature to have intended this as such a healing system, it would be necessary for the patient to be aware of the tenderness. But even more significantly, the same meridians and acupoints exist on all mammals, and most of them do not have the digits, nor the dexterity to be *able* to stimulate acupoints on themselves. For example, a horse, dog or cat (all of whom acupuncture is performed on) would have great difficulty using one of their own hooves or paws to press a very specific acupoint (less than a centimetre in diameter) on themselves. What's more, many of the most powerful acupoints are located on the back, so that even primates would be unable to stimulate these acupoints on themselves.

Acupuncture is a happy accident

It is clear that acupuncture was not designed by evolution as a self-healing system, and therefore could not have been designed as a healing system at all—since such a system could not possibly have evolved over millions of years in anticipation of the day when humans would also evolve and then eventually discover that if they stimulated certain points, healing would take place. This is not tenable. Instead, there are two *accidental* facts that enable the acupuncture system to exist.

The fact that electrical current exists in the body is by design. Electrical charges exist pretty much everywhere in the body, from every cell upwards, and are an essential element that enables cells to function. But there appears to be an extra electrical current that is conducted through the body's connective tissue via semiconduction (p.342). Though its function has not been fully explored, it may serve the purpose of acting as a reservoir of charge to enable cells to perform their normal functions (p.340), in which case it must also exist by design.

However, the fact that an electrical current can adopt information from the organs (or any other tissue) it passes through is *not* by design (p.365). This would happen anyway—accidentally. And the fact that bodily tissue interprets organ information conveyed in this way (on an electromagnetic wave) is almost certainly an accidental arrangement that probably occurred in early evolution but which then (according to the intelligent tissue hypothesis) enabled the bodies of all animals to evolve under the influence of their abdominal organs (p.353).

This process established a resonance between each organ and the tissue along its meridian (p.356). However, this resonance has no physiological purpose today, and was certainly not created to establish the healing mechanism of acupuncture.

It is the combination of these two accidents (that organ information can be conveyed on an electromagnetic wave, and that bodily tissue interprets such organ information) that allows the acupuncture system to exist.

Note that this book defines a meridian as a distal tract of tissue affected by organ function (p.355), which means that the precise paths of the meridians and positions of the acupoints along them were created incidentally and serve no physiological purpose. But when an organ is stressed, it is this same resonance that allows the organ's information (which is accidentally encoded into an electrical wave) to interfere with the function of the local tissue at certain locations on that meridian (due to the tissue interpreting this information), such that the tissue becomes tender or reddened or cold, or such that boils or pain occur (p.369). This arrangement also has no physiological purpose (in fact it is a hindrance, since it impedes the healthy function of that tissue). However, it is this accidental resonance that also permits that location, when stimulated, to be able to correct the corresponding organ malfunction that caused the tenderness or redness, etc.

Acupuncture, though a powerful healing system, is a happy accident.

References and endnotes

Abbreviations used

SW-n: *Su Wen*, Chapter n
LS-n: *Ling Shu*, Chapter n
NJ-n: *Nan Jing*, Section n
fn. footnote
en. endnote

Chapter 1

[1] Hu Hou-hsüan, 1944, p.11a. Cited by Unschuld, 1985, p.21.

[2] Chang Tsung-Tung, 1970, p.69. Cited by Unschuld, 1985, p.21.

[3] Akatsuka Tadashi, quoted in Kanō Yoshimitsu 1980, p.283. Cited by Unschuld, 1985, p.25.

[4] Wilhelm, 1930, pp.32-33. Cited by Unschuld, 1985, p.36.

[5] Unschuld, 1985, p.36.

[6] Ssu-miao, 1965, p.347. Cited by Unschuld, 1985, p.45.

[7] Eichhorn, 1976, p.27. Cited by Unschuld, 1985, p.35.

[8] Unschuld, 1985, pp.54-55.

[9] Unschuld, 1985, p.58.

[10] Yamada, 1979. Cited by Unschuld, 1985, p.63.

[11] Unschuld, 1985, pp.56-61.

[12] Unschuld, 1986, p.3.

[13] *Wu-shih-erh ping fang*, 1979, pp.1-20. Cited by Unschuld, 1985, p74.

[14] Ssu-ma, 1969. Cited by Unschuld, 1985, p.93.

[15] Unschuld, 1985, pp.92-97.

[16] LS-12 states "His outer appearance can be measured. His structures can be followed and pressed with the fingers so as to locate them. Once he has died, he may be dissected to observe his interior appearance. Whether the long-term depots are firm or brittle..." (Unschuld, 2016, p.217). In LS-31, the size, shape and path of the stomach and intestines are given in some detail, which could only have been determined by dissection of a corpse (Unschuld, 2016, pp.355-356). And in NJ-42, the size, shape and dimensions of every organ is given in detail (Unschuld, 1986, pp.416-8). See also Unschuld, 1985, pp.213-215 and 236-238.

[17] Unschuld, 1985, pp.78-79.

[18] In Unschuld's early translations of the *Nan Jing* (1986) and the *Su Wen* (2011), he translates *zang* as "depot" and *fu* as "palace"; whereas in his later translation of the *Ling Shu* (2016), he now translates *zang* as "long-term depot" and *fu* as "short-term repository". The non-medical meaning of *fu* was clear, but its use in the medical context was less easy to translate, and this is reflected in his changed translation of the term. During the late Zhou and early Han dynasty, the meaning of *fu* changed, from "short-term storage facility", to also signify venues of administration, and subse-

quently a palace where an administrator resides. Hence, Unschuld's translation of *fu* as "palace" (see Unschuld, 2011, pp.16-18). In his 2016 translation of the *Ling Shu*, he now prefers the term "short-term repository" instead of "palace" as a translation of *fu* (see Unschuld, 2016, p.13, footnote 11). Whatever his reason for the changed translation, to me, this new choice does seem more suitable, since I previously found the term "palace" misleading. It suggests a more important organ than a depot might represent; whereas the depots (the *zang*, or *yin* organs) are in fact the more important organs.

[19] Unschuld, 2011, Vol I, p.16; or Unschuld, 1985, pp.81-82.

[20] Yang Shang-shan, 1981, pp.63-69. Cited by Unschuld, 1985, p.82.

[21] Unschuld, 1985, p.82.

[22] LS-28 states "…As for the very first origin of all diseases, they all originate from wind, rain, cold and summer heat, from yin and yang [influences (*chi*)], joy and anger, from beverages and food and from living conditions, from being severely scared and from sudden fear. Then blood and [influences] may separate; the yin and the yang [influences] may be destroyed; the conduits and network vessels may have receding [influences], and circulation may even be interrupted, with the vessel paths being impassable…" Unschuld, 2016, p.328.

[23] Tian, 2007.

[24] Unschuld, 2011, Vol I, pp.155-159 (SW-8).

[25] Unschuld, 1985, p.67

[26] Unschuld, 2011, Vol II, pp.244-284 (SW-69).

[27] Unschuld, 1985, p.81.

[28] See Unschuld, 1985, p.71; Unschuld, 2016, pp.603-612 (LS-66); Unschuld, 2016, pp.739-751 (LS-79).

[29] See the commentaries in the Unschuld translation of the *Nan Jing*: Unschuld, 1986.

[30] The evidence to support this hypothesis is described in Chapters 17-20, and the hypothesis is summarized on page 372.

Chapter 2

[1] Unschuld, 1985, pp.71-73. See also Unschuld's introduction to his translation of the *Nan Jing*: Unschuld, 1986. pp.13-14.

[2] Cited by Unschuld, 1986, p.349. The comment was made as a commentary on Section 31 of the *Nan Jing*, when Yü Shu wrote "The *Ling Shu* states 'The upper section of the [*san jiao*] resembles fog'. That is to say, when it passes the influences, that resembles mist gently flowing into all the [meridians]."

[3] Unschuld, 1985, pp.75-78.

[4] In SW-56, it states "When evil settles in the skin, then the interstice structures open. When they have opened, then the evil enters the [collaterals (*luo mai*)] and settles there. When the [collaterals] are full, then it pours into the [meridians]. When the [meridians] are full, then [the evil] enters the [organs] and lodges there." (Unschuld, 2011, Vol II, p.42.)

[5] "Jing" is defined, rather poetically, in LS-30, which states "When the two spirits strike at each other, their union results in the formation of a physical appearance. That which usually precedes the generation of a human body, it is called 'essence'." (Unschuld, 2016, p.351.) The phrase *two spirits strike at each other* is referring to the sexual union of a man and woman. This results in a *physical appearance* (i.e. the start of a foetus), and "that which preceded" this (the merging of the "two spirits"; i.e. the combining of the genetic and "energetic" blueprints of the two people—p.177), this is the essence passed on to the new person.

[6] Cheng X, 1999, p.52.

[7] Unschuld, 2016, p.352 (LS-30).

[8] LS-59 describes the process of "draining" excess influence through various "holes" (Unschuld, 2016, p.538), as do many passages throughout the

Nei Jing. And LS-71 describes the "opening of clogged ditches" in the context of clearing "evil visitors" (pathogens) from the meridians (Unschuld, 2016, p.633).

[9] Unschuld, 2011, Vol I, pp.668-669 (SW-45).

[10] Unschuld, 2011, Vol I, p.586 (SW-39).

[11] Unschuld, 2011, Vol II, pp.40-41 (SW-56). The next sentence following the extract reads "In case it consists of plenty of heat, then this causes the sinews to slacken and the bones to waste, the flesh to melt away, and the protuberant muscles to be destroyed. The body hair stands up straight and breaks." I omitted this because I felt the language, whether it be intended literally or metaphorically, requires too much imaginative interpretation on the part of today's reader to be able to take it seriously. Such imaginative adventures are left to those students who wish to refer to the original texts to make what they can of them.

[12] Unschuld, 2016, p.254 (LS-17).

[13] Unschuld, 2016, p.42 (LS-1).

[14] Unschuld, 2016, pp.766-767 (LS-81).

[15] Unschuld, 2016, pp.401-404 (LS-39).

[16] "...the *Suwen* was not the work of a single author. ...it combines texts written by numerous authors over an extended period of time. However, this *extended period of time* may...have lasted for no more than two centuries." (Unschuld, 2011, p11). "Much of the version [of the *Ling Shu*] known today probably dates back to individual, shorter texts that began to be written between the 2nd and 1st centuries BCE.... The authors of these texts are unknown, as is the individual who, at some point in that time, collected the individual texts into one great work." (Unschuld, 2016, p.1).

[17] Unschuld, 2016, pp.249-251 (LS-16).

[18] Unschuld, 2016, p.555 (LS-60).

[19] Unschuld, 2016, p.565 (LS-62).

[20] Unschuld, 2016, p.447 (LS-47).

[21] Unschuld, 2011, Vol I, p.191 (SW-10).

[22] Cited by Berk, 1986. However, no date is given for the chart. Berk's book translates ancient Chinese Kung-fu texts, the earliest dating from 1591 AD, so it may be assumed that the anatomy charts date from around this period.

[23] Unschuld, 2011, Vol I, p.649 (SW-43).

[24] Unschuld, 2011, Vol I, p.372-376 (SW-21).

[25] Unschuld, 2016, pp.523-4 (LS-56).

[26] Unschuld, 2016, pp.631-632 (LS-71).

[27] Unschuld, 2011, Vol I, pp.584-586 (SW-39).

[28] Unschuld, 2016, pp.259-260 (LS-18).

[29] Unschuld, 1986, p.341.

[30] Cited by Unschuld, 1986, p.343.

[31] Cited by Unschuld, 1986, p.344.

[32] Cited by Unschuld, 1986, pp.343.

[33] Cheng X, 1999, p.41.

[34] Unschuld, 2016, pp.524 (LS-56).

[35] Cited by Unschuld, 2016, p.525, fn.4.

[36] Cited by Unschuld, 2016, p.524, fn.1.

[37] Unschuld, 2016, p.764 (LS-81).

[38] Unschuld, 2016, pp.264-265 (LS-18).

[39] Maciocia, 1989, p.71.

[40] Cheng X, 1999, p.28 and 54. (It should be stated that in editions of my own book previous to June 2017, I also followed this tendency set by today's Chinese medicine textbooks—until I had thoroughly researched the *Nei Jing* and *Nan Jing*.)

[41] —Though they appear to have not considered what the process of "extracting" something from the food or air would involve, in terms of physiological stomach or lung function; or, due to the absence of knowledge of chemistry and of the microscopic anatomy of the organs, the concept of physiology (as we know it—i.e. the chemical breakdown and transformation of substances, and the microscopic workings of the body which perform such things) did not then exist, so it did not even occur to them to ponder such things. That is, as we would think of them. However, they did consider this detail using the notion of "physiology" available to them, which was a metaphorical

one. They considered that such processes consisted of the stomach somehow "cooking" the food, so that the vapours rose from the food (just as happens when cooking in reality), and those vapours were then able to split into their *yin* and *yang* components and circulate the body via the meridians. However, there was no such process imagined with the lungs. It is possible that because the air was already in a vapour-like form, they imagined there was no need for the lungs to process it to transform it into a useable vapour.

[42] Cheng X, p.34, states that the lung "is closely related to the formation of pectoral *chi* [i.e. chest influence], which is formed from the combination of the essential *chi* of water and food, and the clear *chi* inhaled by the lung." This notion does not originate from the *Nei Jing*. On the same page, the book also states that the lung "inhales clear *chi* from the natural environment and exhales waste *chi* from the interior of the body". This function of exhaling waste is also a modern invention, and does not appear in the *Nei Jing* (p.41). (It should be stated that in editions of my own book previous to June 2017, I also followed this tendency set by today's Chinese medicine textbooks—until I had thoroughly researched the *Nei Jing* and *Nan Jing*.)

[43] And I would again make it clear that in editions of my own book previous to June 2017, I also followed this tendency set by today's Chinese medicine textbooks—until I had thoroughly researched the *Nei Jing* and *Nan Jing*.

[44] Unschuld, 1985, pp.75-77.

[45] Friedland, 2009.

[46] Waugh, 2001, pp.60-65.

[47] Waugh, 2001, pp.61-67.

[48] Unschuld, 2016, p.14, Introduction section (includes descriptions of why "blood is blood", etc.).

[49] Unschuld, 2011, Vol I, p.649 (SW-43).

[50] Unschuld, 2016, p.604 (LS-66).

[51] Unschuld, 2011, Vol I, p.337 (SW-19).

[52] Unschuld, 2011, Vol II, p.73 (SW-60).

[53] Unschuld, 2016, pp.604-611 (LS-66).

[54] Unschuld, 2016, p.328 (LS-28).

[55] Unschuld, 2016, pp.603-611 (LS-66).

[56] Unschuld, 2011, Vol I, p.72 (SW-3).

Chapter 3

[1] Porkert, 1974.

[2] Kim, 1963, p.32.

[3] NJ-1 states "When a normal person exhales once, the contents of the vessels proceed three inches; when a normal person inhales once, the contents of the vessels proceed three inches too." (Unschuld, 1986, p.65). This equates to a speed of around one inch per second, which translates to 2.54 centimetres per second, or 152 centimetres per minute. However, is it clear that the statements in this *Nan Jing* section are theoretical and arbitrary, for the following reasons. It also states that the rate of the movement in the vessels is directly linked with the speed of breathing, and that the contents of the vessels perform a cycle of the entire meridian circuit 50 times a day. These two statements are contradictory, since if the breathing rate increased or decreased, then so too would the number of cycles per day completed. But more importantly, these theories suggest that a child's breathing rate ought to be considerably slower than an adult's. Depending on the size difference between the two people compared, a small child's breathing rate may need to be four or six times slower than an adult's, and a baby's rate perhaps ten times slower—so that the contents of the vessels would circulate the person's body 50 times a day, in all cases. These theories make no sense and are not borne out by reality, so can only be wrong—like so many other *Nei Jing* theories, in contrast to their practical observations.

Chapter 4

[1] Betts, 2013, section: 23.6 Accessory Organs in Digestion: The Liver, Pancreas, and Gallbladder.

[2] Berg, 2002, section: 30.2, Each Organ Has a Unique Metabolic Profile.

[3] Betts, 2013, section: 17.9 The Endocrine Pancreas.

[4] Bronte, 2013.

[5] Cesta, 2006.

[6] Note that the correct attribution is also indicated by the *yin-yang* pairing of the meridians (p.348). When the bodily structures were defined during evolution, such pairings were established due to the functional relationships between the organs (Chapter 19). And due to the functional relationship between the pancreas and stomach, the pairing of these organs now makes sense. Whereas there is no conceivable reason why evolution would have paired the stomach and spleen organs, since there is no functional relationship between them (page 208 describes the functional relationship between the heart and small intestine, and page 137, that between the lungs and large intestine). This indicates that the meridian paired with the stomach meridian, should therefore be associated with the pancreas, rather than the spleen. But further, the spleen could not even be considered a *yin* organ; it is part of the lymphatic system, which is a *yang* organ (p.211), therefore evolution would not have paired it with the stomach, which is *also* a *yang* organ.

[7] Unschuld, 1986, p.417 (NJ-42).

[8] Waugh, 2001, p.133.

[9] Clearly it was not known to all, since some authors got the location of key organs wrong, such as the liver, lungs and "pancreas"; see page 270.

[10] Betts, 2013, section: 23.1 Overview of the Digestive System.

[11] "General weakness" (i.e. the four limbs not working) is associated with the pancreas in SW-29 (Unschuld, 2011, Vol I, pp.482-483); and (i.e. "the body feels heavy") in LS-35 (Unschuld, 2016, p.377); and (i.e. "the body and all its limbs feel heavy") in LS-10 (Unschuld, 2016, p.183).

[12] "Emaciation and malnutrition" (i.e. the sinews, muscles and flesh not having the "nourishment" to "live") is associated with the pancreas in SW-29 (Unschuld, 2011, Vol I, pp.482-483). And LS-10 associates "the muscles and the flesh soften" with illness of the pancreas (Unschuld, 2016, p.198).

[13] "Poor appetite" is associated with the pancreas in SW-50 (Unschuld, 2011, Vol I, p.735).

[14] "Abdominal bloating and discomfort" (i.e. "distension and obstruction") is associated with the pancreas in SW-29 (Unschuld, 2011, Vol I, pp.482-483); in SW-10 (Unschuld, 2011, Vol I, p.195); in SW-50 (Unschuld, 2011, Vol I, p.735); in LS-47 (i.e. "accumulation in the lower flanks accompanied by pain" and a "feeling of fullness and tends to develop abdominal swelling) (Unschuld, 2016, pp.452-453); and in LS-10 (i.e. "the abdomen is swollen") (Unschuld, 2016, p.183).

[15] "Excess gas" (i.e. "intestinal flush", which is defined by Wang Bing/Unschuld as "gases"—see fn.10 in following reference) is associated with the pancreas in SW-29 (Unschuld, 2011, Vol I, p.481).

[16] "Loose stools" (i.e. "outflow of undigested food") is associated with the pancreas in SW-29 (Unschuld, 2011, Vol I, p.481).

[17] SW-17 has a quaint description of loose stools: "When the granaries do not keep what they store, in this case the doors are not under control." (Unschuld, 2011, Vol I, p.279).

[18] These signs and symptoms would have been accounted for as follows. When the digestive resources are not transported to every part of the body, this could cause the influence (*chi*) to flow contrary to its normal course, which would account for the abdominal bloating and discomfort, excess gas and loose stools (see p.103).

[19] Unschuld, 2011, Vol I, pp.482-483 (SW-29).

[20] Cheng X, 1999, p.32.

[21] The notion of the "sinews, muscles and flesh" not having the "nourishment" to "live" is associated with pancreas malfunction in SW-29 (Unschuld, 2011, Vol I, pp.482-483); the notion that the "muscles and flesh soften" is associated with pancreas malfunction in LS-10 (Unschuld, 2016, p.198); and SW-10 states that "the correlate of the pancreas is the muscle tone" (Unschuld, 2011, Vol I, p.185).

[22] Cheng X, 1999, p.33.

[23] LS-17 states "When the [influence] of the [pancreas] is in harmony, then the mouth can recognize the five types of grain." (Unschuld, 2016, p.255.) The "influence" of an organ being "in harmony" means that the organ is healthy and hence all its related functions are working well. "Recognizing the five types of grain" implies being able to distinguish all flavours. Therefore the statement means that when the pancreas is healthy, the sense of taste is strong, but when the pancreas is stressed, the sense of taste is weak.

[24] SW-10 states that the pancreas's "splendour appears in the lips" (Unschuld, 2011, Vol I, p.185).

[25] Thorens B, 2010.

[26] Cheng X, 1999, p.33.

[27] LS-60 states that "All diseases are either movements contrary to or movements in accordance with the norms," and it gives many examples of signs and symptoms that represent a movement contrary to the norms, such as a bloated abdomen, noises in the abdomen associated with a feeling of fullness, unending nosebleed, cough, discharges of blood in the urine—most of these signs and symptoms being pancreas related (Unschuld, 2016, pp.552-553).

[28] Waugh, 2001, pp.74-75.

[29] Cheng X, 1999, p.33.

[30] Unschuld, 2016, pp.152-153 (LS-8).

[31] Unschuld, 1986, p.220 (NJ-16). The following sentence is omitted from the extract. "Internal evidence of such an illness is the presence of moving influences right of the navel which, if pressed, respond with firmness and pain." See p.270, which demonstrates that this "abdominal diagnosis" is theoretical only and does not apply in reality.

[32] Unschuld, 2011, Vol I, p.108 (SW-5).

[33] Collins, 1991

[34] SW-17 states "When the speech is feeble and when it takes an entire day before he speaks again, this is [influence] deprivation." (Unschuld, 2011, Vol I, p.279).

[35] LS-10 describes the path of each meridian, then describes the signs and symptoms that may result when each meridian's associated organ is stressed. These include pains at various locations, following the path of the meridian; and in many cases even states that the toe or finger that the meridian ends at may be "useless"; i.e. either too weak or too stiff or painful to be used. In the case of the pancreas, the signs and symptoms include "the stomach duct aches, the abdomen is swollen.... a feeling of tension and pain below the heart... the inner side of their thighs and knees are swollen... the big toe is useless." (Unschuld, 2016, pp.176-184). And LS-13 also describes the path of every meridian and the "diseases" of each meridian; i.e. the signs and symptoms that might occur along the meridian when a "blockage" occurs, or when its associated organ is stressed in some way. (Unschuld, 2016, pp.225-238).

[36] NJ-16 associates "a tendency to ponder" with pancreas "affliction" (Unschuld, 1986, p.220).

[37] Unschuld, 2011, Vol I, p.189 (SW-10).

[38] Unschuld, 2016, p.390 (LS-37).

[39] Unschuld, 2011, Vol I, p.108 (SW-5).

[40] Unschuld, 2011, Vol I, p.57 (SW-2).

[41] Unschuld, 2011, Vol I, pp.480-481 (SW-29).

[42] Leggett, 1994, p.29.

[43] Unschuld, 2011, Vol I, p.188 (SW-10).

[44] Leggett, 1994, p.17.

[45] Leggett, 1994.

[46] The *Nei Jing* theory to explain numbness is described in SW-34, as follows "When the [constructive influence] is depleted, then this results in numbness. When the [defensive influence] is depleted, then this results in a loss of function. When both the [constructive and defensive influence] are depleted, then this results in numbness together with a loss of function," (Unschuld, 2011, Vol I, p.531). It should be noted that "constructive influence" is sometimes regarded as being synonymous with "blood"; see p.185.

[47] SW-40 states "The disease is named blood decay. It is acquired in younger years either because of a massive loss of blood .... and the liver is harmed. Hence, the monthly affair is weak and diminished and fails to arrive," (Unschuld, 2011, Vol I, p.601).

[48] Leggett, 1994, p.28.

[49] Unschuld, 2011, Vol I, p.156 (SW-8).

[50] Unschuld, 2011, Vol I, p.372-376 (SW-21).

[51] Unschuld, 1986, p.347 (NJ-31).

[52] Maciocia, 1989, p.111; Cheng X, 1999, p.39. (It should be stated that in editions of my own book previous to June 2017, I also followed this tendency set by today's Chinese medicine textbooks—until I had thoroughly researched the *Nei Jing* and *Nan Jing*.)

[53] SW-43 associates "vomiting liquid" with illness in the pancreas (Unschuld, 2011, Vol I, p.643). LS-10 associates "food ingested will be thrown up again" along with "the stomach duct aches" with illness of the pancreas (Unschuld, 2016, p.183). It is notable that these signs and symptoms are associated with the pancreas. This is perhaps a result of the *Nei Jing* tendency to consider the stomach and pancreas jointly. However, it should be stated that the attribution of many of the signs and symptoms in this bullet list to the stomach, is a practice of today's Chinese medicine, informed by the knowledge of contemporary anatomy and physiology.

[54] SW-23 states "When the [influence] in the five [*yin* organs] have a disease.... In the stomach it causes [influence] to move contrary to its regular course, it causes hiccup," (Unschuld, 2011, Vol I, p.402).

Chapter 5

[1] SW-13 states "People in antiquity lived [simple lives]... Internally, they knew no entanglements resulting from sentimental attachments, externally, they did not have [the stresses of today]. In this peaceful and tranquil world [they did not get seriously ill]. The people of today are different. Anxiety and suffering encircle their interior.... Also, the people have lost the knowledge how to follow the four seasons... This is why minor diseases inevitably develop into serious problems" (Unschuld, 2011, Vol I, pp.219-223). And SW-14 states "If cravings and desires have no limits, if anxiety and suffering find no end, the essence [influence] will be destroyed, the [constructive influence (*ying chi*)] is impeded, and the [defensive influence (*wei chi*)] vanishes. Hence, the spirit leaves and the disease does not heal" (Unschuld, 2011, Vol I, p.238).

[2] NJ-16 associates "a tendency towards tidy appearance" and "an inclination to become angry" with liver "afflictions" (Unschuld, 1986, pp.219-220).

[3] LS-66 states "Rage harms the liver" (Unschuld, 2016, p.611).

[4] LS-47 associates the following states with a heart condition: "[people] suffer from vexation and tend to be forgetful. They have difficulties to open their heart and say something... They are made to fear by someone else's words" (Unschuld, 2016, p.450). And LS-34 associates the following with heart conditions: "The heart is vexed with closure and [the person is speechless]. Patients

lower the head and silently withdraw" (Unschuld, 2016, p.369).

[5] SW-44 states "In case of a loss, or in case one longs for something but does not get it, then this manifests itself as [shortness of breath and noisy breathing; i.e. it weakens the lungs]" (Unschuld, 2011, Vol I, p.656).

[6] SW-77 states "When a man of noble rank is stripped of his power, even though he was not struck by a [pathogen from outside], his essence and spirit have been harmed inside... [i.e. his 'kidneys' have been harmed by the loss of status]" (Unschuld, 2011, Vol II, p.671).

[7] SW-5 states "If fear causes harm, it harms the kidneys" (Unschuld, 2011, Vol I, p.110).

[8] SW-67 states that "Pensiveness harms the [pancreas]" (Unschuld, 2011, Vol II, p.207).

[9] NJ-16 states "External evidence of [an illness in the pancreas] includes ... a tendency to ponder" (Unschuld, 1986, pp.219-220).

[10] Betts, 2013, pp.508-509, 586-589, p.679.

[11] Ingraham, 2016.

[12] Chun-Xia, 2010.

[13] Pandol, 2010.

[14] Or more accurately: within the "words", since any particular word itself is merely a meaningless sound, and we create the ideas ourselves by finding one of our own past experiences that we think *may* match the words, then associating this past idea of our own with the other person's words. Therefore someone else's words that we hear do not *contain* ideas; it is our own mind that creates the ideas we understand in their words (Kovich, 2009).

Chapter 6

[1] Betts, 2013, pp.1155-1162.

[2] Betts, 2013, pp.1168-1172.

[3] Betts, 2013, pp.1166-1168.

[4] Betts, 2013, pp.1174-1185.

[5] Waugh, 2001, p.309.

[6] Betts, 2013, p.807.

[7] Waugh, 2001, p.309.

[8] Waugh, 2001, pp.307-312.

[9] Clearly, much of the fact-based knowledge expressed in the *Nei Jing* must have been discovered by previous generations—in order to allow the craft to progress to the point where the detailed theories laid out in the *Nei Jing* could be written. SW-67 suggests that all this "groundwork" knowledge was passed down from an ancient ancestor, who is often assumed to be Huang Di, the Yellow Emperor, who reigned almost 3,000 years prior to the *Nei Jing's* compilation. It states "Huang Di sat in the Hall of Light. In the beginning he rectified the mainstay of heaven. He looked down from his elevated seat and observed the eight farthest regions. Having carried out investigations, he established the five constants...." and it goes on to describe the correspondences for each organ (Unschuld, 2011, Vol II, p.189). This does not mean that the knowledge literally originated from the Yellow Emperor, but rather that it was of unknown origin, having been passed down by previous generations. The reference to "Huang Di" was understood to mean a revered but unknown ancestor, rather than any specific person (Unschuld, 2016, p.4). SW-5 (clearly written by a different author to that of Chapter 67) also makes the same suggestion, but this time the suggestion is expressed as though coming from Huang Di himself. It states "Huang Di: I have heard, the sages of high antiquity in discussing and structuring the physical appearance of man, they arranged and distinguished among the [organs], they traced and connected the [meridians] and they combined them to set up the six [pairs of meridians]. In each case they followed the respective [meridians]. The [acupoints] where [the influences (*chi*)] are effused, all their locations have a name...." and it goes on to describe all the same correspondences as Chapter 67 does (Unschuld, 2011, Vol I, p.105). Hence, there is no record of this "practical approach" used to discover all the information the

"ancients" did, but there would have been no other method available. And since the facts have proved so reliable (having stood the test of time to this day), I have assumed that practical observation, unhindered by questionable theories, was the method used to discover these facts.

[10] SW-10 states "When man lies down the blood returns to the liver," (Unschuld, 2011, Vol I, p.191). And see page 35, which discusses this observation.

[11] SW-44 associates liver malfunction with the symptoms of "the sinews become tense and are cramped," (Unschuld, 2011, Vol I, p.655). And NJ-16 includes the symptom of "twisted muscles" as an indicator of liver "affliction" (Unschuld, 1986, p.220).

[12] See endnote 46 in Chapter 4 above.

[13] SW-10 associates "blurred vision" with a liver condition (Unschuld, 2011, Vol I, p.195).

[14] SW-69 associates liver disease with "pain below the two flanks and in the lower abdomen," which is the location where many women feel their period pains (Unschuld, Vol II, p.251). SW-22 associates the following symptom with liver disease "pain below the two flanks and this pain pulls on the lower abdomen," (Unschuld, 2011, Vol I, p.394). And SW-40 associates a weak or absent "monthly affair" with a liver irregularity. The section is in the context of blood deficiency (Unschuld, 2011, Vol I, p.601).

[15] Lautt W, 1976.

[16] SW-70 associates liver disease with the symptoms of "internal tightness" and "propping fullness" (Unschuld, 2011, Vol II, p.288). And LS-10 associates liver disease with a "feeling of fullness in the chest" (Unschuld, 2016, p.196).

[17] NJ-34 states that one of the "transformations" of the liver is "its liquid is the tears". In the commentaries, the meaning of the "transformations" is debated (Unschuld, 1986, p.367; and see pp.367-373 in the same volume for a selection of the commentaries). One interpretation of this association may be that when the liver is stressed, the person's stress is "transformed" into tears.

[18] SW-22, associates liver disease with "a tendency to be angry" and "the patient tends to be fearful, as if someone were about to arrest him." That is, they have paranoid thoughts (Unschuld, 2011, Vol I, p.394).

[19] Cheng X, 1999, p.30.

[20] Unschuld, 2011, Vol I, pp.179-180 (SW-9).

[21] Cited in Unschuld, 2011, Vol I, pp.179-180, fn.66.

[22] Chun-Xia, 2010.

[23] Thorens, 2010.

[24] Unschuld, 2016, pp.552-553 (LS-60).

[25] Unschuld, 2011, Vol II, p.244 (SW-69).

[26] Cited by Unschuld, 2011, Vol II, p.244, fn.21.

[27] Unschuld, 2011, Vol I, p.105 (SW-5).

[28] Wang Bing. Cited by Unschuld, 2011, Vol I, p.105, fn.53.

[29] NJ-16 associates liver illness with the symptoms of swollen and stiff limbs, and "twisted muscles" (Unschuld, 1986, pp.219-220). LS-20 associates the liver with symptoms of "cramp when walking" and "swollen legs" (Unschuld, 2016, p.276). And SW-44 associates liver malfunction with the symptom of "the sinews become tense and are cramped" (Unschuld, 2011, Vol I, p.655).

[30] Unschuld, 2011, Vol I, p.186 (SW-10).

[31] Wang Bing. Cited by Unschuld, 2011, Vol I, p.186, fn.8.

[32] SW-22 associates liver disease with the symptoms of "the eyes become unclear and cannot see anything," (Unschuld, 2011, Vol I, p.394). The phrase "cannot see anything" is doubtless not meant literally, and could be taken as referring to the colours being dimmed, the vision blurred, or visual disturbances of other types. And LS-17 states "The [influence] of the liver passes through the eyes. When the [influence] of the liver is in harmony, then the eyes can distinguish the five colours," (Unschuld, 2016, p.255).

[33] SW-69 states that when the liver has a disease "The eyes are red and have pain; the canthi develop ulcers," (Unschuld, 2011, vol II, p.251).

[34] Deadman, 1989, p.469; or Cheng, 1999, p.81. But see endnote 15 from Chapter 9 below.

[35] McCarley, 2007.

[36] Unschuld, 1986, pp.219-220 (NJ16).

[37] LS-13 describes the pathways of each meridian and the symptoms that occur along the meridian. In the case of the gallbladder meridian (which is where many liver-related symptoms are expressed), these include pains at the hips, the buttocks, the upper sections of the flanks, the neck (with "tense ribbon sinews") and the temples (Unschuld, 2016, p.227).

[38] To explain this symptom, LS-47 states "When the liver is big, then it lies attached to the stomach and presses against the throat," (Unschuld, 2016, p.450). In this chapter, the author uses the theory that an organ's changed size, position and texture may explain its signs and symptoms. This theory was devised when there was little knowledge of the body's internal anatomy. Clearly the theory is wrong, but the important point is that the signs and symptoms being explained must have been discovered through practical observations; therefore, this chapter is a reference to this liver-related symptom of a feeling as though something were pressing against your throat.

[39] NJ-16 associates the symptom of "difficult stools" with "illness in the liver". (Unschuld, 1986, pp.219-220). And a commentary by Yü Shu, written in 1067 stated "When the liver is ill, the influences move contrary to their proper course and fail to descend downward. Hence the stools are difficult to pass." (Cited by Unschuld, 1986, pp.226-227). As with many *Nei Jing* (and *Nan Jing*) theories, the theory itself is not literally true (p.261), though the original observation *is* true—that constipation is sometimes associated with stagnated liver function. An explanation in contemporary physiology could be simply related to the disruption in the liver's function of regulating the production and supply of resources to *all* the organs, including the large intestine. This is also only a theory, though it does seem more credible.

[40] When referring to the commonest abnormality in liver function, the term "stagnation" of its function is used, rather than "poor" function. The term "poor" organ function is a translation of today's Chinese medicine term *deficient chi*. For example, the term "pancreas *chi*" translates as: "pancreas function"; therefore, the term "Pancreas chi deficiency" translates to "poor pancreas function". But when describing liver malfunction, today's Chinese medicine chose to use the term "stagnated *chi*", which translates as "stagnated function"—rather than using the term "poor function". This was because, by observation, the commonest liver malfunction was thought to be characterized by a build up of resources within the liver, accompanied by *stagnated* circulation of those resources around the body, all of which accounted for the many, often powerful, symptoms. Hence, the term "stagnated function" seemed more appropriate than "poor function".

[41] Unschuld, 2011, Vol I, p.189 (SW-10).

[42] Unschuld, 2011, Vol I, p.106 (SW-5). And NJ-34 associates the liver with the sound of shouting (Unschuld, 1986, p.367).

[43] SW-19 states "When [the liver-related movement in the vessels] is greatly excessive, then this causes a person to be forgetful [i.e. confused]; he experiences vertigo and suffers from peak illness [i.e. pain at the peak, or top, of the head]" (Unschuld, 2011, Vol I, pp.323-324).

[44] SW-10 describes the symptoms that result when a blockage of both influences and blood occur in the liver and gallbladder meridians, such as "dizziness and shaking, blurred vision and deafness" (Unschuld, 2011, Vol I, p.195). The de-

scription of "deafness" may be a reference to loud tinnitus.

[45] Cheng X, 1999, pp.315-316.

[46] Cheng X, 1999, p.316.

[47] Waugh, 2001, p.311.

[48] Waugh, 2001.

[49] Unschuld, 2011, Vol I, p.655 (SW-44).

[50] Cited by Unschuld, 2011, Vol I, p.655.

[51] Unschuld, 1986, pp.416-417 (NJ-42).

[52] Cited by Unschuld, 1986, p.421.

[53] Cited by Unschuld, 1986, p.421.

[54] Maciocia, 1989, p.116. Note that this policy of "modernizing" certain *Nei Jing* content is also adopted by other contemporary textbooks, such as Cheng X, 1999, p.38. And it should also be stated that in editions of my own book previous to June 2017, I also followed this tendency set by today's Chinese medicine textbooks—until I had thoroughly researched the *Nei Jing* and *Nan Jing*.

[55] Unschuld, 2011, Vol I, p.156 (SW-8). See also fn.7.

[56] Unschuld, 2011, Vol I, p.182 (SW-9).

Chapter 7

[1] Betts, 2013, pp.1059-1061.

[2] Betts, 2013., pp.990-991.

[3] Waugh, 2001, p.249.

[4] Shelly, 2014.

[5] Waugh, 2001, p.255.

[6] Unschuld, 2011, Vol I, p.278 (SW-17).

[7] Wang Bing. Cited by Unschuld, 2011, Vol I, p.278, fn.24.

[8] Unschuld, 2011, Vol I, p.504 (SW-32).

[9] Wang Bing. Cited by Unschuld, 2011, Vol I, p.504, fn.22.

[10] Maciocia, 1989, p.83 states "When we say that the Lungs govern respiration we mean that they inhale 'pure [*chi*]' (air) and exhale 'dirty [*chi*]'. The constant exchange and renewal of [*chi*] performed by the Lungs ensures the proper functioning of all the body's physiological processes which take [*chi*] as their basis." This whole statement is alien to any of the *Nei Jing* theories of metabolism and is more a statement of contemporary metabolism. And Cheng X, 1999, p.34 states that the lung "exhales waste [*chi*] from the interior of the body." Again, there is nothing in *Nei Jing* metabolic theories that supports this statement. (It should be stated that in editions of my own book previous to June 2017, I also followed this tendency set by today's Chinese medicine textbooks—until I had thoroughly researched the *Nei Jing* and *Nan Jing*.)

[11] Cheng X, 1999, pp.33-34; Maciocia, 1989, pp.83-84.

[12] Unschuld, 1986, p.301 (NJ-24).

[13] Unschuld, 2016, p.764 (LS-81).

[14] In the context of "diseases generated by the lung", LS-10 states "If the [influences] are depleted, the shoulders and the back will feel pain with cold. The patients experience shortness of [influence], so that there is not enough [influence] available for breathing" (Unschuld, 2016, p.178). And in the context of "illness in the lung", NJ-16 lists "shivering from fits of cold and heat" along with various other signs and symptoms (Unschuld, 1986, pp.219-220).

[15] Cheng X, 1999, p.33.

[16] SW-22 associates the signs and symptoms of "the patient pants and coughs and the body is heavy" with "kidney disease" (Unschuld, 2011, Vol I, p.397). The sign of "pants and coughs" is clearly produced by the lung, and today would probably be described as "shortness of breath" or "asthma", particularly of the type where it is hard to breathe in. The symptom of "the body is heavy" (i.e. the patient has poor energy) would be an obvious consequence of not being able to breathe properly.

[17] It was theorized that the lungs circulate defensive influence (see the extract from LS-18 on p.37). Though the *Nei Jing* model of immunity is incorrect (p.44), it is true that the lungs feature many immune aspects that protect us from exter-

nal pathogens (p.123). Therefore we can assume that the association between poor lung function and reduced "immunity" (which is fact based) was discovered through practical observations.

[18] LS-78 states "the lung has an aversion to cold" (Unschuld, 2016, p.731). And NJ-16 states "External evidence of [an illness in the lung] includes a white face, a tendency to sneeze.... The illness, as perceived by the patient, consists of panting and coughing, and of shivering from fits of cold and heat" (Unschuld, 1986, pp.219-220).

[19] LS-4 states "The [chest influence (*zong chi*) rise and leave the face through the nose. They enable smelling" (Unschuld, 2016, p.90). LS-17 states "the [influence] of the lung passes through the nose. When the [influence] of the lung is in harmony, then the nose is able to distinguish bad from good odours" (Unschuld, 2016, p.254). SW-70 associates the lungs with the symptom of a stuffy nose (Unschuld, 2011, Vol II, pp.307-308). And LS-8 states "The lung influence: if depleted, then the nose will be blocked" (Unschuld, 2016, p.153).

[20] SW-70 associates the lungs with the signs and symptoms of sneezing, stuffy nose and nose bleed (Unschuld, 2011, Vol II, pp.307-308). And LS-8 states "The lung influence: if depleted, then the nose will be blocked. The breath [influence] will not flow freely, with shortness of breath [influence]" (Unschuld, 2016, p.153).

[21] Deadman, 1989, p.73 and 95; or Cheng, 1999, p.66.

[22] Waugh, 2001, pp.206-207.

[23] Unschuld, 2011, Vol I, p.185 (SW-10).

[24] Unschuld, 1986, p.301 (NJ-24).

[25] SW-22 associates the sign of flowing sweat with "lung disease" (Unschuld, 2011, Vol I, p.396). And NJ-24 associates the sign of dry skin and hair with poor lung function (Unschuld, 1986, p.301).

[26] Unschuld, 2011, Vol I, p.373-376 (SW-21).

[27] Unschuld, 2016, p.364 (LS-33).

[28] Unschuld, 2011, Vol I, p.279 (SW-17).

[29] Deadman, 1998, pp.517-518.

[30] Rye, 2013, pp.801-805.

[31] SW-23 associates "sadness" with an accumulation of the "five essences" in the lungs. That is, a symptom resulting when the "essence influence" of the five *yin* organs tends to accumulate in a single organ. In other words, overemphasis of that *one* organ, which in this case is the lung (Unschuld, 2011, Vol I, p.404; and see fn.14). And NJ-16 states "External evidence of [an illness in the lung] includes ... grief without joy, and an inclination to cry" (Unschuld, 1986, pp.219-220).

[32] SW-44 states "In case of a loss, or in case one longs for something but does not get it, then this manifests itself as [shortness of breath and noisy breathing]." That is, it weakens the lungs (Unschuld, 2011, Vol I, p.656).

[33] In clinic, I have found that these symptoms are reliably linked to the malfunction of either the kidneys or the lungs; however, I have not found a *Nei Jing* reference to this distinction, which could mean either that the authors did not then make this particular distinction, or that the nature of Chinese medical writing at that time precluded (or discouraged) the recording of such a fine distinction.

[34] Wilkie, 2002.

[35] Farrell, 2011.

[36] Unschuld, 2011, Vol II, p.73 (SW-60).

[37] In the original text, this part simply reads "When the heat is fought". Unschuld's translation adds "When the heat is fought [by the proper *chi*]". But since proper influence is said to be created from chest influence (*zong chi*), which is said to be created by the lungs, I have replaced "by the proper *chi*" with "by the lungs", to more readily capture the intended sentiment.

[38] Unschuld, 2011, Vol I, pp.503-504 (SW-32).

[39] Unschuld, 2011, Vol I, p.575 (SW-38).

[40] Unschuld, 2011, Vol I, p.337 (SW-19).

[41] Ross J, 1985, p.147.

[42] LS-10 states "If the [influences] are depleted, the shoulders and the back will feel pain with cold. The patients experience shortness of [influence], so that there is not enough [influence] available for breathing" (Unschuld, 2016, p.178).

[43] NJ-16 states "External evidence of [an illness in the lung] includes a white face" (Unschuld, 1986, pp.219-220).

[44] SW-17 states "When the speech is feeble and when it takes an entire day before he speaks again, this is [influence] deprivation" (Unschuld, 2011, Vol I, p.279). And LS-33 states "When the sea of [influence] has an insufficiency, then the breath [influence] will be diminished and are not enough to allow one to speak" (Unschuld, 2016, p.364).

[45] SW-32 states "When the lung has a heat disease [i.e. a wind-heat invasion]... sweat leaves the body and the patient feels cold" (Unschuld, 2011, Vol I, p.503). In LS-10, "patients sweating" is associated with a disease of the lungs. (Unschuld, 2016, p.177). And NJ-24 states that when the lung has an illness, "the liquids leave" [through the skin] (Unschuld, 1986, p.301).

[46] LS-8 states "The lung [influence]: if depleted, then the nose will be blocked. The breath [influence] will not flow freely, with shortness of breath [influence]. If replete, then the patient will cough with loud noises, a feeling of fullness in the chest, and breathing with the face directed upwards" (Unschuld, 2016, p.153).

[47] LS-13 describes the pathways of each meridian and the symptoms that occur along them. In the case of the lungs, it is stated that "Its diseases are at the locations passed [by the lung meridian]. They include aching divergences and torn sinews [i.e. muscular pain of various sorts]" (Unschuld, 2016, pp.235-236).

[48] Unschuld, 2011, Vol I, p.189 (SW-10).

[49] Unschuld, 2011, Vol I, p.109 (SW-5).

[50] See endnote 33 in this chapter above.

[51] Unschuld, 2011, Vol II, pp.211-212 (SW-67).

[52] Wang Bing. Cited by Unschuld, 2011, Vol II, p.211, fn.108.

[53] Waugh, 2001, pp.95-104.

[54] Deadman, p.469.

[55] Waugh, 2001, pp.304-305.

[56] Unschuld, 2011, Vol I, p.157; and see fn.10-11.

[57] Unschuld, 2016, pp.377-378 (LS-35).

[58] Unschuld, 2011, Vol I, pp.401-403 (SW-23).

[59] Cited by Unschuld, 2011, Vol I, pp.403, fn.9.

[60] Maciocia states "The main function of the Large Intestine is to receive food and drink from the Small Intestine. Having re-absorbed some of the fluids, it excretes the stool" (Maciocia, p.115). And Cheng states "The main function of the large intestine is to receive the waste material sent down from the small intestine, absorb its fluid content...." (Cheng X, 1999, p.39). (It should be stated that in editions of my own book previous to June 2017, I also followed this tendency set by today's Chinese medicine textbooks—until I had thoroughly researched the *Nei Jing* and *Nan Jing*.)

[61] Cheng X, 1999, pp.309-310.

[62] Ross J, 1985, p.150.

[63] Deadman, 1998, pp.162-163.

Chapter 8

[1] Betts, 2013, Chapter 27.3 Development of the Male and Female Reproductive Systems, p.1309.

[2] Waugh, 2001, pp.343-346.

[3] Klabundle, 2014.

[4] Waugh, 2001, pp.345-346.

[5] Gerich, 2010.

[6] Waugh, 2001, p.344.

[7] Waugh, 2001, p.223.

[8] Jelkmann, 2011.

[9] Betts, 2013, Chapter 26.4 Acid-Base Balance, pp.1265-1272.

[10] Maglione-Garves, 2005.

[11] Tsigos, 2002.

[12] Randall, 2010.

[13] Gerich, 2010.

[14] Jefferies, 1991. Note that when reading scientific papers such as several of those cited here, it becomes apparent that when authors attempt to codify the fine detail of organ hormonal activity, there is probably still more unknown than known, and that the knowledge often shifts as it grows. This is perhaps inevitable in such a comparatively young science. This, on top of other issues, makes the correlating of Chinese medicine organ functions with contemporary physiology a challenge, so that sometimes only approximate correlations can be made. But however inexact the science is, it is sufficient for the purposes of this section, which is to simply correlate Chinese Medicine organs with contemporary ones—without being unduly distracted by mating the fine detail.

[15] Kennedy, 2014.

[16] Barcroft, 1949.

[17] Neave, 2009.

[18] Betts, 2013, Chapter 27 The Reproductive System, pp.1310-1312 and pp.1289-1290.

[19] Celec, 2015.

[20] De Vries, 2009.

[21] Betts, 2013, Chapter 27 The Reproductive System, pp.1300-1308.

[22] Betts, 2013, Chapter 28.4 Maternal Changes During Pregnancy, Labour, and Birth, pp.1342-1344.

[23] Unschuld, 2016, pp.447-463 (LS-47).

[24] Unschuld, 2016, pp.489-493 (LS-50).

[25] Unschuld, 2016, pp.513-514 (LS-54).

[26] See Unschuld, 2011, Vol I, p.130. A line in SW-6 states "The major yang vessel originates from the Extreme Yin hole, and ends in the gate of life," and fn.18, p.130, provides Wang Bing's commentary on this line: "The gate of life stores essence; it is the location of brilliant radiance. It is a name for the two eyes. The major yang vessel originates from the eyes and extends downwards to the feet. Hence its root is in the tips of the toes and its conclusion is in the eyes. The *Ling shu* states: 命門者目也, 'Gate of life is the eye'." See also Unschuld, 1985, p.200.

[27] Unschuld, 1986, p.382 (NJ-36).

[28] See the commentaries cited in Unschuld, 1986, pp.382-386.

[29] Cited by Unschuld, 1986, p.385.

[30] Peking Academy of Chinese Medicine, 1968, pp.174-176. Cited by Unschuld, 1985, pp.202-203.

[31] Cheng X, 1999, p.35. Note that the notion that the influences obtained from our food were able to nourish essence was first introduced in SW-5, and this appears to be the source for the notion of "acquired essence". See Unschuld, 2011, Vol I, pp.98-99 (SW-5).

[32] LS-47 associates the following with inherited poor kidney function: "one easily suffers from lower back pain. He cannot bow down and rise again, and is easily harmed by [harmful influence]" (Unschuld, 2016, Vol I, p.453). Being "easily harmed by harmful influence (i.e. external pathogens)" suggests poor immunity. In LS-47, the theory is applied that our constitution is determined by the size, shape, etc. of the organs we were born with. The above symptoms were attributed to the kidneys being "big". Other variants are the kidneys being "elevated, sunken down, firm, brittle, small, upright, inclined". The theory is clearly untrue (p.156), however the important point is that the symptoms quoted would have been discovered trough practical observations and associated with the kidneys. Hence the symptoms

and organ association are fact based, even if the theory to explain them is not.

[33] Cheng X, 1999, p.36.

[34] Unschuld, 2011, Vol I, pp.36-41 (SW-1).

[35] See Unschuld, 2011, Vol I, p.37, fn.43, which cites a selection of the commentaries.

[36] Wang Bing's commentary on the meaning of "heaven *gui*" states "The controlling vessel and the thoroughfare vessel are both extraordinary [meridians]. When the [influence] of the kidneys is complete and abundant, the thoroughfare and the controlling [meridians] are passed by a flow. The menstrual blood gradually accumulates and moves down when its time comes. The thoroughfare is the sea of blood; the controlling vessel governs uterus and foetus. When both supply each other one may have children." Cited by Unschuld, 2011, Vol I, p.37, fn.43.

[37] LS-10 associates the following symptoms with "excitement" in the bladder and kidney meridians (i.e. indicating a problem with those organs, which results in the symptoms listed; and note that kidney issues are often expressed on the bladder channel): "the nape feels as if it were pulled, the spine aches, the lower back feels as if broken, the hip bones cannot be bent, the hollow of the knees feels like knotted" (Unschuld, 2016, p.188).

[38] LS-10 associates the following signs with kidney malfunction: "the teeth grow long and have stains" (Unschuld, 2016, p.198).

[39] LS-20 associates kidney disease (i.e. "when [harmful influence] is in the kidneys") with the symptoms of "aching bones..., the lower back aches... at times patients feel dizzy" (Unschuld, 2016, p.277).

[40] SW-10 states that "all marrow is tied to the brain" (Unschuld, 2011, Vol I, p.190). This may indicate knowledge, gained from practical observation, of the connection between the strength of kidney function and brain function, particularly in the brain's production of the symptoms of poor short-term memory, poor concentration, and light-headedness.

[41] SW-10 states "Headache and peak illness, this is depletion below and repletion above. The excess is in the [kidney and bladder meridians]. If it is serious, it enters the kidneys" (Unschuld, 2011, Vol I, p.195). "Peak illness" refers to an illness at the peak of the scull. The quote is in the context of a "blockage" of the influences and/or blood in the "meridians". "Depletion below" refers to poor kidney function (Kidney chi deficiency), which causes "repletion above", meaning a pain at the top part of the body; i.e. a headache. When such a blockage is "serious", this could only reflect disrupted function of the related organ, hence the text says "it enters the kidneys". And LS-10 associates the following symptoms with "excitement" in the bladder and kidney meridians (i.e. indicating a problem with those organs, which results in the symptoms listed): "the disease presses into the head and causes pain there [i.e. headache in the whole head], the eyes feel as [if] they were [about] to fall out [i.e. uncomfortable feeling in the eyes]" (Unschuld, 2016, p.188).

[42] SW-21 states "When one bears a heavy load and walks over a long distance, the resulting sweat originates from the kidneys" (Unschuld, 2011, Vol I, p.71). That is, working excessively hard strains the kidneys. This particular sentence makes sense, but when reading the surrounding sentences in the original chapter, some of those make no sense, regarding the concept of the "resulting sweat originating from a certain organ", and the commentators are clearly struggling to make sense of the passages. Therefore this current sentence cannot be taken at face value. However, the logic aside, it does indicate the knowledge of a link between working hard and this weakening the kidneys, which is the important point. One other point to note about this extract is that the author believed that sweat literally emitted from the stressed organ. This is untrue, but again, the sig-

nificant point is the association of the activity with the weakening of the kidney function, which was a fact based observation, even if the theory to explain it is untrue. See pp.163-166.

[43] Unschuld, 2016, p.89 (LS-4).

[44] SW-5 states "the kidneys generate the bones and the marrow," Unschuld, 2011, Vol I, p.110.

[45] SW-10 states "All marrow is tied to the brain." Unschuld, 2011, Vol I, p.190.

[46] Unschuld, 2011, Vol II, pp.91-93 (SW-61).

[47] Wang Bing. Cited by Unschuld, 2011, Vol II, p.93, fn.14.

[48] See page 263, which describes the five phase association of water with kidneys. This association is featured throughout the *Nei Jing*. For example, SW-61 states "The lung causes panting exhalation and the kidneys cause water swelling. The lung causes a [influence] movement contrary to its normal course and the patient cannot lie down" (Unschuld, 2011, Vol II, p.94). And commenting on this, Wang Bing (in 762 AD) stated "The lung causes panting exhalation, [influence] moving contrary to its normal course and inability to sleep because it rules the breathing. The kidneys cause water swelling because they rule the water" (Wang Bing. Cited by Unschuld, 2011, Vol II, p.94, fn.16).

[49] SW-21 states "When one has drunk or eaten to extreme repletion, the resulting sweat originates from the stomach. When one was frightened and has lost essence, the resulting sweat originates from the heart. When one bears a heavy load and walks over a long distance, the resulting sweat originates from the kidneys. When one runs fast and is in fear, the resulting sweat originates from the liver. When one agitates the body and works hard, the resulting sweat originates from the [pancreas]" (Unschuld, 2011, Vol I, pp.371-372). However, note that this passage is capable of metaphorical interpretation. The sweat "originates from" could be interpreted to mean that it is the stress in that organ that caused the person to have raised temperature, which then resulted in them sweating—not that the sweat was literally produced by the stressed organ. Though, on balance, I believe the author regarded the passage to be literally true.

[50] Waugh, 2001, pp.363-364.

[51] Waugh, 2001, p.118.

[52] Betts, 2013, Chapter 21.1 Anatomy of the Lymphatic and Immune Systems; and Chapter 26.1 Body Fluids and Fluid Compartments.

[53] SW-23 associates a disease in "the five [*yin* organs (*zang*)]" (which would include the kidneys) with signs and symptoms in each of the other organs; in relation to the bladder, it states "In the urinary bladder, if [the influence] does not pass freely it causes protuberance illness; if it is unrestrained, it causes involuntary loss of urine" (Unschuld, 2011, Vol I, pp.401-403). And SW-17 states "When the granaries do not keep what they store, in this case the doors are not under control. When the water fountain does not stop, in this case the urinary bladder does not keep what it stores" (Unschuld, 2011, Vol I, pp.279-280). The commentaries cited by Unschuld explain that this passage refers to uncontrollable diarrhoea or incontinence, and that "When the storage is not firm, the responsibility lies with the kidneys. Why? Because the kidney has the two yin [openings; i.e. the openings for urine and faeces] as its orifices. When the kidneys are depleted, they are unable to firmly close these orifices." (Cited by Unschuld, 2011, Vol I, p.280, fn.28).

[54] LS-10 associates the following sign and symptom with kidney malfunction "the breath [influence] is insufficient [i.e. shortness of breath] and this causes fear" (Unschuld, 2016, p.189). And SW-22 associates the signs and symptoms of "the patient pants and coughs and the body is heavy" with "kidney disease" (Unschuld, 2011, Vol I, p.397). The sign of "pants and coughs" is clearly produced by the lung, and today would probably be described as "shortness of breath" or

"asthma", particularly of the type where it is hard to breathe in. This sign was observed to be produced by "kidney disease", implying that the kidneys assist the lungs to breathe. The symptom of "the body is heavy" indicates poor energy, which would be an obvious consequence of not being able to breathe properly.

[55] In SW-22, the times of each organ's peak activity was stated, but this was calculated using five phase theory and the results were consequently untrue (p.269). It was not until over a millennium later that the correct times were calculated, which today's clinical observations confirm to be accurate (p.379).

[56] Cheng X, 1999, p.36.

[57] LS-33 states "When the sea of bone marrow has an insufficiency, then the brain revolves, and there are noises in the ears" (Unschuld, 2016, p.365). Here, "the brain revolves" could be understood to be referring to either vertigo or loss of balance.

[58] LS-17 states "the five [*yin* organs (*zang*)] internally always communicate with the seven orifices.... The [influence] of the kidneys passes through the ears. When the [influence] of the kidneys is in harmony, then the ears can hear the five tones" (Unschuld, 2016, pp.254-255). When an organ was described as being "in harmony", this meant that it was functioning correctly. In other words, for the hearing to be healthy, it was noticed that the kidneys needed to function well. LS-29 states "One inspects the ears to find out whether their hearing ability is good or bad, and from this one may recognise [the health of the kidneys]" (Unschuld, 2016, p.349). And LS-30 states "when the essence are lost the ears are deaf" (Unschuld, 2016, p.353).

[59] Unschuld, 2016, p.349 (LS-29).

[60] Unschuld, 2016, p.365 (LS-33).

[61] LS-30 states "when the essence are lost the ears are deaf" (Unschuld, 2016, p.353).

[62] This particular illustration is, admittedly, hit and miss, but this reflects the way people respond to pharmaceuticals, which is a very personal thing and is certainly hit and miss, so that no reliable observations could be made from any of the undesirable (and usually unpredicted) effects of such remedies. However, in my own experience of patients who have been affected in this way, there is a strong correlation between the loss of balance, along with other kidney-related signs, and the taking of a particular pharmaceutical—even where the drug was not intended to affect the patient's kidney function.

[63] Deadman, 1989, p.331 and 251; or Cheng X, 1999, p.75.

[64] SW-67 says of the kidneys "Its state of mind is fear. Fear harms the kidneys" (Unschuld, 2011, Vol II, p.210). SW-5 states "If fear causes harm, it harms the kidneys" (Unschuld, 2011, Vol I, p.110). NJ-16 states "External evidence of [an illness in the kidneys] includes a black face and a tendency to be fearful" (Unschuld, 1986, pp.219-220). And SW-23 associates "fear" with an accumulation of the "five essences" in the kidneys. That is, a symptom resulting when the "essence influence" of the five *yin* organs tends to accumulate in a single organ. In other words, overemphasis of the kidney function (Unschuld, 2011, Vol I, p.404; and see fn.14).

[65] SW-21, states "When one bears a heavy load and walks over a long distance, the resulting sweat originates from the kidneys" (Unschuld, 2011, Vol I, p.371). That is, working excessively hard stresses the kidneys. And LS-4 states "When one uses all his strength to lift something heavy... this will harm the kidneys" (Unschuld, 2016, p.89).

[66] Unschuld, 2011, Vol II, pp.667-671 (SW-77).

[67] SW-10 states "The kidneys long for salty flavour" (Unschuld, 2011, Vol I, p.188), meaning that when the kidneys are weak, the person craves salt because salt tends to benefit the kidneys.

[68] Lewis, 2017.

[69] SW-61 associates kidney dysfunction with swelling in the lower part of the body, which it terms a "*fu*-swelling" (Unschuld, 2011, Vol II, pp.91-92); see page 163, which quotes the *Nei Jing* theory that aims to explain the sign, then assess the validity of the theory.

[70] Loss of balance is not usually included as a kidney-related symptom in today's Chinese medicine textbooks, but I have included it for the following reasons. Apart from the clear association with old age, whose signs and symptoms are mainly due to poor kidney function, it can also be experienced earlier in life in people with poor kidney function; and I have also encountered clear evidence of loss of balance being induced when a person's kidney function is impeded as one of the unwanted effects of taking a pharmaceutical that adversely affects the kidneys.

[71] SW-22 states that "In the case of a kidney disease... Sweat flows during sleep.... Patients suffer from coolness because of receding [influence]" (Unschuld, 2011, Vol I, p.397). That is, the patient may feel cool during the day, but with occasional hot flushes.

[72] LS-10 associates the following signs and symptoms with kidney malfunction: "heat in the mouth, and dry tongue... the lower side of the feet is hot and aches" (Unschuld, 2016, p.189). And SW-44 describes the disease of "heat recession". One of its causes is given as "A person with this disease must have frequently entered the women's chambers drunk to intoxication". The chapter then states "...and when the [influence] of the kidneys is weak, the *yang* [influence] dominates alone. Hence, it is therefore that the hands and the feet are hot." (Unschuld, 2011, Vol I, p.669). The passages are in the context of the effects of wine on us, and it theorizes about how those effects are produced. However, the important point is that it associates the symptoms of hot hands and feet with weak kidney function. It also states that one cause of the condition is having sex too often, which is one key way of weakening the kidney function.

[73] SW-22 states that "In the case of a kidney disease... the body is heavy... patients dislike wind.... Patients suffer from coolness because of receding [influence]; their sentiments are unhappy" (Unschuld, 2011, Vol I, p.397).

[74] SW-70 associates disruption of normal kidney function with "The *yin* (i.e. the sexual organ) is limp; its [influence] is weakened massively and it does not rise. It does not function." (Unschuld, 2011, Vol II, pp.335-336).

[75] Unschuld, 2011, Vol I, p.189 (SW-10).

[76] Unschuld, 2011, Vol I, p.110 (SW-5).

[77] SW-10 states "The kidneys long for salty flavour" (Unschuld, 2011, Vol I, p.188)

[78] Leggett, 1994, p.17.

[79] This acupoint is not traditionally listed for treating the kidneys but I have found it to be extremely effective, particularly on occasions when some of the key kidney acupoints seem ineffective, such as Kidney-6 (*Zhaohai*) or Kidney-3 (*Taixi*). Its effect is probably due to the "six channel" *shaoyin* association of the heart and kidneys, in the same way that Pericardium-6 (*Neiguan*) can be used to treat the liver (p.397).

[80] Cheng X, 1999, pp.35-36.

[81] The concept of "kidney essence" being replenished by the food we eat, and the essence then going on to stimulate the function of the digestive organs, in a cyclic manner, was referred to in SW-5, which states "Flavour turns to physical appearance. Physical appearance turns to [influence]. [Influence] turns to essence. Essence turns to transformation. Essence is nourished by [influence]. Physical appearance is nourished by flavour. Transformations generate essence. [Influence] generates physical appearance" (Unschuld, 2011, Vol I, pp.98-99). See also Cheng X, 1999, p.35.

[82] Commenting on NJ-66, Yang K'ang-hou (in 1098) wrote "...The location between the two

kidneys is called 'great sea'; another name is 'submerged in water'. Inside of it is the spirit-turtle. It exhales and inhales the original influences.... The two kidneys are distinguished by their storing of the essence... The essence consists of immaterial influences; it constitutes man's source and root..." (Cited by Unschuld, 1986, pp.567-568). See also, Cheng X, 1999, p.35.

[83] Maciocia, p.40.

[84] Maciocia, p.40; but see my caveat in endnote 10 of Chapter 9 below.

[85] Betts, 2013, Chapter 25.2 Gross Anatomy of Urine Transport.

[86] Waugh, 2001, p.345.

[87] "Regional rectifier" has several possible interpretations, one being an "administrative region", another being a person responsible for identifying and classifying all males considered qualified for government office (See Unschuld, 2011, Vol I, p.158, fn.14). These organ descriptions in SW-8 are metaphorical, so, over two thousand years later, they do not lend themselves to literal interpretation. However, the quote ends by stating "the body liquids are stored in it," so that it is safe to assume this was considered to be the bladder's sole function—that of storing liquids prior to excretion.

[88] Unschuld, 2011, Vol I, p.158 (SW-8).

[89] In *Nei Jing* or *Nan Jing* passages, such phrases as "the upper opening of the bladder" usually refer to acupoints. These were regarded as "holes" or "openings" through which influences may be released or affected. Hence, anatomy was usually considered more in terms of the location of an organ's acupoints, rather than the physical location of the organ in the torso. This certainly seems to be the case in most passages discussing the *san jiao*.

[90] Unschuld, 1986, p.347 (NJ-31).

[91] Cited by Unschuld, 1986, p.351.

[92] Cheng X, 1999, p.41.

[93] Unschuld, 2016, p.266 (LS-18).

Chapter 9

[1] Waugh, 2001, pp.79-109.

[2] Unschuld, 2016, pp.631-632 (LS-71).

[3] Unschuld, 2011, Vol I, p.208 (SW-10).

[4] Ma Shi. Cited by Unschuld, 2011, Vol I, p.208, fn.25. Note that the statement "Of the five *yin* organs, only heart and lung are located above the diaphragm" is not literally true, since the pancreas is also clearly located above the diaphragm. But this issue is more one of interpretation. The *Nei Jing* notions of the anatomical organs were often vague, and sometimes completely wrong (p.270), so that such statements should not be interpreted literally in terms of contemporary anatomy. They sometimes relate to the location of acupoints rather than to that of the anatomical organs; or are sometimes merely theoretical—and often misguided. However, the original *Su Wen* passage may have been expressing a practical observation. When either the lungs or heart "have a disease", shortness of breath is one possible symptom. In other words, the person's "nose is not free", meaning they are unable to breathe freely through their nose. If this is what the *Su Wen* author meant, then clearly this was based on a practical observation, which was therefore factual, but the expression of his observation is a little vague. Then (some 1,700 years later), in order to attempt to clarify the statement, Ma Shi then produced his own theory. Unfortunately *his* clarifying statement does not seem to make sense. He attributes the symptom to the fact that both the heart and lungs are the only *yin* organs located above the diaphragm. Leaving aside the anatomical inaccuracy, his statement still does not make sense, since the function of the diaphragm is unrelated to the ability to breathe freely through the nose. This seems to imply that Ma Shi believed that one of the diaphragm's functions was to enable us to breathe freely through the nose. This would then explain his comment, though, of course, his theory is un-

true. However, in his own mind, his explanation would have clearly accounted for the symptom.

[5] Zhang Zhenyu. Cited by Unschuld, 2011, Vol I, pp.208-209, fn.25.

[6] Unschuld, 1986, p.358 (NJ-32).

[7] However, in 762 AD (about a millennium after the *Nei Jing* was compiled), Wang Bing was still clearly of the opinion that blood and "constructive influence" were two separate substances. Commenting on a line in SW-4, he states "This refers to the [meridians]. They are the passage ways through which the [constructive and defensive influence], the blood and the [influence] flow." (Unschuld, 2011, Vol I, p.83, fn.2).

[8] Cited by Unschuld, 1986, p.359. Commenting on *Nan Jing*, Section 32.

[9] Waugh, 2001, p.95.

[10] Maciocia, 1989, p.71; Cheng X, 1999, p.28. (It should be stated that in editions of my own book previous to June 2017, I also followed this tendency set by today's Chinese medicine textbooks—until I had thoroughly researched the *Nei Jing* and *Nan Jing*.)

[11] Unschuld, 2011, Vol I, p.178 (SW-9).

[12] Wang Bing. Cited by Unschuld, 2011, Vol I, p.178, fn.61.

[13] LS-34 associates the following with heart conditions: "The heart is vexed with closure and the person is speechless. Patients lower the head and silently withdraw," (Unschuld, 2016, p.369). And in NJ-34, the sound associated with the heart is "talk" (Unschuld, 1986, p.367).

[14] The *luo-connecting* meridian. See Deadman, 1989, p.210.

[15] I say that such meridian links are "supposed", or theoretical only, for the following reason. Such meridians (such as an internal meridian that connects the heart to the tongue, etc.) could not be detected in the same way that the meridians on the skin can be (and note that meridians are defined in this book as a "tract of distal tissue affected by organ function"—p.355). It is possible that such "tracts" may exist internally, but I think it is most likely that the *Nei Jing* authors noticed the associated between the heart and tongue (and the liver and the eyes, etc.), and to account for this, they simply assumed that there must therefore be a "meridian" (i.e. an artery-like tube) that connects the organ directly to the related sense; but that, in fact, no such meridian really exists.

[16] SW-23 states "The locations where the five essences collect: When essence [influence] collects in the heart, joy results" (Unschuld, 2011, Vol I, p.404). Wu Kun (in 1984) commented on this line: "As long as the essence [influence] of the five [*yin* organs (*zang*)] are stored in their respective [*yin* organ], no disease results. But when they unite and agglomerate within one single [*yin* organ], then they are [harmful influences] causing a repletion there" (Wu Kun. Cited by Unschuld, 2011, Vol I, p.404, fn.14). In other words, when the heart function is dominant in the person, this produces these tendencies in their personality: inappropriate smiling or laughter; inappropriate cheerfulness. And LS-8 states "The heart [influence]: if depleted, then the patient will be grieved. If replete, then he will laugh without end" (Unschuld, 2016, p.152).

[17] Joshi, 2011.

[18] Borreli, 2016.

[19] SW-43 states "In the case of a heart block, the vessels are not passable. When the patient is vexed, then there is a drumming below the heart [i.e. palpitations]. There is fiercely rising [influence], and the patient pants [i.e. shortness of breath]. The throat is dry and the patient tends to belch. When receding [influence] moves up, then the patient has fear" (Unschuld, 2011, Vol I, p.642). The term "vexed" is open to interpretation; it may mean constantly angered, distressed, disturbed, annoyed, confused, worried, or tormented.

[20] SW-69 associates the following signs and symptoms with the heart being harmed: "body

heat and a vexed heart, racing pulse, a feeling of being excited, feeling chilled, speaking incoherently, the heart aches [i.e. palpitations]; panting and coughing, sweating during the night; thirst and confusion" (Unschuld, 2011, Vol II, pp.253-254). The chapter is somewhat metaphorical. It compares a supposed climatic situation to the conditions within the body, and the above signs and symptoms are said to arise when a person's Fire phase has been harmed. Though the chapter is metaphorical and somewhat theoretical, it is assumed that the knowledge of the symptoms mentioned was obtained from practical observations.

[21] LS-43 associates the following signs and symptoms with the heart "a vexed heart, short of breath, cannot sleep peacefully" (Unschuld, 2016, p.377).

[22] The symptom of "dyslexia" is added by myself, derived from my own observations; I have found no mention of this in the *Nei Jing*.

[23] LS-47 associates the following states with heart conditions "Such persons suffer from vexation and tend to be forgetful. They have difficulties to open their heart and say something.... They are easily made to fear by someone else's words" (Unschuld, 2016, p.450). Interestingly, this chapter explains these symptoms by using the theory that an organ may vary physically (such as whether it is small, big, elevated, sunken, firm, brittle, or stands upright), and that these variations account for the various symptoms the organ may produce. They theory is untrue (p.156), but the important point is that the various symptoms would have been previously discovered from practical observations, which associated them with the heart. So, even though the author's explanatory theory is untrue, the symptoms are fact based.

[24] These are the signs and symptoms of "Yin deficiency", which include hot flushes during the day, night sweats, a sensation of heat on the soles and palms, dry mouth and constant thirst. They were referenced in this book's Chapter 8, in relation to the kidneys (endnotes 71 and 72), though the same signs and symptoms would occur when any other organ is affected by "Yin deficiency".

[25] LS-10 describes the path of each meridian and then describes the symptoms that may result when each meridian's associated organ is stressed. These include pains at various locations, following the path of the meridian; and in many cases even states that the toe or finger that the meridian ends at may be "useless"; i.e. either too weak or too stiff or painful to be used. In the case of the heart, the symptoms include "dry throat, thirst, desire to drink, pain in the heart; pain, aching or stiffness anywhere on the path of the heart meridian" (Unschuld, 2016, pp.176-185).

[26] SW-22 states "In the case of a heart disease, there is pain in the chest.... There is pain between breast, back, shoulder, and shoulder blades. There is pain inside of both arms" (Unschuld, 2011, Vol I, p.394).

[27] SW-70 associates the following signs and symptoms with the heart "laughing, craziness and absurd behaviour" (Unschuld, 2011, Vol II, pp.314-316). The chapter is metaphorical, and the current extract is in the context of the climactic conditions of "fire-red sunlight" and "summer heat" and the "transformations" caused. That is, it relates to the Fire phase, which corresponds to the heart (though it cites the related organs as being "the heart and the lung"). Though the chapter uses a metaphorical approach, relating climatic conditions to those in the body, it is assumed that the knowledge of all the signs and symptoms cited was originally discovered through practical observations.

[28] SW-9 states "[The heart's] effulgence is in the face" (Unschuld, 2011, Vol I, p.178). And SW-10 states "The correlate of the heart is the movement in the vessels; its splendour appears in the face and manifests itself in a red complexion" (Unschuld, 2011, Vol I, p.185).

[29] Unschuld, 2011, Vol I, p.189 (SW-10).

[30] SW-10 states "The heart longs for bitter flavour" (Unschuld, 2011, Vol I, p.187).

[31] Ross J, 1985, p.127

[32] Ross J, 1985, p.130.

[33] Cheng X, 1999, p.304.

[34] Ross J, 1985, p.130.

[35] Ross J, 1985, p.129.

[36] Ross J, 1985, p.134.

[37] Unschuld, 2011, Vol I, p.157 (SW-8).

[38] Wang Bing. Cited by Unschuld, 2011, Vol I, p.157, fn.11.

[39] Unschuld, 2016, p.266 (LS-18).

[40] Betts, 2013, Chapter 23.5 The Small and Large Intestines.

[41] Unschuld, 1986, p.347 (NJ-31).

[42] Cited by Unschuld, 1986, p.351.

[43] Cited by Unschuld, 1986, p.351.

[44] Cited by Unschuld, 1986, p.354.

[45] Maciocia, p.114. (It should be stated that in editions of my own book previous to June 2017, I also followed this tendency set by today's Chinese medicine textbooks—until I had thoroughly researched the *Nei Jing* and *Nan Jing*.)

[46] Maciocia, p.114. (Same caveat as above.)

[47] Unschuld, 2016, p.267 (LS-18).

Chapter 10

[1] Unschuld, 1986, p.310 (NJ-25).

[2] Cited by Unschuld, 1986, pp.310-316.

[3] Waugh, 2001, pp.130-131.

[4] Waugh, 2001, pp.379-382.

[5] Waugh, 2001, pp.132-135.

[6] Waugh, 2001, p.300.

[7] Waugh, 2001, p.67.

[8] This does not include the brain and uterus, which are associated with two of the *extra* meridians (beyond the twelve main meridians), in this case the Du and Ren meridians.

[9] This relationship is known as the "six channel theory" in Chinese medicine—where, since the pericardium and liver meridians are consecutive, the pair can be regarded as a single meridian (the *jueyin*); therefore acupoints on the one meridian can affect the organ associated with the other meridian (p.397).

[10] Unschuld, 2011, Vol I, p.89 and 158 (SW-4 and SW-8).

[11] Unschuld, 2016, pp.259-267 (LS-18).

[12] Unschuld, 1986, p.310 (NJ-25).

[13] Cited by Unschuld, 1986, pp.312-315.

[14] Unschuld, 1986, p.347 (NJ-31).

[15] Unschuld, 1986, p.395 (NJ-38).

[16] Unschuld, 1986, pp.395-396.

[17] Cited by Unschuld, 1986, p.396.

[18] Unschuld, 1986, pp.560-561 (NJ-66).

[19] See Ellis, 1989, pp.306-307, where a total of 29 alternative names are given for this single acupoint, Ren-4 (*Guanyuan*).

[20] Cited by Unschuld, 1986, pp.567-68.

[21] Cited by Unschuld, 1986, p.568.

[22] Beijing, 1980, pp.28-29.

[23] Cheng X, 1999, p.40.

[24] Cheng X, 1999, p.40.

[25] Unschuld, 2011, Vol I, pp.37-41 (SW-1).

Chapter 11

[1] Unschuld, 2016, pp.604-611 (LS-66). The quoted passage then goes on to describe the progress of the pathogen through the various sections of the body, with the signs and symptoms produced at each.

[2] Unschuld, 2016, pp.322-323 (LS-27).

[3] Unschuld, 2016, pp.766-767 (LS-81).

[4] This notion is suggested by the evidence above; or at least, it is an alternative way of explaining the above phenomena. But if this alternative explanation *were* correct, it would be a simple and elegant idea that would account for most, if not all, meridian-related phenomena in acupuncture treatments.

[5] Unschuld, 2011, Vol I, p.640 (SW-43).

[6] Unschuld, 2016, p.604 (LS-66).

Chapter 12

[1] Unschuld, 2011, Vol I, pp.220-222 (SW-13). From the original, I have changed "did not have the physical appearance of stretching towards officialdom" to "were not stressed by the demands of society and the workplace".

[2] Unschuld, 2016, pp.533-534 (LS-58).

[3] Unschuld, 2011, Vol I, pp.229-230 (SW-13).

[4] Zhang Jiebin, 1957. Cited by Unschuld, 2011, Vol I, pp.230, fn.34.

[5] Pharmaceutical intervention is not a natural phenomenon, so is not considered here. Once a patient is taking strong pharmaceuticals, so that their body no longer has chemical autonomy, all natural healing would be impeded to some degree. This usually produces an unclear symptom picture in the patient (one that does not resemble the patterns observed over thousands of years in Chinese medicine), and any improvements in organ function which the acupuncture treatment produces may lapse after a day or two. This effect is similar to the "re-programming" effect that a patient's mind has when the patient stubbornly continues harmful mental habits despite the acupuncture treatment normalizing their physical organ functions. After a few days, the old pattern of organ malfunction would start to re-establish. The difference between this and the effect of pharmaceuticals, is that the patient whose treatment is being blocked by their own insistence on repeating harmful mental habits, would still have a clear symptom picture that makes perfect sense in Chinese medicine. However, their "mental block" to treatment would make permanent progress in their treatment challenging.

[6] Unschuld, 2016, pp.344-345 (LS-29).

[7] Unschuld, 2011, Vol II, p.671 (SW-77).

[8] Wang Bing. Cited by Unschuld, 2011, Vol II, p.671, fn.36.

[9] Unschuld, 2011, Vol I, pp.53-56 (SW-2).

[10] Unschuld, 2011, Vol I, p.72 (SW-3).

[11] SW-22 states "The liver rules in spring... The heart rules in summer... The lung rules in autumn... The Kidneys rule in winter." Unschuld, 2011, Vol I, p.383 (SW-22).

[12] SW-29 states "The [pancreas], that is the soil. It governs the centre. Throughout the four seasons it tends the four [*yin* organs (i.e. liver, heart, lungs, kidneys)]. In each season it is entrusted with government for 18 days; it cannot rule an entire season by itself." Unschuld, 2011, Vol I, p.483 (SW-29).

Chapter 13

[1] These are paired organs in Chinese medicine "six channel theory" (p.397), so that acupoints belonging to one can often have a strong effect on the other organ; and when the function of one of the paired organs is low, this often affects the other organ. It is as though they share the same resources. In this case, the Ren-14 (*Juque*) pain was due to poor heart function (induced by his emotional concerns—that is, the breaks in his connections with his loved ones, which weakened his heart function). And due to the "six channel" cooperation between the heart and kidneys, and also the fact that he had poor kidney function as well—when his heart needed to draw on this shared "pool of resources", this depleted the resources available to his kidneys and so worsened his kidney-related signs—one of which was the empty-headedness which coincided with this Ren-14 pain.

[2] Gascoigne, 2003.

Chapter 14

[1] Unschuld, 1985, p.58.

[2] Unschuld, 2011, Vol I, pp.83-93 and pp.106-110 (SW-4 and SW-5).

[3] Maciocia, pp.18-19.

[4] Unschuld, 1986, p.485.

[5] Cited by Unschuld, 1986, p.490.

[6] Unschuld, 1986, p.492.

[7] Cited by Unschuld, 1986, p.493.

[8] Cited by Unschuld, 1986, pp.493-494.

[9] Cited by Unschuld, 1986, p.494.

[10] Unschuld, 2011, Vol I, pp.287-393 (SW-22).

[11] Wang Bing. Cited by Unschuld, 2011, Vol I, p.393, fn.85.

[12] Zhang Jiebin. Cited by Unschuld, 2011, Vol I, p.393, fn.85.

[13] Unschuld, 1986, pp.219-220 (NJ-16).

[14] Cited by Unschuld, 1986, p.226.

[15] Cited by Unschuld, 1986, pp.229-230.

[16] Waugh, p.250.

[17] Commenting on SW-9, Wang Bing states "Spring corresponds to wood; wood dominates soil. Late summer corresponds to soil; soil dominates water. Winter corresponds to water; water dominates fire. Summer corresponds to fire; fire dominates metal. Autumn corresponds to metal; metal dominates wood. This is the normal [course]. Late summer was added to the four seasons; hence the text speaks of the so-called mutual domination of the seasons on the basis of the five agents. The so-called 'late summer' is the sixth month." (Cited by Unschuld, 2011, Vol I, p.171, fn.32). And SW-22 states "The [pancreas] rules in late summer." Commenting on this, Wang Bing states " 'Late summer' is to say: the sixth month." And Lin Yi et al. state "The Quan Yuanqi edition states 'The [pancreas] rules during all four seasons. The sixth month is the place when the fire rules. Now, because the [pancreas] rules the centre and because the sixth month is in the middle of the twelve months, in the half of a year, it is therefore that the [pancreas] rules during the sixth month.' " (Cited by Unschuld, 2011, Vol I, pp.384-385). However, see endnote 12 of Chapter 12 above, which states that the pancreas rules in the final 18 months of each season.

[18] Unschuld, 2011, Vol I, pp.106-110 (SW-5).

[19] Unschuld, 2011, Vol I, pp.185-186 (SW-10).

[20] Wang Bing. Cited by Unschuld, 2011, Vol I, p.185, fn.4.

[21] Wang Bing. Cited by Unschuld, 2011, Vol I, p.186, fn.7.

[22] Wang Bing. Cited by Unschuld, 2011, Vol I, p.186, fn.10, 13, 14.

[23] Unschuld, 2011, Vol II, pp.131-132 (SW-63).

[24] Unschuld, 2011, Vol I, p.311 (SW-34).

[25] Unschuld, 2016, p.330 (LS-28).

[26] Cited by Unschuld, 2016, p.376, fn.10.

[27] Deadman, p.519 and p.523.

[28] Deadman, p.523.

[29] In this book, the explanation for acupuncture's effects in such situations is that when an organ is stressed, this can cause the tissue at its related acupoints to also malfunction—including tissue at the sense organs, tongue, vocal cords and throat. This explains the tenderness that appears at such acupoints in this situation. And (according to the intelligent tissue hypothesis—p.372) by stimulating such acupoints, this encourages the organ to cancel out the malfunction in itself that caused the distal tenderness (or malfunction of tissue), which then corrects the distal signs and symptoms. This hypothesis provides a plausible explanation using concepts from contemporary anatomy and physiology.

[30] Unschuld, 2016, p.755 (LS-80).

[31] Unschuld, 2016, p.758 (LS-80).

[32] Cited by Unschuld, 2016, p.759, fn.15.

[33] Unschuld, 2016, p.329 (LS-28).

[34] Unschuld, 2016, p.333 (LS-28).

[35] Unschuld, 2016, p.264 (LS-18).

[36] Kovich, 2018b.

[37] Unschuld, 2011, Vol I, pp.110-117 (SW-5).

[38] Hu Tianxiong, 1991. Cited by Unschuld, 2011, Vol I, p.111, fn.70.

[39] Chaurasia, 1976.

[40] Reiss, 1997.

[41] UCLA, 2004.

[42] Unschuld, 2016, p.413 (LS-41).

[43] Kovich, 2016.

[44] Unschuld, 2011, Vol I, pp.434-435 (SW-26).

[45] Waugh, 2001, p.366.

[46] Unschuld, 2016, pp.40-41 (LS-1).

[47] Cheng X, pp.347-349.

[48] Unschuld, 2016, p.43 (LS-1).

[49] SW-13 states, "When the people of later generations treated a disease, then this was different. The treatments were not based in the four seasons. They no longer knew of the significance of sun and moon. They did not recognize whether the [influence] moved contrary to or followed its regular course. When a disease had already assumed physical manifestation, they wished to use fine needles to treat the exterior of the patient and decoctions to treat his interior. Uneducated practitioners behave very aggressively, believing they can launch an attack. Before the old disease has ended, a new disease emerges in addition.... The most essential in treatment is the following: Not to miss movement in the vessels and complexion, and to make use of them without confusion, that is the grand rule of treatment. If acting contrary to and acting in compliance with the norms are reversed, and if tip and root do not match, in the course of the treatment the healer loses his spirit, just as in government the ruler loses his country." (Unschuld, 2011, Vol I, pp.227-229). And NJ-16 describes various methods of examining the "movement in the vessels", then states "Today, everybody selects but one of these methods and considers his choice to be correct. How can one distinguish what are correct and incorrect diagnostic techniques?" (Unschuld, 1986, p.219).

[50] Unschuld, 2016, pp.36-37 (LS-1).

[51] Unschuld, 2016, p.37, fn.4-5.

[52] Unschuld, 2016, p.73 (LS-2).

[53] Deadman, p.29.

[54] Unschuld, 2011, Vol I, pp.733-735 (SW-50).

[55] Unschuld, 2016, p.79 (LS-3).

[56] While writing this passage, it occurs to me that in all these routine experiences, I have failed to make a note of which acupoint or meridian I was needling each time this scenario occurred. I think this is because I have only now started to analyse this in detail, so it did not occur to me to notice which meridian, and hence organ, was involved each time.

[57] Unschuld, 2016, pp.402-403 (LS-39).

[58] Waugh, 2001, p.303.

Chapter 15

[1] Unschuld, 2011, pp.274-275 (SW-17).

[2] Unschuld, 1986, p.65 (NJ-1).

[3] Cited by Unschuld, 1986, pp.70-71.

[4] See the commentaries cited by Unschuld, 1986, pp.66-78.

[5] Cited by Unschuld, 1986, p.77.

[6] Slomianka, 2009.

[7] Blausen.com staff, 2014.

[8] Cited by Unschuld, 1986, pp.69-70.

Chapter 16

[1] SW-4 states "The conduits have five winds." Wang Bing (in 762) commented on this line, saying "This refers to the [meridians]. They are the passage ways through which the [constructive and defensive influence], the blood and the [influence] flow." And Zhang Jiebin (in 1957) also commented on this same line, saying "This refers to the [meridians]. The 'five winds' are the winds of the five [*yin* organs (*zang*)]." (Unschuld, 2011, Vol I, p.83, fn.2).

[2] This description is in the context of viruses and bacteria. The Chinese medicine pathogen of *dampness* is a separate scenario. In this case, the *dampness* is produced by poor pancreas function. Simplistically, the state could be imaged as the

blood having become too "soupy", since the digestion is weak; and it is this "soupiness" that is considered the pathogen. But see page 76 for a more detailed explanation.

[3] Deadman, pp.398-399.

Chapter 17

[1] Voll, 1975.
[2] Ahn, 2007.
[3] Kim, 1963.
[4] Kim, 1965.
[5] Fujiwara, 1967 (Japanese). Cited by Soh, 2013.
[6] Soh, 2013.
[7] Jiang, 2002.
[8] Lee BC, 2004a.
[9] Lee BC, 2004b.
[10] Lee KJ, 2004.
[11] Shin, 2005.
[12] Lee BC, 2005.
[13] Johng, 2007.
[14] Cho, 2004.
[15] Lee BC, 2010.
[16] Kwon, 2012.
[17] Sung, 2008.
[18] Kim, 1963, pp.9-10.
[19] Kim, 1965, pp.15-16.
[20] Kim, 1965, p.31.
[21] The diagrams in this chapter are reproduced from Kim's 1963 and 1965 books.
[22] Kim, 1965, p.13 and 30.
[23] Kim, 1965, p.23.
[24] Kim, 1965, p.34.
[25] Kim, 1965, p.63.
[26] Kim, 1963, p.11.
[27] Kim, 1965, p.11.
[28] Kim, 1965, p.34.
[29] Kim, 1965, p.31.
[30] Kim, 1965, p.64.
[31] Kim, 1965, p.40.
[32] Kim, 1965, p.73.
[33] Kim, 1965, p.97.
[34] Kim, 1965, pp.80-81.
[35] Kim, 1965, pp.90-94 and 34.
[36] Kim, 1965, p.94.
[37] Kim, 1965, p.95.
[38] Sung, 2005.
[39] Kim, 1965, p.35.
[40] Kim, 1965, p.55.
[41] Kim, 1965, p.60.
[42] Kim, 1965, p.61.
[43] Cai, 2013.
[44] Serisawa, 1978.
[45] Oleson, 1980.
[46] Rosenblatt, 1981
[47] Sullivan, 1985.
[48] Saku, 1993.
[49] Kovich, 2018d.
[50] Kovich, 2018b.
[51] Betts 2013. Chapter 23 - The Digestive System, p.1106.
[52] Kovich, 2018c.
[53] Kovich, 2018e.
[54] Kovich, 2018f.
[55] Kovich, 2018b.

Chapter 18

[1] Urone, 2012, p.240.
[2] Betts, 2013, pp.42-54.
[3] Urone, 2012, pp.694-700.
[4] Betts, 2013, section: 3.2 The Cytoplasm and Cellular Organelles.
[5] Szent-Gyorgyi, 1941.
[6] Oschman, 2016.
[7] Gascoyne PRC, 1981.
[8] Becker, 1985, pp.192-202.
[9] Becker, 1985, pp.58-59.
[10] Sinyukhin. Cited by Becker, 1985, p.61.
[11] Becker, 1985, pp.150-154.
[12] Illingworth, 1980.
[13] Becker, 1985, pp.88-91.
[14] Becker, 1985, p.90.
[15] Cheng N, 1982.
[16] Alvarex, 1983.

[17] Baker, 1997.
[18] Becker, 1961.
[19] Becker, 1985, p.101 and 107.
[20] Becker, 1985, p.90.
[21] OpenStax, 2014.
[22] Becker, 1985, p.237.
[23] King, 2016.
[24] Lee BC, 2010.
[25] Chen E, 2008.
[26] Chen EY, 1998 (Chinese). Cited by Chen E, 2008.
[27] Chen EY, 2000 (Chinese). Cited by Chen E, 2008.
[28] Liu F, 2000 (Chinese). Cited by Chen E, 2008.
[29] Oschman, 2009.

Chapter 19

[1] Unschuld, 2011, Vol I, p.89 (SW-4); and Unschuld, 2011, Vol I, pp.95-126 (SW-5).
[2] Unschuld, 2011, Vol I, p.89 (SW-4).
[3] Kovich, 2018a.
[4] Wang X, 2012.
[5] Han, 2009.

Chapter 20

[1] Urone, 2012, pp.652-656.
[2] Burr, 1944-49. Cited by Becker, 1985, pp.84-84.
[3] Inyushin, 1978 (Russian). Cited by Freeman, 2008, p.568.
[4] Urone, 2012, p.734.
[5] Urone, 2012, pp.768-772.
[6] Park, 2009. Image reproduced with kind permission.
[7] Kuphaldt, 2006, p.491.
[8] Hasgall, 2015.
[9] Urone, 2012, pp.954-956.
[10] Urone, 2012, pp.956-957.
[11] Urone, 2012, pp.956-958.
[12] It is possible that this is achieved simply by the stimulation causing the local tissue to relax. This effect can be readily noted in clinic. When a patient has stiff muscles at any location, whether on a meridian or not, and an acupuncture needle is inserted, the tissue normally relaxes immediately.
[13] Longhurst, 2010.
[14] Langevin, 2002a and 2002b.
[15] Kim, 1963, p.32.
[16] Zhang WB, 2008.

Appendix B

[1] Liu Z, 1999, p.43.

Appendix C

[1] See the patient example I described in an online article, where the patient had a life-long lump on the liver-region of his tongue, which swelled in response to liver-related stress (Kovich, 2017).

Appendix D

[1] Royal Society of Chemistry, 2004.
[2] Waugh, 2001, p.306.
[3] Waugh, 2001, pp.301-303.
[4] McGinness, 1974.
[5] Shirakawa, 1977.

Appendix F

[1] Longhurst, 2010.
[2] Gabe, 1969.
[3] Kim, 1965.
[4] Langevin, 2002a.
[5] Langevin, 2002b.
[6] Kim, 1963, p.32.
[7] Kim, 1963, pp.31-33.
[8] Ling, 2016, Chapter 9.2 Model of Conduction in Metals, pp.391-395.

Glossary

[1] Unschuld, 2011, Vol I, pp.394 (SW-22).
[2] Unschuld, 2016, p.276 (LS-20).
[3] Unschuld, 2016, pp.176-208 (LS-10).
[4] Unschuld, 2016, p.177 (LS-10).
[5] Unschuld, 2016, p.178 (LS-10).
[6] Unschuld, 1986, pp.219-220 (NJ-16).

Bibliography

Alvarex OM, Mertz PM et al 1983. The Healing of Superficial Skin Wounds is Stimulated by External Electrical Current. *Journal of Investigative Dermatology.* 81:144-148.

Ahn AC, Martinsen ØG 2007. Electrical Characterization of Acupuncture Points: Technical Issues and Challenges. *Journal of Alternative and Complementary Medicine,* 13(8),817-824. doi:10.1089/acm.2007.7193

Baker LL et al 1997. Effects of Electrical Stimulation on Wound Healing in Patients with Diabetic Ulcers. *Diabetes Care.* March 1997; 20:405-41.

Barcroft H, Konzett H 1949. On the actions of noradrenaline, adrenaline and isopropyl noradrenaline on the arterial blood pressure, heart rate and muscle blood flow in man. *The Journal of Physiology.* 110(1-2):194-204.

Becker RO 1961. Proof that the direct electrical currents in the salamander are semiconducting in nature. *Science.* 134:101-102.

Becker RO 1985. *The Body Electric, Electromagnetism and the foundation of life.* New York, NY: Harper.

Beijing 1980. *Essentials of Chinese Acupuncture.* Beijing: Foreign Languages Press (this is an English translation of *Zhongguo Zhenjiuxue Gaiyao.* 1964).

Berk WR (ed.)1986. *Chinese Healing Arts, Internal King-Fu.* Burbank, CA: Unique Publications.

Berg JM, Tymoczko JL, Stryer L 2002. *Biochemistry. 5th edition.* W H Freeman: New York. Available from: https://www.ncbi.nlm.nih.gov/books/NBK22436/

Betts JG, Desaix P, Johnson E, Johnson JE, Korol O, Kruse D et al 2013. *Anatomy and Physiology.* Houston, TX: OpenStax, Rice University. Freely available at https://openstax.org/details/books/anatomy-and-physiology (page numbers refer to the downloadable pdf edition).

Blausen.com staff 2014. Blausen gallery. Wikiversity Journal of Medicine. doi:10.15347/wjm/2014.010. ISSN 20018762.

Borreli L 2016. Can An Organ Transplant Change A Recipient's Personality? Cell Memory Theory Affirms Yes. *www.medicaldaily.com* <http://www.medicaldaily.com/can-organ-transplant-change-recipients-personality-

cell-memory-theory-affirms-yes-247498> (Accessed May 09 2016)

Bronte V, Pittet MJ 2013. The spleen in local and systemic regulation of immunity. *Immunity*. 39(5):806-818. doi:10.1016/j.immuni.2013.10.010.

Burr H 1944-49. Various articles. *Yale Journal of Biological Medicine*. 1944, 16; 1942, 14; 1947, 19; 1949, 21.

Cai DJ, Chen J, Zhuang Y et al 2013. Review and comment on the Relationship between Primo Vascular System and Meridians. *Evid Based Complement Alternat Med.* 2013:279176.

Celec P, Ostatníková D, Hodosy J 2015. On the effects of testosterone on brain behavioral functions. *Frontiers in Neuroscience*. 9:12. doi:10.3389/ fnins.2015.00012.

Cesta MF 2006. Normal Structure, Function, and Histology of the Spleen. *Toxicologic Pathology*. 34(5): 455-465. doi:10.1080/01926230600867743.

Chang Tsung-Tung 1970. *Der kult der Shang-Dynastie im Spiegel der Orakelin-schriften*. Wiesbaden.

Chaurasia BD, Mathur BB 1976. *Eyedness*. Acta Anat (Basel). 96(2):301–5. doi:10.1159/000144681.

Chen E 2008. The Structure of Liquid Crystal Energy Band of Meridian. *Journal of Accord Integrative Medicine*. 4(3):139-146.

Chen EY, Shen LY, Dang RS, Cheng HS, Cai DH, He WQ et al 1998. Relation of connective tissue and concentrated area of Calcium element at acupoints below the neck of Gallbladder Meridian. *Shanghai Journal of Acupuncture and Moxibustion*. 17(2):36-37.

Chen EY, Dang RS, Cheng HS, Shen LY, Liu F, Gong J 2000. Blood vessels and calcium distribution in Waiqiu (GB 36). *Shanghai Journal of Acupuncture and Moxibustion*. 19(1):34-36.

Cheng N et al 1982. The effects of electric currents on ATP Generation, protein synthesis, and membrane transport in rat skin. *Clin Orthop Relat Res*. Nov-Dec;(171):264-72.

Cheng X (ed.) 1999. *Chinese Acupuncture and Moxibustion, Revised Edition*. Beijing, China: Foreign Languages Press.

Cho SJ, Kim BS, Park YS 2004. Threadlike structures in the aorta and coronary artery of swine. *Journal of International Society of Life Information Science*. 22:609-611.

Chun-Xia Yi et al 2010. The role of the autonomic nervous liver innervation in the control of energy metabolism. *Biochim Biophys Acta*. Apr; 1802(4): 416–431.

Collins 1991. Collins English Dictionary. Collins London.

Deadman P 1998. *A Manual of Acupuncture*. Hove, UK: Journal of Chinese Medicine Publications.

De Vries GJ, Södersten P 2009. Sex Differences in the Brain: the Relation between Structure and Function. *Hormones and behavior*. 55(5):589-596. doi:10.1016/j.yhbeh.2009.03.012.

Eichorn Werner 1976. *Die alte chinesische Religion und das Staatskultwesen*. Leiden.

Ellis A, Wiseman N, Boss K 1989. *Grasping the Wind*. Brookline, Massachusetts: Paradigm Publications.

Farrell AP (ed.) 2011. *Encyclopaedia of Fish Physiology, from Genome to Environment*. Elsevier, Academic Press.

Filshie J, Cummings M 1999. Western medical acupuncture. in: *E Ernst, A White*

(Eds.) Acupuncture: A Scientific Appraisal. Oxford: Butterworth-Heinemann:31-59.

Freeman LW 2008. *Mosby's Complementary & Alternative Medicine: A Research-Based Approach, 3rd Edition.* St Louis, Missouri: Mosby Elsevier.

Friedland G 2009. Discovery of the function of the heart and circulation of blood. *Cardiovascular Journal of Africa.* 20(3):160.

Fujiwara S and Yu SB 1967. Bonghan theory morphological studies. *Igaku noAyumi.* 60: 567-577 (Japanese).

Gabe IT, Gault JH, Ross J, Mason DT, Mills CJ, Schillingford JP et al 1969. Measurement of Instantaneous Blood Flow Velocity and Pressure in Conscious Man with a Catheter-Tip Velocity Probe. *Circulation.* 40:603-614. doi:10.1161/01.CIR.40.5.603.

Gascoigne S 2003. *The prescribed drug guide, a holistic perspective.* Clonakilty, Ireland: Jigme Press.

Gascoyne PRC, Pethig R, Szent-Gyorgyi A 1981. Water structure-dependent charge transport in proteins. *Proceedings of the National Academy of Sciences.* 78:261-265.

Gerich JE 2010. Role of the kidney in normal glucose homeostasis and in the hyperglycaemia of diabetes mellitus: therapeutic implications. *Diabetic Medicine.* 136-142. doi:10.1111/ j.1464-5491.2009.02894.x.

Han HJ, Sung B, Ogay V, Soh KS 2009. The flow path of alcian blue from the acupoint BL23 to the surface of abdominal organs. *Journal of Acupuncture and Meridian Studies.* 2(3):182-189.

Hasgall PA, Di Gennaro F, Baumgartner C, Neufeld E, Gosselin MC, Payne D et al 2015. Database for thermal and electromagnetic parameters of biological tissues. *ITIS Foundation.* Version 3.0, Sep 1. doi: 10.13099/VIP21000-03-0. www.itis.ethz.ch/database.

Hu Hou-hsüan 1944. Yin-jen chi-ping kao. *Chia-ku-hsüan Shang-shih lun-tsung.* Cheng-tu.

Hu Tianxiong 胡天雄, *Su wen bu shi* 素问补识. Beijing 北京: Chinese Medical and Pharmaceutical Science and Technology Press 中国医药科技出版社 1991.

Illingworth CM and Barker AT 1980. Measurement of electrical currents emerging during the regeneration of amputated finger tips in children. *Clin. Phys. Physiol. Meas.* 1:87.

Ingraham P 2016. *Organ Health Does Not Depend on Spinal Nerves* (2016, Mar 18). Retrieved Aug 26, 2016, from https://www.painscience.com/articles/spinal-nerves-and-organs.php

Inyushin VM 1978. Elements of a theory of the biological field. Alma-Ata, Kazakhstan. Kazakh State Department for Higher and Special Academic Education (Russian).

Jefferies WMK 1991. Cortisol and immunity. *Medical Hypotheses.* 34(3):198-208.

Jelkmann W 2011. Regulation of erythropoietin production. *The Journal of Physiology.* 589(Pt 6):1251-1258. doi:10.1113/ jphysiol.2010.195057.

Jiang X, Kim HK, Lee BC, Choi C, Soh KS, Cheun BS et al 2002. Method for observing intravascular Bonghan duct. *Korean J Orient Prevent Med Soc.* 6:162-166.

Johng HM, Yoo JS, Yoon TJ, Shin HS,1 Lee BC, Lee C et al 2007. Use of magnetic nanoparticles to visualize threadlike structures inside lymphatic vessels of rats. *Evid Based Complement Alternat Med.* Mar; 4(1):77-82.

Joshi S 2011. Memory transference in organ transplant recipients. *NAMAH, Journal of New Approaches to Medicine and Health* Apr;19,1 <https://www.namahjournal.com/doc/Actual/Memory-transference-in-organ-transplant-recipients-vol-19-iss-1.html>. (Accessed May 09 2016)

Kanō Yoshimitsu 1980. "Isho ni mieru ki-ron." In *Ki no shisō*. Onozawa Seiichi et al. (ed.), pp.280-313.

Kennedy R 2014. Cortisol (Hydrocortisone). *The Doctors' Medical Library*. Web 3 April 2014. < http://www.medical-library.net/content/view/1401/41/ >.

Kim BH 1963. *On the Kyungrak System*. Pyongyang, Korea: Medical Science Press (English).

Kim BH 1965. *Kyungrak System and Theory of Sanal.* Pyongyang, Korea: Medical Science Press (English). Also available in a 2016 edition: *Kyungrak System and Theory of Sanal.* Bristol, UK: CuriousPages Publishing.

King D 2016. Neurons and Support Cells. *SIU Med* (Southern Illinois University School of Medicine). http://www.siumed.edu/~dking2/ssb/neuron.htm#3 Retrieved 9 Oct 2016.

Klabundle RE 2014. Blood Volume. *Cardiovascular Physiology Concepts.* http://www.cvphysiology.com/Blood Pressure/BP025. Updated Apr 25 2014.

Kovich F 2009. *The Trouble with Conversation.* Bristol, UK: CuriousPages Publishing.

Kovich F 2016. Practice insight into the issue of whether to needle on both sides. *CuriousPages.com/tcm.* Retrieved June 15 2017 from www.curiouspages.com/sketchbook/TCMissueNeedleOnBothSides.php.

Kovich F 2017. An unusual tongue anomaly. *CuriousPages.com/tcm.* Retrieved July 21 2017 from http://www.curiouspages.com/sketchbook/TCMunusualTongueAnomaly.php

Kovich F 2018a. A new definition of an acupuncture meridian. J Acupunct Meridian Stud 2018; doi: https://doi.org/10.1016/j.jams.2018.05.001

Kovich F 2018b. The stomach's communication with its related acupoints, and the "intelligent tissue" hypothesis. J Acupunct Res 2019;36(1): 21-27. doi: https://doi.org/10.13045/jar.2018.00409

Kovich F 2018c. The impedance profile of acupuncture points. J Acupunct Res 35(3): 104-107; doi: https://doi.org/10.13045/jar.2018.00080

Kovich F 2018d. The Daily Variance in Impedance at Acupuncture Points. J Acupunct Res 2018; 35(4): 176-181. doi: https://doi.org/10.13045/jar.2018.00122

Kovich F 2018e. The lungs' real-time states are reflected in the tissue at its related acupuncture points. J Acupunct Res 2019;36(2):88-91. doi: https://doi.org/10.13045/jar.2019.00045

Kovich F 2018f. Possible insights into the respiration pacesetter mechanism derived from observations at acupuncture points. Mendeley Data 2019, v1 http://dx.doi.org/10.17632/bh8xmpfs48.1

Kuphaldt Tony R 2006. *Lessons In Electric Circuits, Volume II – AC, Sixth Edition.* Available free from https://www.ibiblio.org/kuphaldt/electricCircuits/

Kwon BS, Chang MH, Yu SS, Lee BC, Ro JY, Hwang S 2012. Microscopic nodes and ducts inside lymphatics and on the surfaces of internal organs are rich in granulocytes and secretory granules. *Cytokine*. Vol.60, no.2:587-592.

Langevin HM, Yandow JA 2002a. Relationship of acupuncture points and meridians to connective tissue planes. *Anatomical Record*. 269(6):257–265.

Langevin HM, Churchill DL, Wu J, Badger GJ, Yandow JA, Fox JR et al 2002b. Evidence of connective tissue involvement in acupuncture. *The FASEB Journal*. 16(8):872–874.

Lautt W, Greenway C 1976. Hepatic venous compliance and role of liver as a blood reservoir. *American Journal of Physiology*. 231:292-295.

Lee BC, Baik KY, Johng HM, Nam TJ, Lee J, Sung B et al 2004a. Acridine orange staining method to reveal the characteristic features of an intravascular threadlike structure. *Anat Rec (New Anat)*. 278B:27-30.

Lee BC, Park ES, Nam TJ, Johng HM, Baik KY, Soh KS 2004b. Bonghan ducts on the surface of rat internal organs. *Journal of International Society of Life Information Science*. 22:455-459.

Lee BC, Yoo JS, Baik KY, Kim KW, Soh KS 2005. Novel threadlike structures (Bonghan ducts) inside lymphatic vessels of rabbits visualized with a Janus Green B staining method. *Anat Rec B New Anat*. Sep; 286(1):1-7.

Lee BC, Eom KH, and Soh KS 2010. Primo-vessels and Primo-nodes in Rat Brain, spine and sciatic nerve. *J Acupunct Meridian Stud*. Jun; 3(2):111-5.

Lee KJ, Kim SY, Jung TE, Jin D, Kim DH, Kim HW 2004. Unique duct system and the corpuscle-like structures found on the surface of the liver. *Journal of International Society of Life Information Science*. 22:460-462.

Leggett D 1994. *Helping Ourselves, A guide to traditional Chinese Food Energetics*. Devon, England: Meridian Press.

Lewis JL 2017. *Hyponatremia, Professional Version*. MSDManuals.com. Accessed July 11 2017. <http://www.msdmanuals.com/en-gb/professional/endocrine-and-metabolic-disorders/electrolyte-disorders/hyponatremia>

Ling SJ, Sanny J, Moebs W 2016. *University Physics Volume 2*. Houston, TX: OpenStax, Rice University. Freely available at https://openstax.org/details/books/university-physics-volume-2 (page numbers refer to the downloadable pdf edition).

Li Zhengdong, Wang Xiuzhen 1987. 李正东, 王秀珍. *Nei jing* teng tong ji zhi quan shi 《内经》疼痛机制诠释. *Zhong yi yao xin xi* 中医药信息 6, 1-3.

Liu F, Chen EY, Dang RS 2000. Distribution of vessel and calcium on tibial margin of leg interosseous membrane. *Academic Journal of Second Military University*. 21(8):759-760.

Liu Zheng-cai, Hua Ka 1999. A Study of Daoist Acupuncture & Moxibustion. Boulder, CO: Blue Poppy Press.

Longhurst JC 2010. Defining meridians: a modern basis of understanding. *Journal of Acupuncture and Meridian Studies*. 3(2):67–74.

Ma Shi 马莳, *Huang Di nei jing su wen zhu zheng fa wei* 黄帝内经素问注证发微.

(Written in 1586.) Beijing 北京：科学技术文献出版社 1999. Normally cited according to Cheng Shide et al.

Maciocia G 1989. *The Foundations of Chinese Medicine*. Edinburgh, UK: Churchill Livingstone.

McCarley RW 2007. Neurobiology of REM and NREM sleep. *Sleep Medicine*. 8:302-330.

McGinness J, Corry P, Proctor P 1974. Amorphous Semiconductor Switching in Melanins. *Science*. 183(4127):853-5.

Maglione-Garves CA, Kravitz L, Schneider S 2005. Cortisol connection: Tips on managing stress and weight. *ACSM's Health & Fitness Journal*. 9(5):20-23.

Neave N, O'Connor DB 2009. Testosterone and male behaviours. *The Psychologist*. 22:28-31.

Oleson TD, Kroening RJ, Bresler DE 1980. An experimental evaluation of auricular diagnosis: the somatotopic mapping of musculoskeletal pain at ear acupuncture points. Pain 1980;8:217-219.

OpenStax 2014. Anatomy & Physiology. OpenStax CNX. Jul 30, 2014 http://cnx.org/contents/14fb4ad7-39a1-4eee-ab6e-3ef2482e3e22@6.27.

Oschman JL 2009. Charge transfer in the living matrix. *Journal of bodywork and movement therapies*. 13,215-228.

Oschman JL 2016. The Living Matrix Connective Tissue Concept. *www.energy-medicine.org*. Accessed 10 Oct 2016.

Pandol SJ 2010. *The Exocrine Pancreas*. San Rafael (CA): Morgan & Claypool Life Sciences. Regulation of Whole-Organ Pancreatic Secretion. Available from: https://www.ncbi.nlm.nih.gov/books/NBK54132/

Park SH, Lee BC, Choi CJ et al 2009. Bioelectrical study of bonghan corpuscles on organ surfaces in rats. *J Korean Phys Soc*. Aug; 55(2):688-693. (Image reproduced with kind permission.)

Peking Academy of Chinese Medicine 1968. *Chung-i ko-chia hsüeh-shuo chiang-i*. Hong Kong.

Porkert M 1974. *The theoretical foundations of Chinese medicine*. Massachusetts institute of technology. MIT Press.

Randall M 2011. The Physiology of Stress: Cortisol and the Hypothalamic-Pituitary-Adrenal Axis. *Dartmouth Undergraduate Journal of Science*. Fall 2010.

Reiss MR 1997. "Ocular dominance: some family data". Laterality. 2(1):7–16. doi:10.1080/713754254.

Rhee PL, Lee JY, Son HJ, Kim JJ, Rhee JC, Kim S et al 2011. Analysis of pacemaker activity in the human stomach. J Physiol. Dec 15; 589(Pt 24): 6105–6118.

Rosenblatt S 1981. The Electrodermal Characteristics of Acupuncture points. Am J Acupunct 1981;10:131-137. Cited by Sullivan SG, 1985.

Ross J 1985. *Zang Fu The Organ Systems of Traditional Chinese Medicine*. Edinburgh, UK: Churchill Livingstone.

Royal Society of Chemistry 2004. Carbohydrates. *Chemistry for Biologists*. http://www.rsc.org/Education/Teachers/Resources/cfb/Carbohydrates.htm. Updated Nov 2004. Accessed Apr 25 2017.

Rye C, Wise R, Jurukovski V et al 2013. *Biology*. Houston, TX: OpenStax, Rice University. Freely available at https://openstax.org/details/books/biology (page numbers refer to the downloadable pdf edition).

Saku K, Mukaino Y, Ying H, Arakawa K 1993. Characteristics of reactive electropermeable points on the auricles of coronary heart disease patients. *Clinical Cardiology.* 16:415-19.

Schaefer B 1965. Changes in the Leadership of the Korean Workers Party and the Government of North Korea. *History and Public Policy Program Digital Archive, SAPMO-BA, Berlin, DY 30.* 1965, July 12. http://digitalarchive.wilsoncenter.org/document/111822. Accessed Oct 1, 2016.

Serisawa K 1978. An Approach on Meridians and Acupuncture Points in Modern Medicine. J Comprehensive Rehabilitation 1978, 11:789. Cited by Sullivan SG, 1985.

Shelly, Maire P 2014. *Editorial: The upper airway - the forgotten organ.* PubMed Central (PMC) at the U.S. National Institutes of Health's National Library of Medicine. Web 17 Apr 2014 <http://www.ncbi.nlm.nih.gov/pmc/articles/PMC137263/>.

Shin HS, Johng HM, Lee BC, Cho SI, Soh KS, Baik KY 2005. Feulgen reaction study of novel threadlike structures (Bonghan ducts) on the surfaces of mammalian organs. *Anat Rec.* 284B:35-40.

Shirakawa H, Louis EJ, MacDiarmid AG, Chiang CK, Heeger AJ 1977. Synthesis of electrically conducting organic polymers: halogen derivatives of polyacetylene. *Journal of the Chemical Society.* Chemical Communications. (16):578.

Sinyukhin AM. Nature of the variation of the Bioelectric potentials in the regeneration process of plants. Lomonosov State University, Moscow.

Slomianka L 2009. Blue Histology - Vascular System. *School of Anatomy and Human Biology - The University of Western Australia.* http://www.lab.anhb.uwa.edu.au/mb140/corepages/vascular/vascular.htm. Accessed 19 Oct 2016.

Soh KS 2009. Bonghan Circulatory system as an Extension of Acupuncture Meridians. *J Acupunct Meridian Stud.* Jun; 2(2):93-106. (See section 5.2)

Soh KS, Kang KA, Ryu YH 2013. 50 Years of Bong-Han Theory and 10 Years of Primo Vascular System. *Evidence-Based Complementary and Alternative Medicine.* 587827. doi:10.1155/2013/587827

Sullivan SG, Eggleston DW, Martinoff JT, Kroening RJ 1985. Evoked electrical conductivity on the lung acupuncture points in healthy individuals and confirmed lung cancer patients. *American Journal of Acupuncture.* 13(3):261-66.

Sung B, Ogay V, Yoo JS, Yu HS, Lee BC, Chung C et al 2005. UV-A induced activation of Bonghan granules in motion. *Journal of International Society of Life Information Science.* 23(2):297-301.

Sung B, Kim MS, Lee BC, Yoo JS, Lee SH, Kim YJ et al (2008). Measurement of flow speed in the channels of novel threadlike structures on the surfaces of mammalian organs. Naturwissenschaften. 95:117–124.

Sung B, Kim MS, Lee BC et al 2008. Measurement of flow speed in the meridians of novel threadlike structures on the surfaces of mammalian organs. *Naturwissenschaften.* Vol.95, no.2:117-124.

Ssu-ma Ch'ien (ed.) 1969. *Shih-chi.* Chung-hua Shu-chü. Hong Kong.

Ssu-miao S 1965. *Chien-chin i-fang.* Taipei.

Szent-Gyorgyi A 1941. Towards a New Biochemistry. *Science.* 93:609-11.

Thorens B 2010. Central control of glucose homeostasis: the brain-endocrine pancreas axis. *Diabetes Metab.* Oct;36 Suppl 3:S45-9. doi: 10.1016/S1262-3636(10)70466-3.

Tian J 2007. Electroacupuncture combined with flash cupping for treatment of peripheral facial paralysis—a report of 224 cases. *J Tradit Chin Med.* Mar;27(1):14-5.

Tsigos C, Constantine GP et al 2002. Hypothalamic–pituitary–adrenal axis, neuroendocrine factors and stress. *Journal of Psychosomatic Research.* 53(4):865-871. doi:10.1016/ S0022-3999(02)00429-4.

UCLA 2004. Left And Right Ears Not Created Equal As Newborns Process Sound, Finds UCLA/UA Research. *ScienceDaily.* Retrieved June 14, 2017 from www.sciencedaily.com/releases/2004/09/040910082553.htm

Unschuld P 1985. *Medicine in China: A History of Ideas.* Berkeley, CA: University of California Press.

Unschuld P 1986. *Nan-Ching, the Classic of Difficult Issues.* Berkeley, CA: University of California Press.

Unschuld P, Tessenow H 2011. *Huang Di nei jing su wen: An Annotated Translation of Huang Di's Inner Classic – Basic Questions.* Berkeley, CA: University of California Press.

Unschuld P 2016. *Huang Di Nei Jing Ling Shu.* Oakland, CA: University of California Press.

Urone PP, Hinrichs R, Dirks K, Sharma M 2012. *College Physics.* Houston, TX: OpenStax, Rice University. Freely available at http://cnx.org/content/col11406/latest (page numbers refer to the downloadable pdf edition).

Voll R 1975. Twenty years of electroacupuncture diagnosis in Germany: A progress report. *Am J Acupunct.* 3:7-17.

Wang Bing 王冰 (ed.), *Huang Di nei jing su wen* 黄帝内經素問 (ed. 762 AD). Taipei 台北: 国立中国医药研究所影印明嘉靖顾从德本 1960.

Wang X, Shi H, Shang H, Su Y, Xin J, He W et al 2012. Are Primo Vessels (PVs) on the Surface of Gastrointestine Involved in Regulation of Gastric Motility Induced by Stimulating Acupoints ST36 or CV12? *Evidence-based Complementary and Alternative Medicine : eCAM.* 2012:787683. doi:10.1155/2012/787683.

Waugh A, Grant A 2001. *Ross and Wilson, Anatomy and Physiology in Health and Illness, ninth Edition.* Edinburgh, UK: Churchill Livingstone.

Wilhelm Richard 1930. Li Gi. Das Buch der Sitte des Älteren und Jüngeren Dai. Jena.

Wilkie MP 2002. Ammonia excretion and urea handling by fish gills: present understanding and future research challenges. *J Exp Zool.* Aug 1;293(3):284–301. doi:10.1002/jez.10123

Wu Kun 吳崐: *Nei jing su wen Wu zhu* 内经素问吴注. Jinan 济南: Shandong kexue jishu chubanshe 山东科学技术出版社 1984.

Wu-shih-erh ping fang 1979. Annotated edition by anonymous committee. Peking.

Yamada Keiji 1979. The formation of the Huang-Ti Nei-Ching. *Acta Asiatica.* 36:67-89.

Yang Shang-shan 1981. *Huang-ti nei-ching t'ai-su.* Peking.

Zhang Jiebin 张介宾, *Lei jing* 類經. Beijing 北京: Renmin weisheng chubanshe 人民卫生出版社 1957.

Zhang WB, Tian YY, Li H, Tian JH, Luo MF, Xu FL et al 2008. A discovery of low hydraulic resistance channel along meridians. *JAMS Journal of Acupuncture and Meridian Studies*. 1(1):20–28.

Zhang Zhenyu 张珍玉 1984. Du *Nei jing* zha ji (4) 读《内经》札记(四). *Shan dong zhong yi xue yuan xue bao* 山东中医学院学报.

Zhang Zhicong 张志聪 (=Zhang Yin'an 张隐庵), *Huang Di nei jing su wen ji zhu* 黄帝内经素问集注, or *Su wen ji zhu* 素问集注. Taipei 台北: Wenguang tushu youxian gongsi yingyin 文光图书有限公司影印 1982.

Glossary of today's Chinese medicine disease terms

Introduction

Disease names used in the *Nei Jing*

Most of the disease names in the following glossary were not used in the *Nei Jing*, but were adopted more recently in Chinese medicine. The *Nei Jing* (and *Nan Jing*) is a large collection of scripts from different authors, so that there was no uniformity in the terms used. However, there was a general approach to describing organ disease. This was, in effect, to simply list the possible signs and symptoms that may occur when an organ was "diseased", but not to give the disease (or syndrome) a specific name.

An organ "disease"

In Chapter 22 of the *Su Wen*, a list of possible signs and symptoms is given for a "disease" in each of the organs. No specific disease names are given; instead only the generic term of "disease" is used.

> **Extract from *Su Wen*, Chapter 22**
> In the case of a liver disease, there is pain below the two flanks and this pain pulls on the lower abdomen. The disease lets that person develop a tendency to be angry. In the case of depletion, the eyes become unclear and cannot see anything; the ears cannot hear anything. The patient tends to be fearful, as if someone were about to arrest him.[1]

"The case of depletion" is mentioned (in other words, when the liver condition led to a depleted state; or, when a state of depletion already existed), but this is only mentioned in the context of being a possible explanation for some of the liver-related symptoms ("the eyes become unclear and cannot see anything"), and is not suggested as a "disease" in its own right.

The presence of "evil influence" in the organ

Chapter 20 of the *Ling Shu* defines "disease" as being the result of "evil" (or "harmful") influence being present in the affected organ. In other words, again, it is mentioned that an organ is "diseased", and the possible signs and symptoms are listed. But no name is given to the organ's condition. It was thought sufficient to (in effect) merely state that the organ had a condition.

> **Extract from *Ling Shu*, Chapter 20**
> When [harmful influences] are in the liver, then the patient will feel pain in the upper flanks. His centre is cold, and malign blood is inside. When he walks, his joints tend to cramp. At times his legs are swollen.[2]

And the passage uses the same approach to describe the state of "disease" in the other four *yin* organs (*zang*).

An organ's meridian being "excited"

Chapter 10 of the *Ling Shu* describes the paths of all the meridians, and states that when any of these "vessels are excited", this results in signs and symptoms in the related organ.[3] In other words, the fact that an organ has a disease is detected in the "movement" in its meridian (i.e. the "organ pulse" in today's Chinese medicine terms), and a list of possible signs and symptoms is suggested. And the signs and symptoms themselves are termed a "disease".

For example, the chapter states "These are diseases generated by the lung: cough with rising [influence], panting and thirst, vexed heart, a feeling of fullness in the chest, pain and receding [influence] at the frontal edge inside the soft parts of the upper arms. Heat in the palms."[4]

The passage does, though, go on to mention some symptoms that may occur depending on whether the influences are "exuberant" or "depleted" (i.e. whether the "lung pulse" is either full or weak). It states "When the [influences] abound in exuberance, the shoulders and the back will feel pain with wind. Patients sweat and urinate frequently, but only small quantities. If the [influences] are depleted, the shoulders and the back will feel pain with cold. The patients experience shortness of [influence], so that there are not enough [influences] available for breathing."[5] But here, still, there is no mention of a disease name. Instead, the passage suggests that the diagnostic method (taking the patient's pulses, in this case) can sometimes indicate that certain signs or symptoms may be prevalent. But the "disease" is not called "Lung chi exuberance" or "Lung chi depletion" for example. Instead, this particular *Nei Jing* author simply regards all signs or symptoms as being the "disease". In other words, at this time, no specific disease terms were known to this author to describe these lung conditions, so he simply lists the signs and symptoms.

An organ having an "illness" or being "afflicted"

In the *Nan Jing*, which is slightly later than the *Nei Jing*, the same general approach was still used. In the following example, an organ is described as having an "illness" (which is detectable in the "movements" in its meridian; i.e. the "organ pulse" in today's terms), and the possible signs and symptoms are listed. Apart from this, no specific disease name was used.

> **Extract from *Nan Jing*, Section 16**
> Consider feeling a movement in the vessels that is associated with an illness in the lung. External evidence of such an illness includes a white face, a tendency to sneeze, grief without joy, and an inclination to cry.... The illness, as perceived by the patient, consists of panting and coughing, and of shivering from fits of cold and heat. If this evidence is

present, the lung is afflicted. If it is not present, the lung is not afflicted.[6]

Today's approach

The above simple, straightforward approach coincides with this book's approach, which is to simply state that an organ's function is poor, and to cite the possible signs and symptoms that might result. This has the added bonus that it also makes sense to today's readers outside of Chinese medicine.

However, in today's Chinese medicine, many terms have been adopted that were not used by the *Nei Jing* authors—where an organ's malfunction is now divided into several syndromes, depending on whether certain states recognised in Chinese medicine are also present (such as *heat*, *dampness*, deficiency, stagnation, and so on). These syndromes, and the related terms, are described below.

Glossary of today's Chinese medicine disease terms

blood Blood was considered to be a nourishing substance made from liquids that the digestion extracted from the diet. It was considered to flow in the "meridians" (p.29), along with *chi* (see below), and to be self-propelling. In other words, the heart was not thought to have the function of circulating the blood, as it is known to today (p.42).

Blood deficiency Since blood is manufactured by the digestion, when the digestion is weak, or the diet inadequate, this may cause poor quality blood ("Blood deficiency"), which may produce any of the signs and symptoms listed on page 83. In contemporary terms, the same condition is known as anaemia.

Blood stagnation Some conditions were thought to involve an accumulation of blood in the "meridians" (p.29) and collaterals, where the flow was either sluggish or had ceased. Today, this is known as "Blood stagnation", and is associated with sharp, stabbing sensations, as in sciatica. However, this notion is conceptual only; the blood does not literally flow in the "meridians", therefore it is not able to stagnate there, and there are other explanations for such symptoms (p.219).

chi This term was first used in a medical context in the *Nei Jing*. And it was understood to mean a vapour-like substance that circulates in the "meridians", in much the same way that mist drifts through the air. The vapour was thought to contain the essence of the substance it originated from—such as food, wind, cold, and so on. It thus communicated the influence of that substance to every part of the body, either nourishing it (in the case of food influence) or damaging it (in the case of wind or cold influence).

This whole notion is conceptual only, since we now know that *chi* does not really exist in the body (pp.40-47). However, it forms the core of all *Nei Jing* thinking about how the body works, so that, even though the notion is conceptual only, it is important to understand it as the *Nei Jing* authors did, so that their other thinking can also be understood as they intended it.

In this book the term is translated as "influcnce". However, in today's Chinese medicine, this term is often translated as energy, using a contemporary concept to replace the intended one. But the concept of energy, as we know it, was unknown to the *Nei Jing* authors and is incompatible with their notions of metabolism. See Chapter 3 (p.49), which discusses the varying notions of *chi* through the history of Chinese medicine.

Chi deficiency — This term is usually applied to an organ, as in "Heart chi deficiency". In this case, it means that the organ function is poor (or has a lack of "resources") which causes the organ to produce various signs or symptoms (p.27). The term is also sometimes used generally, in which case it means that the person has low energy and would have signs or symptoms such as slow movements, slow speech, a quiet voice, a pale complexion, cold flesh, and they would feel the cold and generally appear fragile.

collateral — See meridian.

damp — *Dampness* results in us when the digestion, particularly the pancreas function, is poor. Simplistically, it could be imagined as the "soup" of nutrients in the blood being too "thick"—or remaining unprocessed long after we had eaten. And this state may lead to various signs or symptoms, hence *dampness* is regarded as a pathogen (p.76).

damp heat — When *dampness* has been present in the body for some time, this often produces signs or symptoms of *heat* (see below), and this condition would then be referred to as *damp heat* (p.181). The signs and symptoms could include redness, itching, dry skin, or such conditions as burning on urination (known as "thrush" in contemporary terms).

Damp heat in the pancreas — This condition is a worsening of "Pancreas chi deficiency", and only usually occurs after the pancreas function has been poor for some time. In this case, *dampness* (see *damp* above) would have usually also been present for some time, which has then generated *heat* (see below), to produce *damp heat*. Hence, there would be signs or symptoms of "Pancreas chi deficiency" (p.74), plus signs of *damp heat*, such as bright yellow face, eyes and skin, with scanty, yellow urine (p.82).

Damp heat in the spleen See "Damp heat in the pancreas" (above).

deficient This term may be applied in many situations. When applied to a pulse, it would signify a weak, thin, or "empty" pulse, which would indicate that the function of the related organ was poor, which would tend to produce weak signs or symptoms related to that organ. For example, if the person had a cough, it would be a weak, quiet cough, rather than a strong, loud one.

Or the term could be applied to substances, such as blood (see "Blood deficiency"), or *chi* (see "Chi deficiency"), meaning that those substances were deficient in some way, which could produce various signs or symptoms.

Or the term could be applied to a person, meaning the person was a "deficient-type person". Such a person would tend to be quiet, withdrawn, fragile, and have low energy, poor stamina, and a weak constitution, and would tend to suffer deficient-type conditions.

Disharmony of the liver and spleen This is another term for "Liver invading spleen", or, as it is known in this book, "Liver invading pancreas" (see below).

essence This term is usually used in relation to the "kidneys". It was not used consistently by the *Nei Jing* authors (p.25), but in today's Chinese medicine it is used in various contexts, including the constitution passed on to us from our parents (p.156); the part played by the "kidneys" in regulating and enabling the function of the other organs (p.159); etc. Other terms are also used in these contexts, such as *jing*, original influence (*yuan chi*), kidney *yang* , and so on (p.177).

It should be noted that none of these substances literally exist. Rather, they are theoretical notions used to attempt to explain the kidney functions. However, in contemporary physiology, all these theoretical substances are strongly analogous to the hormonal activity of the three kidney-related structures (p.177). It is said that "kidney essence" includes a *yin* and *yang* part, with the *yin* part producing various effects, and the *yang* part producing other effects. In other words, the *yin* part (kidney *yin*) has certain functions which (in contemporary physiology) equate to the functions that some kidney-related hormones have; while the *yang* part (kidney *yang*) has other functions which (in contemporary physiology) equate to the functions that other kidney-related hormones have.

excess This term may be applied in many situations. When applied to a pulse, it would signify a strong, "full" pulse, which would indicate that the function of the related organ was in an "excess" state, which would tend to produce strong signs and symptoms related to that organ. For example, if the person had a cough, it would be a strong, loud cough, rather than a weak, quiet one.

Or the term could be applied to a person, meaning the person was an "excess-type person". Such a person would tend to be loud, active, outgoing, with quick movements and an apparent excess of energy. They would tend to have good stamina and a strong constitution, and would tend to suffer excess-type conditions (i.e. with powerful signs and symptoms).

fire This is another term for *heat* (see *heat* below).

heat *Heat* refers to all bodily signs and symptoms of unusual warmth, redness, dryness, or itching. *Heat* is considered a pathogen (i.e. can cause us harm), but in this case the pathogen is usually generated from within, rather than "invading" us from outside (p.307).

Heart chi deficiency This term means that the function of the heart is poor, producing a selection of the signs and symptoms from list "A" on page 196.

Heart blood deficiency This term means that the function of the heart is poor (as in "Heart chi deficiency"), and that the patient also has poor quality blood (or "Blood deficiency"), which has affected the heart. Hence, they would tend to have the basic signs and symptoms of "Heart chi deficiency" (see above), plus extra symptoms produced by their heart, due to the poor nourishment of the heart tissue. Such symptoms are of a mental nature and could include any from those from list "B" on page 196.

Heart fire This refers to poor heart function (or "Heart chi deficiency"), but with signs and symptoms of *heat* being present as well. Hence, the signs and symptoms would include those of "Heart chi deficiency" (see above), plus symptoms of *heat* which are produced by the heart. These would tend to be a selection of the mental symptoms listed under "Heart blood deficiency" above, only the symptoms would be more pronounced, such as a greater degree of emotional upset, anxiety, unease, restlessness, stronger panic attacks, and dreams of a more disturbing nature.

The tip of the tongue would be noticeably red, the heart pulse "full" or "surging", and the skin would tend to be red around key heart acupoints, such as Heart-7 (*Shenmen*) and Heart-8 (*Shaofu*). And acupoints such as Heart-3 (*Shaohai*) would tend to be notably tender when pressed.

Heart yin deficiency This term refers to poor heart function (or "Heart chi deficiency"), but with symptoms of "Yin deficiency" being present as well. Hence, the signs and symptoms would include those of "Heart chi deficiency" (see above), plus a selection of the symptoms from list "C" on page 196, which are the general symptoms of "Yin deficiency" and, in this case, are being produced by the heart.

influence This book translates *chi* as "influence" (see *chi* above).

jing This is an alternative term for *essence* (see *essence* above).

Kidney chi deficiency This term means that the function of the kidneys is poor, producing a selection of the signs and symptoms from list "A" on page 174.

Kidney essence deficiency This term means that the function of the kidneys is poor, but that the signs and symptoms also include those related to *essence* (see above). Hence the signs and symptoms would include a selection of those from list "A" on page 174, and also some from list "E".

Kidney failing to receive chi This term means that the function of the kidneys is poor, but that the symptoms also include those related to the kidney effect of assisting the lungs to breathe in. Hence the signs and symptoms would include a selection of those from list "A" on page 174, and also some from list "B".

Kidney jing deficiency This is an alternative name for "Kidney essence deficiency" (see above).

Kidney yin deficiency This term means that the function of the kidneys is poor, but that the symptoms also include those or "Yin deficiency" (see below) which are being produced by the kidneys. In other words, the *yin* of the kidneys has been affected, which produces these extra symptoms. Hence the signs and symptoms would include a selection of those from list "A" on page 174, and also some from list "C".

Liver chi stagnation This term means that the function of the liver is stagnated, producing a selection of the signs and symptoms from those listed on page 113.

Liver blood deficiency This term means that the function of the liver has been affected by "blood deficiency" (see above), which causes the liver to produce a selection of the signs and symptoms from those listed on page 116.

Liver fire This term refers to the condition of stagnated liver function, but with signs and symptoms of *heat* also being produced by the liver, such as hot flushes, dizziness, vertigo, redness and pain of the eyes, burning sensation in the liver region, bitter taste in the mouth, dry mouth, irritability, yellow urine and constipation. And the tongue would be red with a yellow coating; and the pulse "wiry" and rapid.

Liver invading pancreas This term means that the function of the liver is stagnated, and that this has also affected the function of the pancreas. Hence the signs and symptoms would include a selection of those of stagnated liver function (p.113), and also of poor pancreas function (p.74).

The term derives from the *Nei Jing* five phase theory, in which the phase of Wood (liver) was thought to have a "control" or "domination" relationship with the phase of Earth (pancreas), such that when the liver was in excess and the pancreas was deficient, the liver tends to take advantage of this weakness and "invades" the pancreas. Though the syndrome is real, this *Nei Jing* theoretical explanation is conceptual only (p.103).

Liver invading spleen See "Liver invading pancreas".

Liver invading stomach This term means that the function of the liver is stagnated, and that this has also affected the function of the stomach. Hence the signs and symptoms would include a selection of those of stagnated liver function (p.113), and also of poor stomach function (p.85). See the comments under "Liver invading pancreas" on the derivation of this term in five phase theory, which comments also apply to "Liver invading stomach".

Liver yang rising This term refers to a condition in the liver, where "Liver chi stagnation" is present, but the more *yang* symptoms of "Liver chi stagnation" have now become even more pronounced, resulting in a selection of the symptoms listed on page 117, such as frequent bouts of angry shouting, violent rages, and migraines and headaches with severe pain.

Lung chi deficiency This term means that the function of the lungs is poor, producing a selection of the signs and symptoms from those listed on page 143.

Lung yin deficiency This term means that the function of the lungs is poor, and that the *yin* of the lungs has been affected, which causes the lungs to also produce the symptoms of "Yin deficiency" (see below). Hence the signs and symptoms would include a selection of those of "Lung chi deficiency" (p.143) and also of "Yin deficiency" (listed on page 199).

meridians and collaterals In the *Nei Jing*, there was considered to be a single circulatory system, known as the "meridians and collaterals". At that time, these terms meant the following. The collaterals were the superficial veins that were used for bleeding (p.31). The "meridians" were the deeper, main vessels of this circulatory system, and the collaterals were thought to branch off from them.

However, these "meridians" were thought to be artery-like tubes, but having different routes to the arteries known today (p.29). It was thought that the *pathways on the skin* (which is what we today think of as the meridians) were merely a "shadow" of these deeper, artery-like tubes, and hence, that the "meridians" (these deep tubes) took the same paths as those *pathways on the skin*. Therefore, the "meridians" referred to by the *Nei Jing* were imaginary vessels, since no such artery-like tubes existed on those paths.

Further, both blood and "influences" (*chi*) were thought to flow together through the "meridians" and collaterals; and these substances were thought to be self-propelling. That is, the heart was not thought to have the pump-like function that it is known to today (p.29).

Pancreas chi deficiency — This term means that the function of the pancreas is poor, producing a selection of the signs and symptoms from those listed on page 74.

Pancreas yang deficiency — This condition is a worsening of "Pancreas chi deficiency", and only usually occurs after the pancreas function has been poor for some time. Hence the signs and symptoms are similar to those of poor pancreas function, only they are more severe—such as extreme lack of energy, with the body feeling heavy; excessive feeling of coldness, particularly in the limbs, and an aversion to cold; undigested food in watery stools (p.82).

phlegm — This term refers to a "thickening" of the *dampness* pathogen (see *dampness* above), and is a more severe pathogen than mere *dampness*. It only usually occurs after *dampness* has been present for some time (p.202).

Phlegm misting the mind — This term refers to a heart condition. The condition results after *dampness* (see *damp* above) has been present for some time, which then results in *phlegm* (see above), which impedes the function of the heart. This also impedes the mental functions of the heart, which produces symptoms such as those in list "E" on page 196 (also see page 202).

Spleen chi deficiency — See "Pancreas chi deficiency".

Spleen yang deficiency — See "Pancreas yang deficiency".

Stomach chi deficiency — This term means that the function of the stomach is poor, producing a selection of the symptoms listed on page 85.

Stomach heat/fire — This term means that the function of the stomach is poor, but that the signs and symptoms also include those of *heat* (see above), which are being produced by the stomach. Hence the signs and symptoms would include a selection from those listed on page 85, and also signs and symptoms such as redness or spots anywhere along the stomach meridian; bad breath, usually with a burnt odour; a sensation of heat rising up the Ren meridian on the chest (usually called "heart burn"); and acid reflux.

The tongue would tend to be red in the centre (or generally), with a yellow coat; and the stomach pulse would be full or surging.

wind In the *Nei Jing*, this term was most often used to describe the literal wind outside, which was considered to be a pathogen that was capable of penetrating the body and causing harm. But the term was also used to refer to the movement of the influences (*chi*) from a particular organ, as in "liver *wind*", "heart *wind*", and so on.

In today's Chinese medicine, the term *wind* is also used to describe any phenomena in the body characterized by sudden movement. These include the internal signs produced by a "wind invasion", such as sneezing and shivering, but also such phenomena as trembling and facial tics (p.307).

Wind cold invasion This term would equate to a common cold or influenza in today's terms. It refers to poor lung function, caused by an airborne pathogen of some type. The symptoms could include sneezing, cough, build up of mucous, nasal obstruction, watery nasal discharge, possible fever and chills, aching body, an aversion to wind and drafts, and headache. This would be termed a "wind cold invasion", since most of the symptoms do not include pronounced signs of *heat* (see above). But if the signs and symptoms also includes thirst, yellow mucous, sore throat, sweating, rapid pulse, and a red tongue with a thin yellow coat—this would be termed a "wind heat invasion", since these signs and symptoms include pronounced signs of *heat* (p.139).

Wind heat invasion This term refers to a "wind invasion" that includes pronounced signs of *heat*, such as those mentioned in "Wind cold invasion" above.

Yang deficiency This term refers to a worsening of the state of "Chi deficiency" (see above). Therefore the symptoms produced would be the same as those in "Chi deficiency", only more severe—such as extreme lack of energy, with the body feeling heavy; excessive feeling of coldness, particularly in the limbs, and an aversion to cold (p.82).

yin and *yang* In terms of the organs, *yin* refers to the health of the organ fabric, while *yang* refers to the functioning of the organ. For a general definition of *yin* and *yang*, see page 345.

Yin deficiency This condition describes the situation where the tissue of the organs is not healthy which causes it to produce heat. This results in symptoms such as low grade fever during the day (hot flushes); night sweating; feeling a sensation of heat on the soles of the feet and palms of the hands; and a dry mouth, or feeling constantly thirsty (p.199).

Index

A

B

F

G

M

N

O

P

Q

R

S

T

U

V

W

X

Y

Z

Also available from CuriousPages

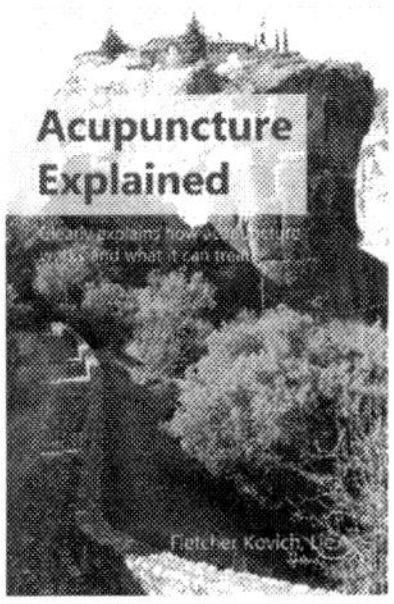

Acupuncture Explained
Fletcher Kovich
The book is a reduction of *Acupuncture Today and in Ancient China*. It does not include the academic content, such as the many references to the *Nei Jing*, and other citations; and also leaves out other selected content. It contains only the content necessary to enable the general reader to fully understand what acupuncture is, how it works and what it can treat. It is an ideal book to recommend to patients, and would enable them to understand every aspect of the treatment and their condition, including any mental or emotional cause.

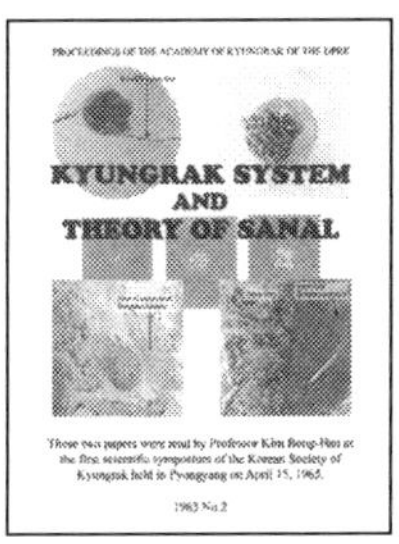

Kyungrak System and Theory Of Sanal
Bong-Han Kim
In 1962, Bong-Han Kim published the first scientific evidence of the structures that underlie the acupuncture meridians. After three years of further research he published the present book, which is a complete account of his findings.

The book describes a range of completely new anatomical structures, including node-like structures at the acupoints, connected with fine vessels which extend to the internal organs, and also exist within blood and lymph vessels and throughout the nervous system. These structures circulate embryonic-like cells which transform into the various cells required by our body's organs and tissues. And the purpose of the entire system is said to be the continuous repair and regeneration of key cells in our organs and elsewhere.

Please visit **www.curiouspages.com/books** for details of free sample downloads, full details of the above books, and a complete list of books available.

Made in the USA
Monee, IL
13 September 2026

62975593R00260